A
MODEL
FOR THE
COUNTRY

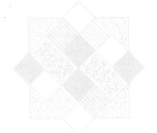

A
MODEL
FOR THE
COUNTRY

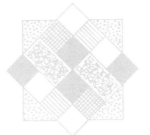

The Founding
and Pioneering
First Half-Century of
Penn Foundation

PHILIP RUTH

A Model for the Country: The Founding and Pioneering
First Half-Century of Penn Foundation

Copyright © 2005 by Penn Foundation, Inc.
807 Lawn Avenue, Sellersville, PA 18960.

International Standard Book Number: 0-9741020-4-0 (original)
                                        978-0-9741020-4-7 (converted)
Library of Congress Control Number: 2005903700

Design and publication services by PMT, Ltd., Harleysville, PA 19438

Printed in the United States of America.

This book has been brought to publication with the generous
assistance of T.H. Properties, Harleysville, PA,
and Univest Corporation, Souderton, PA.

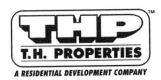

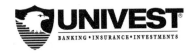

"If I were to select a half-dozen community mental health centers that nearly approach the dream I dreamed, not only would Penn Foundation be included, it would be one of the top three. Not only is it the only one of its kind in Pennsylvania; it is a model for the country and the world. Go on to bigger dreams; go on and on and on."

— ROBERT H. FELIX
Founder of the National Institute of Mental Health and Dean of the University
of St. Louis Medical School, addressing Penn Foundation staff and supporters at
the Foundation's Tenth Anniversary celebration, October 5, 1965

Contents

Foreword

Penn Foundation's story begins in the late 1940s when a remarkable man, Dr. Michael Peters, a physician on the staff of Grand View Hospital and practicing medicine in Telford, Pennsylvania, developed a concern for patients in his medical practice who were presenting with psychiatric symptoms. Dr. Peters treated those that he could, but he believed strongly that his patients and others with psychiatric illness could be better served if they were treated by someone trained in the medical specialty of psychiatry.

Dr. Peters shared his vision for a psychiatric service with a number of successful local businessmen who agreed that this was needed for the community served by Grand View Hospital. This small group of men, not yet formally organized (that would come several years later), decided that Dr. Norman Loux, a native of the Indian Valley who was practicing psychiatry at the renowned Butler Hospital in Rhode Island, would be the right person to begin this psychiatric service.

The selection of Dr. Loux to start the psychiatric practice that would become Penn Foundation for Mental Health, and then to lead its development, turned out to be providential. In many ways Dr. Loux has been the kind of Level 5 leader described in the book *Good to Great* by Jim Collins. "It is very important to grasp that Level 5 leadership is not just about humility and modesty," Collins wrote. "It is equally about ferocious resolve, an almost stoic determination to do whatever needs to be done to make the company great." Those of us who know Dr. Loux and have had the privilege of working with him know him to be a humble person who has been completely dedicated to the success of the organization he helped create.

Penn Foundation's story is one of people with a shared vision responding to community need by developing and then offering the best in behavioral health services. This vision, which began with Dr. Peters and was further developed by Dr. Loux, has inspired the Penn Foundation staff for fifty years. It led to the development of a wonderfully innovative Day Treatment Program. It led Penn Foundation to become one of the first community mental health centers in the nation. Over the years it has led to the development of other programs that were clearly needed by our community. When the deinstitutionalization movement began, Penn Foundation established housing programs and other supports for people who had been hospitalized previously in state hospitals and who would now be expected to live in the community. As other community needs were identified, additional programs were developed, including the Employee Assistance Program, Drug and Alcohol Services, Mental Health and Retardation Case Management, and Pastoral Services.

The vision to offer the very best in behavioral health services will continue to guide our growth and development. Our staff will continue to respond to new developments in the field of Mental Health and Substance Abuse. Advances in psychiatric medication afford us the opportunity to focus on providing assistance to people recovering from illness. In the next half-century, our goal will be full integration of these persons into the community.

Penn Foundation's story has been one of vision and challenge, opportunities and threats, and of people who share the vision to offer a needed service to the community and who are committed to the success of the organization. Our first fifty years have given us a wonderful foundation to build upon as we look to serve our community in the next fifty years.

John Goshow
President and CEO
Penn Foundation, Inc.

Preface

A book published in 1983 under the title *If We Can Love: The Mennonite Mental Health Care Story* recounted the establishment by Mennonite groups of eight mental health centers across the United States and Canada between 1949 and 1967. Each of these centers, according to the authors of their brief histories, arose through the efforts of a unique group of promoters, and within its own peculiar set of circumstances. And yet, as the book's editor and other contributors made clear, running through the individual stories were unifying threads of religious conviction, unflagging resolve, and a tradition of serving one's neighbors.

The fifth-oldest mental health organization discussed in this chronicle was the Penn Foundation for Mental Health, organized in Souderton, Pennsylvania in 1955, and relocated a year later to a permanent campus in neighboring West Rockhill Township, just west of Sellersville Borough. "Penn Foundation," as the organization became widely known and was later renamed, had recently observed its Twenty-Fifth Anniversary when *If We Can Love* was published in 1983. Happily, more than half of the founders were *still* around to celebrate the reaching of that milestone. Indeed, some of them still held positions on the Board of Directors.

Fast forward another quarter-century and, remarkably, some of those founders are still around, a few of them even contributing as emeritus Board members to the organization they helped establish half-a-century earlier. In looking back over the origins and evolution of Penn Foundation, they concluded with the current administration that the time had come to have the story of this pioneering institution told in greater detail than ever before, especially insofar as several progenitors would be available to help the author frame the overarching themes and identify the qualities that inspired no less an authority than the founder of the National Institute of Mental Health to describe Penn Foundation in 1962 as "a model for the country and the world."

They handed the assignment of writing Penn Foundation's history to a regional historian with no more than a layman's acquaintance with psychiatry, health care, or business administration. I had, however, recently teased out the stories of several service-oriented institutions enjoying fiftieth anniversaries, each of them having sprouted in the mid-twentieth century from a hotbed of Anabaptist conviction and Pennsylvania German culture within southeastern Pennsylvania's Franconia Mennonite Conference. Penn Foundation, I eventually discovered, was yet another florescence of this astonishing energy, but with a collection of participants and challenges that set it apart from its contemporaries in ways that I found—and I hope my readers will find—fascinating.

Philip Ruth
Lower Salford Township
March 11, 2005

1

A NEED PERCEIVED

The morning of Thursday, October 20, 1955 dawned clear and cool in the southeastern Pennsylvania railroad town of Souderton. Sunlight wakened hues of red, gold, and orange in the thinning trees and bushes that lined the tidy streets of the industrious Montgomery County borough. Out of the procession of cars and trucks gliding down Broad Street toward its intersection with Main at the center of town, a car separated itself, turned into the parking lot between the railroad station and the Union National Bank, and slipped into one of the few vacant parking spots. A minute passed, and then a young man—clean-shaven, slightly built, eyes squinting behind a pair of glasses—emerged from the car, swung the door closed, and began walking slowly across the parking lot, back to the intersection of Broad and Main. The man's pace picked up slightly as he crossed Broad Street, but it slowed again as he continued down the Main Street sidewalk, in the direction of "the Hollow," Souderton's commercial core. On his left he passed the People's Bank, Gid Haas's restaurant and pool hall, and Yocum & Godschalk's general store. These establishments clearly held no interest for him. He didn't lift his gaze from the sidewalk in front of him until he reached the end of the block, where West Chestnut Street intersected Main Street. Here he turned the corner onto West Chestnut and began scrutinizing the buildings on either side of the street, largely hidden behind veils of gaudy foliage. Several doors down, across the street from a State liquor store, the man spotted what he was looking for: a brick two-story dwelling with a sign attached that read "19 West Chestnut Street."

Coming to a stop on the sidewalk in front of the State store, the man took a deep breath, pulled off his glasses, bowed his head, and began rubbing his eyes. He was alone on the sidewalk, and there were no cars rolling down West Chestnut Street at that moment, so there didn't appear to be anyone around to see him and wonder what he was doing lingering in the shade across from 19 West Chestnut Street. He gave his eyes an extended rubbing, then donned his glasses, glanced up and down the empty street, and walked over to the door of the house he had identified as his destination. A notice pinned to the door invited him to enter the building without knocking. The man let himself into the foyer of the house, where he was greeted by a slender, neatly dressed woman who had been busy behind a desk when he entered. She introduced herself as Miss Horwood, Dr. Loux's assistant. He told her his name was David, and she confirmed that Dr. Loux was awaiting his arrival. The doctor would be with him in a minute, as soon as he completed a telephone call. David sat down on an old parlor chair in the waiting area.

Within moments, a man in his mid-thirties, with short black hair, dark-rimmed glasses, and a friendly, professorial air about him, opened the door to a room at the far end of the waiting room and came out to greet David warmly. He introduced himself as Doctor Loux, and indicated he was glad Dr. Moyer had referred David for a visit. He was looking forward to providing David with whatever help he could, he said, ushering the young man into a room furnished with a desk and chair, a couch, and an overstuffed chair. David sat down on the couch, Dr. Loux seated himself in the overstuffed chair, and a few minutes later David was telling his story.

He had grown up on his family's dairy farm. His mother used to read him fairy tales at bedtime, and from them he learned that Good always triumphed over Evil, and Good People eventually lived happily ever after. He always imagined his life would unfold like a fairy tale. He would grow up working with his father on the farm, then marry the girl-next-door and walk with her into the sunset.

But that wasn't what had happened at all.

A couple of years ago, his father had sold off the farm's dairy cows and, with winter coming on, David found himself with a lot more free time on his hands. He started worrying about his relationship with his girlfriend. They had talked about marriage, but the more they talked, the more David came to feel that marriage would be a mistake. He didn't know how to tell his girlfriend this, but he knew the longer he put it off the harder it would get. When he finally broke up with her, he felt like dirt. He figured he had not only let her down, he had disappointed his whole family. He felt so bad he just wanted to shut himself off from everyone. The feelings became so overwhelming that he sometimes thought about killing himself. When his friends talked about their plans for the following summer, David thought "This time next year, I'll be dead." Then he stopped thinking even that far into the future. He often had so little energy that he just lay in bed all morning. Some days he stayed in bed through the afternoon. His parents got so worried about him they made him go to Dr. Moyer. Dr. Moyer talked to him for a long time, then told him he thought David could get the help he needed from one of his colleagues, Dr. Norman Loux, who had grown up in the Souderton area and had gone into the medical profession with a specialization in psychiatry. Dr. Loux had recently moved back to the area and he had been seeing patients for a couple of weeks in one of Dr. Moyer's offices. He would soon be moving into his own office in a house on Souderton's West Chestnut Street. Dr. Moyer would give him a call and set up a time for David to go see him. And that's how David came to be here, in Dr. Loux's new office on this Thursday morning in mid-October—though, he had to admit, he almost didn't come. It felt like he was dragging a couple of feedbags behind him.

Dr. Loux smiled at David and assured him he had done well to make this effort. The doctor would do everything he could to help David get through this tough time. Things might look pretty hopeless, but Dr. Loux had seen people in similar circumstances find ways out of their depression with professional help. For the first time in months, David didn't immediately think to himself, "What's the point? I'm a failure, and I'm just getting what I deserve." There was something in Dr. Loux's gentle manner and his obvious concern for David that kindled a spark of hope. Perhaps there was light at the end of this long tunnel, after all.

Does the story of the Penn Foundation for Mental Health begin here, with the entrance of the *first* patient into the organization's *first* facility for the *first* session of treatment offered by the organization's *first* paid employees? One could make a case that everything leading up to this inaugural occasion was merely prologue. It is also noteworthy that a meeting held in the afternoon or evening of this red-letter day—Thursday, October 20, 1955—at 19 West Chestnut Street was the first gathering of the organization's founders official enough to warrant the recording of minutes (a sheet of typewritten notes compiled at this "informal and exploratory" session constitute the earliest document in Penn Foundation's collection of meeting minutes).

A problem with picking up the story of Penn Foundation at this momentous juncture is that the two employees involved in the first patient visit to 19 West Chestnut Street a half-century ago—Dr. Norman Loux and his secretary-assistant Ruby Horwood—cannot recall who the patient was, nor on which day in October 1955 (let alone at what specific time of that day) the patient made his or her visit. Records documenting this initial treatment session have been lost in the shuffle of administrative house-cleanings. And even if recollections and records *were* able to identify Penn Foundation's first official client, that information would remain confidential. The foregoing description of "David's" visit to 19 West Chestnut Street in the fall of 1955 only represents an encounter that *could* have marked the commencement of services by the organization eventually known as "The Penn Foundation for Mental Health, Inc."

And therein lies another narrative complication. As of October 20, 1955, Penn Foundation was not yet a corporate entity. It had no official Board of Directors. It didn't even have a name. Several more weeks would pass before a Board was appointed and an organizational name was adopted. The securing of a corporate charter was still nine busy months in the future.

It must also be acknowledged that the arrival of the organization's first client at 19 West Chestnut Street in October 1955 was the culmination of a process that had been underway for a number of years, even decades. That process included the recent relocation of Dr. Loux and his young family from Providence, Rhode Island to the Souderton area. The stage for *that* pivotal event had been partly set a year earlier (in the summer of 1954) when Dr. Loux submitted to a group of Souderton area businessmen—at their request—his proposal for an "organization through which to provide psychiatric service for our community." The impetus behind Dr. Loux's submission of this proposal in the summer of 1954 had been a series of conversations and brainstorming sessions conducted informally in and around Souderton by a handful of concerned citizens and doctors at nearby Grand View Hospital, who had become convinced that their community's mental health needs should be met through the delivery of homegrown-but-expert psychiatric care. Of course, the delivery of that care by Dr. Norman Loux would not have been conceivable if Dr. Loux had not decided—back in January 1949—to switch from general medicine to psychiatry. Then again, his rationale for making this professional shift had been formulated in response to what he had witnessed and heard about the state of mental health care in the United States for several years, during World War II and its aftermath.

The irrepressible Dr. Peters

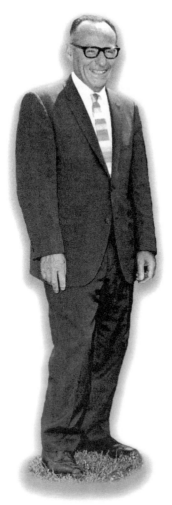

Looking back even further, one finds at least some of the groundwork for Penn Foundation being laid by a man who knew nothing of Norman Loux, the Souderton area, or Grand View Hospital until he was in his late twenties. This was the irrepressible Dr. Michael A. Peters, known to friends as "Pete." Born in 1908 to Italian Catholic parents in Utica, New York, Dr. Peters went on to graduate from Manhattan College in 1930, then move to Philadelphia to pursue an internship and residency in internal medicine at Hahnemann Medical College. What this young doctor lacked in physical

New York native Dr. Michael A. Peters (1908–1994) opened an internal medicine practice in Telford in September 1937 and—among many other medical and civic initiatives—began laying the groundwork for a pioneering community mental health center. When this photograph of "Pete" was taken at a Penn Foundation groundbreaking ceremony in August 1968, the irrepressible internist had been serving as Grand View Hospital's Chief of Medicine for twenty-one years.

stature he more than made up for in energy, intellect, and sociability. He was soon serving as Hahnemann's first Chief Resident of Medicine.

As part of his training in internal medicine, Dr. Peters spent four months studying psychiatry at the Allentown State Hospital in Rittersville, Pennsylvania. "I lived there and made rounds every day," he recalled in a 1990 interview. "Fortunately for me, at that time the State of Pennsylvania was paying the psychoanalyst in the area—Dr. Leo Madow—to come up every Wednesday and give an eight-hour course on psychoanalysis. That was the beginning of my interest in psychiatry."

By the summer of 1937, Dr. Peters had completed some postgraduate studies in cardiology and internal medicine at Massachusetts General Hospital, and he was back at Hahnemann casting about for a venue to open his own practice. He had become friends with fellow resident J. Harvey Sigafoos, the product of a predominantly Pennsylvania Dutch community twenty miles "upcountry" from Philadelphia ("Pennsylvania Dutch" being the popular term for Pennsylvania German). "In the wintertime, I used to go and visit him at his house in Colmar [on the Bucks-Montgomery County border]," Dr. Peters told an interviewer in 1990, continuing:

> On weekends during the summer we went to his bungalow up at Sumneytown [in northern Montgomery County]. One day in the summer of 1937, Carroll Proctor [a radio-repairman and civic activist in Telford, a borough adjoining Souderton on the Bucks-Montgomery County border] went up and met Mrs. Sigafoos in Sumneytown. He said they needed a doctor in Telford. Dr. Sigafoos was supposed to be finishing up his residency at Hahnemann, so would he come up and practice in Telford? Mrs. Sigafoos said, "Dr. Sigafoos is going to stay on as a resident in anesthesia, but his friend Dr. Peters is finishing up. Maybe he'd be interested."
>
> So that's how I ended up going to Telford to have a look, and I decided to start my [internal medicine] practice there. I started in Dr. [John K.] Hedrick's old place, at Third and West Broad Streets. Dr. Hedrick was still there, but he was an invalid. I moved in with him and his wife, and they were glad to see a young fellow come to live with them who turned out to be a doctor. My first few patients were some of Dr. Hedrick's old patients. It wasn't long before I was on my way

successfully. That's when I learned a lot about the need for psychiatry.

I remember my second day here in September 1937, Dr. [Clarence A.] Paulus said to me, "We've got to send a patient up to [Allentown State Hospital in] Rittersville. We've got to have a lawyer and two doctors to get him admitted." So I went along with Dr. Paulus, Dr. [Clyde R.] Flory, and lawyer [Robert H.] Grim. When we got to where the patient was, I stayed in the car to wait while the other doctors and the lawyers went to do all the talking to the family of the patient, who was completely psychotic. I could hear all the people that were there to see what was going on saying, "Well, they doctored too strong! The medicine made him the way he is." And, of course, I began to wonder, "What kind of community am I getting into here? How could they believe 'the medicine is too strong'?"

We went along as the family took the patient up to Rittersville. It wasn't very difficult to admit a patient to a psychiatric institution in those days. I could see right away that psychiatry was being practiced here [in the Souderton area], but the people themselves didn't understand it. Instead of thinking of psychosis as an illness, they blamed it on the medicine being "too strong." They couldn't see that there could be other factors in mental illness, such as inter-personal relationships. The people who came to see me about psychiatric illness didn't talk in psychiatric terms. They called it "notion," as if the patient was just mixed up in his thinking. That was sort of belittling the illness.

The other terminology used was "nerves." People who had a lot of anxiety, who couldn't sleep, or they were shaky and nervous, they'd say, "My nerves are bad." That was a common thing. Because I was psychiatrically oriented, I recognized "nerves" as the minimal depressions that we commonly see in practicing medicine.

Connections with Grand View Hospital

The year he opened his practice in Telford, Dr. Peters joined the medical staff of Grand View Hospital, Bucks County's first hospital, established in 1913 a few miles up the North Pennsylvania Railroad in

West Rockhill Township, just west of Sellersville Borough. Dr. Peters was the institution's first academically-trained internal medicine specialist. "Hospitals in those days were surgically oriented," he recalled late in his life, continuing:

> There was hardly any orientation to medicine. All the doctors did was surgery and tonsillectomies, and occasionally a cataract. There just wasn't room in a community hospital for the treatment of patients medically, except for pneumonia and typhoid fever. We started to treat those kinds of patients because typhoid fever was debilitative to the families at home, plus there was the danger of cross-infection. And with pneumonia we began to use serum.
>
> Back then, people thought you went to the hospital to die. I remember one patient practically passing out in my office when I said he had to go to the hospital to have a ruptured appendix operated on. He said. "You mean I'm going to die!?" That was how hospitals were regarded, as places of terminal care. There weren't medical patients going to the hospital. There weren't patients going in for study. They were going there for surgery. And, of course, a lot of the surgery didn't turn out very well.
>
> Everybody thought that I was coming up here [from Philadelphia] to be a country doctor. I didn't have that idea. My idea was to help [Grand View] hospital continue to departmentalize, the way it is today. I thought we should have much stronger departments of medicine and surgery, obstetrics and GYN, pediatrics, ear, nose and throat, anesthesia, general surgery. At that time, family doctors did all the work in the hospital. There was a problem with that. It wasn't so much a question of training; it was that they just weren't available. They were working in their offices, while their patients were lying up in the hospital. I felt that you had to have people in the hospital most of the day, and on call—close by—at night.

Dr. Peters quickly impressed his colleagues at Grand View as a man whose medical expertise was effectively complemented by social vision. "Pete" earned the confidence of patients and neighbors with equal swiftness. The communal embrace he enjoyed was all the more remarkable in that this diminutive Italian from central New York State brought with him to Telford very little experience with "Pennsylvania Dutch" (actually Pennsylvania *German*) culture, which in 1937 still flavored virtually every aspect of life in northern Montgomery County and west-central Bucks County, an area sometimes referred to as "the Bux-Mont region." The landscape in this part of southeastern Pennsylvania was a crazy quilt of family farms, anchored here and there by knots of rural commerce such as Telford and Sellersville. The largest of these towns—most of which had seceded from their surrounding townships and been incorporated as boroughs in the second half of the nineteenth century—hugged the economic and social lifeline of the North Pennsylvania Railroad, which is why the surrounding corridor was sometimes referred to (non-intuitively) as "the North Penn area." Many North Penn residents and their neighbors in the wider Bux-Mont region could trace their ancestral roots back to Mennonite, German Reformed, Lutheran, or German Baptist immigrants, the earliest of whom had arrived in the New World around the turn of the eighteenth century. More than two hundred years later, descendants of these agriculturally minded and religiously devout pioneers were scattered across America, but a dominating majority remained in the Bux-Mont region, where conversations between old-timers in the late 1930s was still more likely to be conducted in "Pennsylvania Dutch" than in English. "When I came here, I had some difficulty with the language," Dr. Peters recalled in 1990:

> That was my first problem. I remember a lot of my older patients came with interpreters, because they couldn't speak English well enough. They understood me when I talked to them, but they couldn't communicate back to me. The other thing I had a hard time getting used to was the way they lived, which was entirely different than I did. I was a young fellow, a bachelor, who did everything, including smoking. It was interesting, though, that although they were rigid in their own standards, they were very accepting of other people. I never heard anything derogatory said about blacks or about Jewish people, like I did in the city. The people here accepted me, even though I was not one of them. I remember being invited to dinner during my first week here by Robert Kulp, who was caretaker at the Rockhill Mennonite [Retirement] Home. I was invited around to a lot of places because I was a bachelor.

That's how I began to learn about scrapple and panhaas and chicken pot pie and all those things, which we didn't have up in my part of the world.

I came from a Catholic background, but I regularly went to the United Church of Christ [formerly German Reformed] in Telford because of Dr. Hedrick. He used to tell me "That's the church to go to." I joined the Sunday School orchestra there. I played the violin and became a real good member of the church. That was around 1938. I joined the church officially in 1946, after I was married.

Dr. Peters soon learned that religious morés went hand-in-glove with Pennsylvania Dutch culture in the Bux-Mont region, which was home in the 1930s to two-dozen "Old Mennonite" and "New Mennonite" congregations, more than a dozen German Reformed (later United Church of Christ) congregations, an equal number of Lutheran congregations, a handful of Brethren in Christ congregations, and just a few non-Protestant congregations. Especially among the predominant "Old Mennonites" of the two-hundred-year-old Franconia Mennonite Conference, church life, tradition, and agriculture combined to form a social epoxy holding together families, congregations, and communities. Looming over all religious activities for Franconia Conference Mennonites were the bishops, a select few ministers who had been elevated through ordination to powerful positions of oversight. It was the responsibility of these men to steer congregations within their geographic districts through the turbulent waters of a changing and sin-prone world. All questions concerning religious doctrine or discipline among Franconia Mennonite Conference congregations were ultimately resolved through decisions handed down by these patriarchs. If change came to the Mennonite Church of the Bux-Mont region during the mid-twentieth century, it would have to come either *through* these men, or *around* them.

Given the stereotypical view of mid-twentieth-century Mennonite bishops as heavy-handed enforcers of conservatism, it comes as something of a surprise to learn that one of these men actually helped convince Dr. Peters that a psychiatric department at Grand View Hospital was sorely needed, and that a community generally suspicious of newfangled approaches to age-old problems would not simply dismiss psychology as secular clap-trap. Dr. Peters was highly intrigued when he learned that Bishop Jonas Mininger of Harleysville, one of the few local ministers still preaching at least occasionally in German, had sent some members of his congregation at Plains "to a psychiatrist in Philadelphia when they got to the point where he just felt that they needed it." As Dr. Peters would later relate, "I could see that the groundwork for psychiatry was beginning to show itself right there." Harold Mininger, a grandson of Bishop Mininger, and one of Penn Foundation's charter Board members, offered this assessment of his grandfather's motives:

> Among Mennonites at that time, the minister—and especially the bishop—was the person people looked up to for stability. These men felt very responsible for anything that happened in their congregations that wasn't "uplifting." They were involved in a caring mission. Everybody was. Our people had a very deep commitment to care for each other, and they did it in many ways. But when somebody got that "notion," nobody knew what to do with it. They didn't understand it. Sometimes if the family couldn't deal with it, they hid it in the closet, because they were ashamed of it. There was a lot of shame connected with mental illness. There was really nobody outside the family they would have thought they could talk to about such a problem, except the minister or the bishop. And for those men, mental illness was the first thing they encountered that they really couldn't help with. They were frustrated that they couldn't meet those needs in their congregations.

It was apparently this frustration that led Souderton Mennonite Church pastor Jacob M. Moyer to seek Dr. Peters' counsel soon after the doctor set up shop in Telford. "He called me up and said he wanted to see me—not professionally, but after office hours," Dr. Peters later recalled. "He wanted to talk to me about something. So I said, 'Sure, come on over.' I wasn't that busy in those days. So he came over to talk to me and he said he had been hearing about psychiatry, but he didn't really know what it was. He wanted to know if there was 'anything to this psychiatry.' Was it really something *good*? Well, with me just having started my practice and having recently had training in psychiatry, we had a long talk about what psychiatry was, what it could do, and how important it was. Now, I'm sure I didn't convert him into a real evangelist for psychiatry, but I'm sure he began to *understand* it!"

Dr. Peters was also winning converts in his daily practice, as he related in 1990:

> I saw a lot of people who were depressed, and a lot of people with anxiety, which I'm sure was part of their depression. We didn't have the so-called remedies that they have today. We didn't know too much about the chemicals in the brain; how to either dissipate them or build them up. And our remedies were the bromides and the barbiturates. Of course, the bromides used to build up and become very toxic, so we used them very sparingly. Sometimes we gave depressed people a therapeutic dose of alcohol.
>
> My experience up to that time was that everybody—the population as a whole—has periods of depression, sometimes worse than others. There are times when people are a little low; other times they're very low. There are lots of variations. Depression was throughout the community, and not only here. It was the same way when I was in Philadelphia. But I did notice one thing here that was different. People talked about it within their extended families. They recognized the problem. Patients would tell me about other patients they were related to, and they'd say "Oh, so-and-so was like this," and "So-and-so was like that," meaning "mentally ill." The person might have been down to Norristown State Hospital or up to Allentown State Hospital, because there were no psychiatrists to go to in those days. And the families didn't hide it among themselves.
>
> I saw a lot more depressed women than men. Men would hide it better. I can still think of several markedly depressed older women who improved after I went to visit them, and got to talk with them alone. When they were alone—with no family members around—they could tell me about a lot of things that brought their depression on. I remember an old lady I used to go see in Telford who was terribly depressed. One day she said to me, "I want to talk to you alone the next time you come to my house." So the next time I went over there, I told the woman's daughter-in-law to leave us alone, that we wanted to talk in private. When we were alone the woman told me she was very unhappy that she was being

moved—first to the son for three months, then to the daughter for three months, and then to a daughter-in-law for three months. She said, "I'm too old for all this moving around and packing up. Why don't they send me to the Mennonite Home and let me stay there where I can be with my peers?" So I talked to her son, and of course he gave me hell. He said, "Look, I'll take care of my mother!" I said, "Well, if that's the case, then do what she wants!" So that settled that. The point is, I saw a lot of depressed people, and many of them knew they were depressed. They just didn't know what to do about it.

Dr. Peters had been practicing in Telford and promoting departmentalization at Grand View Hospital for just over four years when Japanese fighter pilots bombed the American naval base at Pearl Harbor on December 7, 1941, and a shaken America plunged into its second World War in a quarter-century. Business-as-usual was suspended indefinitely for millions of Americans, most dramatically for those men and women who uprooted themselves to go serve in the Armed Forces. Dr. Peters enlisted in the Army and wound up exercising his medical expertise as a chief of contagions section and the chief of medicine section for an eighteen-month term of service. During that time he was put in charge of a medical ward at Fourth Service Command in Atlanta, Georgia, next-door to a psychiatric ward overseen by no less a personage than Karl Augustus Menninger, co-founder of the pioneering Menninger Sanatorium in Topeka, Kansas, and widely regarded as the "dean of American psychiatry." "Dr. Karl" had been summoned by the Government to help stem the tide of war-related trauma casualties eroding the Nation's fighting capacity. At the Fourth Service Command he recognized in the young chief of medicine in the neighboring ward an uncommon awareness of the psychiatric aspects of health care. "Menninger said to me, 'Look, why don't you move over to the psychiatric division?'" Dr. Peters told an interviewer in 1990. "He says, "I'm the Chief of Psychiatry for the whole Fourth Service Command, and I could really use you.' Of course, I didn't want to do that. I said. 'Look, I'm the medical consultant for the Command, and I'm perfectly happy seeing psychiatric patients for their *medical* problems alone.' So I turned him down. But I was exposed to *a lot* of the psychiatry in the Army, and when I came home, everybody—doctors as well as patients—began to talk in terms of psychiatry. There was so much being made of psychiatric illnesses, because of the war. That was the hot topic."

Few persons in the Bux-Mont region turned a more attentive ear to psychiatric discussions in the years following World War II than a young general practitioner in Souderton named Norman Landis Loux. A seventh-generation German-American Mennonite on both the Loux and Landis sides of his family, Norman had charted a course in early adulthood more adventurous than most of his peers at Rosenberger's one-room school on the southern outskirts of Souderton, who eschewed formal education after six or eight grades in order to devote their energies to farming. Norman envisioned a different future for himself. In September 1937, at the age of eighteen, he enrolled as a boarding student in Eastern Mennonite High School in Harrisonburg, Virginia. He earned his high school degree there over the course of the next two-and-a-half years, and then decided to stay in Virginia to complete a two-year Associate Degree in biology at Eastern Mennonite College. During his time in the Old Dominion State, Norman was smitten by a fellow boarding student named Esther Elizabeth Brunk, whom he married in June 1941. The newlyweds moved to Goshen, Indiana in the summer of 1942 so Norman could continue his pursuit of a B.A. degree in biology at Goshen College, a relatively liberal Mennonite institution of higher education. Seven breathless months later, with his requirements for a B.A. degree fulfilled, Norman brought Esther back with him to Souderton, where the couple moved in with Norman's parents. Here they lived for the next few years,

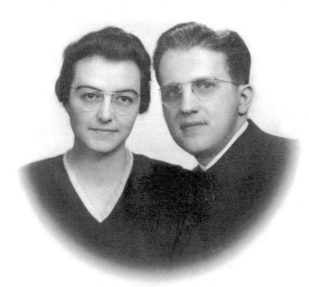

A seventh-generation German-American Mennonite on both sides of his family, Norman Landis Loux (b. 1919) ventured forth from his Franconia Township farming community as a young man to pursue a career in medicine. While earning an Associate Degree in biology at Eastern Mennonite College in Harrisonburg, Virginia, he met and eventually married (in June 1941) Virginia native Esther Brunk.

as Norman commuted by train to Philadelphia while working toward a degree in general medicine at Hahnemann Medical College. In the months following World War II, Norman served his internship under none other than Dr. Michael Peters, who was spending part of his week teaching internal medicine at Hahnemann. "Pete" quickly became a mentor for his young Bux-Mont neighbor. Whenever their schedules permitted, the men shared a ride to or from Philadelphia so they could exchange ideas. The relationship took another step forward in the summer of 1947 when Norman completed his training at Hahnemann and—having just turned twenty-eight—joined the family practice of Mennonite doctor Paul M. Nace in Souderton.

During what turned out to be a sixteen-month career as a general physician, Dr. Loux came to see that "the most important issues in the family practitioner's office revolved around people with emotional problems" (as he told an interviewer in 1999). Dr. Peters put it this way: "Norman was quick to recognize that most of his patients were really in need of psychiatric care rather than pills." "But psychiatry was the area of medicine I knew *least* about," Dr. Loux recalled recently. "That stimulated my interest in getting more training. It was very reassuring to have someone like Dr. Peters support my growing interest."

Also feeding into Dr. Loux's ruminations on a potential career shift were the heart-rending stories and descriptions he heard from his Mennonite brothers and sisters who had spent time during the recent war serving as attendants in state mental hospitals. When the Selective Service had reluctantly agreed in 1941 to allow drafted members of historic peace churches—Mennonites, Brethren, and Quakers—to legally register as conscientious objectors to military service and fulfill their duties through noncombatant "Alternative Service" of "national importance," the first of an eventual host of 37,000 COs were dispatched to 152 Civilian Public Service Camps across the country. Most male COs were housed in the barracks of former Civilian Conservation Corps or Forest Service camps, where they were put to hard unpaid labor planting trees, building roads, and constructing dams in remote locations. Other "conchies" (as they were sometimes called by unsympathetic countrymen) built sanitary facilities for hookworm-ridden communities, ran medical clinics in areas of rural poverty, cared for juvenile delinquents, conducted agricultural experiments, and worked on soil conservation projects.

For many COs, these tasks did not rise to the level of "work of national importance," which they had been promised by law, so they pressed for more significant assignments. Some COs were eventually permitted to serve as guinea pigs in dangerous, even life-threatening, medical experiments designed to find cures for malaria, infectious hepatitis, atypical pneumonia, and typhus. Others undertook hazardous tours of duty as smoke jumpers, fighting fires in national parks in Montana, Idaho, and Oregon. Still others were dispatched to state mental hospitals where staffs had been severely depleted by war-time exigencies. COs ended up serving in forty-one mental institutions in twenty states, and at seventeen training schools for "mental deficients" in a dozen states.

Many lives were changed through the experiences of more than three-thousand conscientious objectors thrust into the chaos of America's understaffed mental institutions in the mid-1940s. Descriptions of deplorable physical conditions and barbaric treatment of "inmates"—a desperate state of affairs exacerbated by a shortage of care-givers and a surfeit of war-related trauma victims—filtered back to the families and congregations of the COs, about half of whom were Mennonites. Surely, something had to be done *immediately* to relieve this suffering, and then long-term reform had to be enacted which would guarantee humane care and treatment for persons afflicted with mental illness. It has been suggested that the postwar movement particularly among Mennonites to establish benevolent and progressive "mental health" institutions was also fueled by a desire to make a major contribution to society, something "Alternative Service" had held them back from accomplishing during the war years.

Norman Loux listened to Mennonites who served in such miserable human warehouses as Philadelphia State Hospital ("Byberry"), New Jersey State Hospital in Greystone Park, and, closer to home, Norristown State Hospital. The young Souderton doctor read—along with the rest of the nation—a shocking article published in the May 6, 1946 issue of *Life Magazine* under the headline "Bedlam 1946, Most U.S. Mental Hospitals Are a Shame and Disgrace," which drew upon narrative data and photographic documentation culled from conscientious objector experiences during the last years of the war. He was aware that the collectors of the information published in the *Life Magazine* article—Quaker founders of the Mental Hygiene Program of the Civilian Public Service—had stepped up their efforts after the war and reorganized as the National Mental Health Association, with headquarters in Philadelphia. He followed discussions among Mennonite CPS veterans as they sought to clarify the role their church should take in providing mental health care. He noted how "the emphasis on humane custodial care" urged by private citizens was

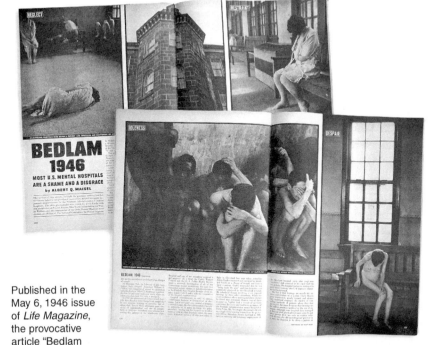

Published in the May 6, 1946 issue of *Life Magazine*, the provocative article "Bedlam 1946" drew upon narrative data and photographic documentation culled from conscientious objector experiences during the last years of World War II to notify the nation that "Most U.S. Mental Hospitals Are a Shame and Disgrace."

being complemented in the medical community by "a greater appreciation for treatment possibilities." War-time had provided "an excellent climate in which to do investigative work in psychiatry," he told an interviewer in 1999. "Psychiatrists who went into the service had their attitudes changed. They began to see that mental illness could be treated and cured. They could see where the actual nature of an illness was changed. Patients responded to treatment for depression. Schizophrenics got better, some even overcoming their delusions."

As Dr. Loux's interest in psychiatry became known in wider Mennonite circles, his counsel was solicited by organizers of mental health institutions. Late in 1946 he accompanied representatives of the Mennonite Central Committee (MCC)—a relief, service, and peace agency of North American Mennonite and Brethren in Christ churches—on a trip to the National

Mental Health Association headquarters in Philadelphia to discuss the establishment of a "rest home for Mennonites needing mental care" on a recently-vacated CPS base in Leitersburg, Maryland (this facility would open its doors in January 1949 as "Brook Lane Farm," the first of three Mennonite mental "rest homes" established under the 1947 MCC master plan for mental health care). In the summer of 1948, members of the recently-organized Lancaster Mennonite Hospitals Board of Trustees met with Dr. Loux to hear his views on the establishment of a private mental hospital in the Lancaster area (three years later, this institution would begin serving the public under the name "Philhaven").

And then there were the persistent urgings of Dr. Peters. Recently appointed Chief of Medicine for Grand View Hospital, "Pete" took every opportunity to impress upon his protégé the community's need for a medically-astute psychiatrist. His colleagues at Grand View Hospital were equally anxious to have this critical service provided in the region. So it came to pass that after sixteen months of general practice in Souderton, Dr. Loux decided at the relatively young age of twenty-nine to pursue a career in psychiatry. "One of my teachers at Hahnemann—an orthopedic surgeon—heard I was interested in psychiatry," he has reported. "He said, 'You ought to go up to Butler Hospital in Providence, Rhode Island. My nephew, David Wright, is up there. He's the administrator of the hospital, and he's a psychiatrist. That's the place you should go.' That was the first time I had heard of Butler. I went up there for a visit, and it was a very sophisticated place, another world for this Pennsylvania Dutch farm boy. But I liked it, so we went up there."

2

"PSYCHIATRY OFFICE OPENED IN SOUDERTON"

Transported in January 1949 with his wife Esther and three-month-old daughter Elizabeth to "another world" in Providence, Rhode Island, Norman Loux enrolled in the residency training program at Butler Hospital, a nonprofit voluntary-admission hospital for emotionally ill patients. The 140-bed establishment had just celebrated a century of cutting-edge psychiatric care and treatment. After twenty-one months of training at Butler, Dr. Loux relocated with his family to New Haven, Connecticut to undertake a one-year fellowship at Yale University's School of Medicine, in the Department of Psychiatry and the Child Study Center. The year in New Haven was made possible by a stipend provided by officials of Butler Hospital, who hoped Dr. Loux would return to Butler when he completed his study at Yale. These hopes were rewarded in the fall of 1951, as Dr. Loux moved his family back to Providence around the time that his number came up in the draft for military service in the year-old Korean War. When he registered as a conscientious objector to war, Dr. Loux was assigned by the Selective Service director for Rhode Island—who happened to be a director of Butler Hospital—to perform alternate service at Butler, where a number of other COs had already been assigned. During his second stint at Butler, Dr. Loux served first as Chief of Service, then as Clinical Director, and finally as Assistant Superintendent.

In New England, Dr. Loux trained under some of the psychiatric profession's leading lights, the brightest among them being Dr. Gregory Zilboorg, Butler's Director of Research and Training and Associate Clinical Professor of Psychiatry at New York State University. "Dr. Zilboorg was a Russian Jew, a very distinguished man who wore his hair long before people wore their hair long," Dr. Loux recalled in a 1999 interview:

He was a prolific writer [most notably *A History of Medical Psychology*, 1941] and he was well-known throughout the world. Of course, I didn't know that at the time, but I was impressed anyway. When we met, he said, "I'm so glad to see you. I knew you were coming to train here. I know you're a Mennonite. The Mennonites and the Quakers saved my life in Russia during the Revolution." That would have been in 1918-19. Dr. Zilboorg became my mentor and was a tremendous help to me in many, many ways. That was remarkable, because I was up there like a babe in the woods. Through him I met so many important people, in ways I couldn't have engineered myself. I got to know Daniel Blain, for example, who was president of the American Psychiatric Association and a very powerful man in American psychiatry. I met [Lancaster County native] Kenneth Appel, who was professor of psychiatry at the University of Pennsylvania, a very distinguished man who had been president of the American Psychiatric Association. He became a great friend, and gave [Penn Foundation] lots of help.

Then there was Milton Senn, who was Director of the Child Study Center at Yale School of Medicine. He was extremely helpful. And Dr. [Fredrick "Fritz" C.] Redlich, who was the professor of psychiatry at Yale. Leo Bartemeier was just an outstanding man, a psychiatrist and a professor at the University of Maryland. Dr. Francis Braceland was president of the American Psychiatric Association. Howard Rome was the psychiatrist at Mayo Clinic, and also a President of the American Psychiatric Association. Dana Farnsworth was the psychiatrist for students at Harvard University. Robert Felix, who was the Director of the National Institute of Mental Health, became a very close friend. These were all people I got to know through Dr. Zilboorg and through Butler Hospital. I had intimate contact with professors of various religious backgrounds—Jewish, Catholic, Protestant—and I was surprised by how supportive they were of me, in helping me integrate psychological understanding into my religious background.

I didn't plan these meetings. They just sort of fell into place. It was interesting that all of these people put an emphasis on my Mennonite background and the influence Mennonites were having in the mental health field. They didn't know that much about Mennonites, but they knew that Mennonites were humanitarians. They knew about the COs in the mental hospitals. That was the start.

Of all the occupational relationships Dr. Loux established in New England, none bore greater fruit than the connection he made with Ruby Horwood, an unmarried Canadian woman equipped with a Master of Library Science degree from the University of Toronto. "I had been working as a branch librarian at the Providence Public Library in 1951 when I went to Butler to set up its medical library," Ruby told an interviewer in 2000, continuing:

> I also served as a research assistant to Dr. Zilboorg. I worked very closely with the clinical staff at Butler, setting up appointments for Dr. Loux, updating mailing lists, serving as secretary of the Board of Trustees. Eventually, a lot of my work had nothing to do with the library. I was great friends with the medical director and Dr. Loux, who was the clinical director. He was regarded at Butler as a very caring physician—very popular with the nurses and liked by the patients. I had a house on the campus next-door to Dr. Loux's house. I really spent quite a bit of time with his family, having dinner with them and that kind of thing.

Ruby remembers that Dr. Loux retained a strong connection to the southeastern Pennsylvania community of his "growing-up years." She was involved in arranging his frequent visits back home—where his mother's health was deteriorating—and she made appointments for long-time patients and friends from the Bux-Mont region to consult with him in Providence. That is how she met the inimitable Dr. Michael Peters, who, while taking a course at Harvard University, made a side trip to drop in on his young colleague at Butler. During his two-day visit, Dr. Peters pressed home the point that psychiatric services were still desperately needed in the Souderton area. If Dr. Loux would only return home to provide those services, he could expect to be welcomed with open arms. He would receive all the assistance he needed from the doctors at Grand View, as well as a handful of area businessmen and community leaders who had been sensitized to psychiatry's healing potential.

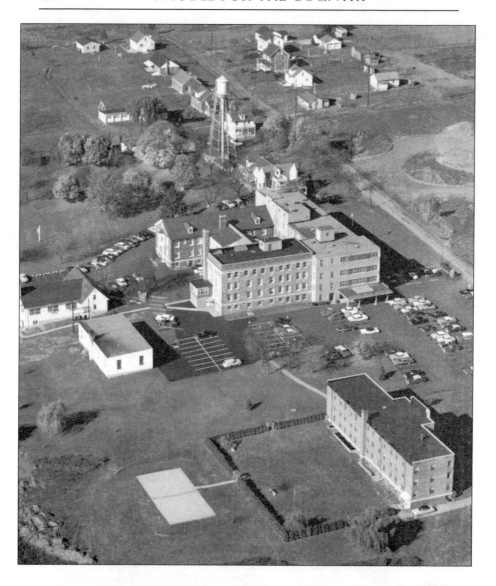

Grand View Hospital was established in 1913 in a two-story frame building along the west side of Lawn Avenue in Bucks County's West Rockhill Township, just west of Sellersville (the original structure is visible in this northward-looking aerial view on the water tower's immediate right). A much larger stone building was erected in 1917, and substantial additions were dedicated in 1919, 1939, and 1956. By the time this picture was taken in 1961, the Hospital campus also included a Nurses Home for the School of Nursing (in the right-hand foreground), opened in 1951.

Laying groundwork in the Bux-Mont region

Dr. Loux was left to ponder his colleague's compelling invitation, while Dr. Peters returned to Pennsylvania to rub the other side of the coin. In his capacities as private practitioner, Chief of Grand View Hospital's Department of Medicine, teacher at Hahnemann Hospital, and community activist, Dr. Peters had frequent opportunities to share with movers and shakers in the Bux-Mont region his dream of community-based psychiatric services. Among the many ears he filled were those of Charles H. Hoeflich, a Philadelphia National Bank officer who had moved to a farm in central Bucks County and joined Hilltown Township's Blooming Glen Mennonite congregation. Charles later remarked on Dr. Peters' strategy: "He went up to Providence to do a little selling, and then, having done a little selling on the *supply* side, he came back to Pennsylvania to create demand on the *use* side. He talked to builders, to bankers, to insurance men, to lawyers, discussing psychiatry with us as though we were wise in the field."

Three other businessmen with whom Dr. Peters had promising exchanges were also middle-aged members of the Blooming Glen Mennonite congregation. The oldest was Mahlon A. Souder, a Grand View Hospital board member who turned fifty in 1952. Mahlon made his living as a "commission merchant" (colloquially known as a "market man," "huckster," or "butter-and-egg man"), selling farm produce door-to-door in Philadelphia and its suburbs, and as an independent insurance broker and agent for State Farm Insurance. Eight years his junior was Roland M. Detweiler, President of I.G. Rosenberger Farm Store in Silverdale, Hilltown Township. The youngest was Paul F. Souder—still in his late thirties—the proprietor of a turkey hatchery in Sellersville, and a part-time insurance agent. All of these men had known Norman Loux in his youth, and all of them had been sensitized—either first-hand or through friends, family members, or employees—to the therapeutic benefits of psychiatric treatment. Dr. Peters singled them out for his most intensive lobbying.

Roland Detweiler was an easy mark, as he was one of Dr. Peters' patients. Four decades after the fact, Dr. Peters recalled:

> I was examining Roland in my office one day. I spent more time talking about starting a mental health center than I did on examining him. I felt a little guilty about that, but I felt I had to do it. And he was all for it. He said he would go out

and take care of his part [in drumming up support]. Well, one day in Philadelphia, when I was teaching at Hahnemann, I stopped into the Reading terminal to get my shoes shined, and who should walk over to me but Paul Souder. And he says, "Dr. Peters, I heard you're talking about starting some psychiatric program up in our area. Count me in! I'm all for it." I was pleased. Then I got word that some people had approached Charlie Hoeflich with the idea. And Charlie said to them, "It really sounds like something we need, but what does Dr. Peters up at Grand View Hospital think about it?" And they said, "Well, he's the guy that's starting it!" So Charlie got very involved.

Actually, Dr. Peters had no intention of "starting" a mental health center through his own efforts. "I always had in mind that one day Norman Loux would come back to the area and start to practice psychiatry," he reflected late in his life. "I had no idea *how* he would do this. I figured he would work that out himself. I remember talking to him as time went on and getting a little distressed when he said he didn't think he was coming back because the [Mennonite] church wanted him to go to some other state to start up a program, maybe a big hospital for the care of the mentally ill. And of course I tried to convince him that he was born and raised here and that he owed it to his community to come back." "He raised a little guilt," Dr. Loux later acknowledged.

Dr. Peters had other ways of applying pressure. Among the Bux-Mont laymen who had expressed interest in helping establish a community mental health center, he let it be known that the only man for the Director's job was Norman Loux. Charles Hoeflich recalls getting together with some of his Blooming Glen Mennonite Church brethren to "pray for direction as to how we should move." He continues:

I knew "Pete" thought highly of Norman. So we decided we'd find out more about this Norman Loux ourselves. I called the President of the Rhode Island Hospital National Bank and I asked him if he knew Dr. Loux. Yes, indeed he did know Dr. Loux! It was like turning on a faucet of praises. Then I happened to be with Will Menninger [Administrator of the Menninger Clinic and brother of "Dr. Karl" Menninger] in Philadelphia, and I asked him if he knew a man named

Dr. Norman Loux. He said, "Indeed I do!" I said, "What could you tell me about him?" He said, "Charlie, that man will be one of the ten brightest psychiatrists in this country." I reported back to the other men on these conversations. There was no question: we weren't going to search anywhere else for someone to get our psychiatric facility off the ground.

Intensive lobbying

Now it was a matter of convincing Dr. Loux—still ensconced in his job as Assistant Superintendent of Butler Hospital—to pull up his tent pegs and make a pilgrimage with his wife, daughter, and newborn son to southeastern Pennsylvania. The most memorable of the lobbying efforts mounted during the first half of 1954 occurred when Dr. Loux traveled home in June to spend some time with his mother, who had been stricken with leukemia. Dr. Peters had gotten wind of Dr. Loux's impending visit, and he put out the word among his fellow lobbyists that an opportunity was at hand. The phone lines buzzed. "When I got to my parents' house," Dr. Loux remembers, "My dad said, 'I don't know what's happening. There are *dozens* of phone calls coming in for you, from people who want you to get in touch with them.' It was all these men calling to tell me they were expecting me to move back to the Souderton area."

Among the callers was construction contractor Harold Mininger, who would become one of Penn Foundation's charter Board members and one of its principal supporters. Harold could attest to pleas he had been hearing from members of the medical community, as he recalled during a recent interview:

> I remember Dr. [Arthur] Wise, who was a family doctor [in Souderton], telling me, "Harold, somebody has to help us." I'd be wondering what he meant. And he'd say, "We see a lot of patients that we shouldn't be seeing. We're not trained to help them.' He'd tell me how so many people were coming to him and putting their faith in him and he wasn't prepared to help them. He wasn't trained for it and he wished he could see something happen. He'd say, "Somebody should be the motivating force to make another kind of treatment available that would meet these needs." He meant "psychiatric treatment," of course.

Stirred by the barrage of entreaties, Dr. Loux became more specific in his conversations with Dr. Peters, who later reported:

> I recall him saying he would give [the idea of establishing a mental health facility in the Bux-Mont area] serious consideration, but that he had certain expectations or requirements. "First of all," [Dr. Loux] said, "I can't practice psychiatry as an individual. I would need a team around me. Secondly," he said, "it should be an institution from which everything having to do with mental health emanates. For example," he said, "We should have communications with the local judges, the local police, the local school teachers, the local doctors, and the local lawyers, and so on." He said, "Everything that has to do with psychiatry should emanate from this particular place." And here, what he was doing—although I didn't recognize it at the time—was describing what later turned out to be the programs that were needed by a community mental health service.

A seminal proposal

Dr. Peters suggested that Dr. Loux expand on his ideas in writing so they could be shared with interested parties, particularly persons who might serve as organizers, fundraisers, and trustees of a Bux-Mont mental health center. In the summer of 1954, thirty-five-year-old Norman Loux typed up and submitted an eight-page summary of his "reflections concerning the establishment of an organization through which to provide psychiatric service for our community." The first half of this paper constituted an overview of psychiatry's evolution during the previous century, culminating in the post-World War II consensus that "the greatest emphasis should not be placed on **custodial** care, important though this aspect of the total care of the mentally ill continues to be, [but on] the **understanding, treatment**, and even **prevention** of emotional illness." In the second half of his paper, Dr. Loux laid out "suggestions concerning the basic requirements in the establishment of a community psychiatric service":

> (1) It requires a nucleus of people who have a vision of the needs for and the possibilities of developing such a psychiatric service.

(2)   It requires a sound organization with a master plan, which is simple but clear as to its basic principles.

(3)   Physical facilities which are intelligently attuned to the needs spelled out by the master plan. The following seem to me to be the basic physical facilities that will be needed.

A.   Facilities for the care of people who are acutely emotionally ill, to such a degree that they cannot remain in the community. These facilities must be of a very special type with accommodations ranging from those which are adapted to the care of those patients who are most disturbed to those which are adapted to those patients who are again nearly ready to take their place in the community.

B.   Facilities for an active out-patient service. In my estimation, it would be important that the physical facilities be attuned to a program where the greatest portion of the work is done among those people who do not need to be hospitalized but who would be receiving care and treatment while living in the community.

C.   Facilities to carry on clinical research. It is my conviction that a service rendering first-class psychiatric care cannot be developed without the simultaneous development of a clinical research program, no matter how modest in scope. It is true that the major ingredient of clinical research comes from the efforts of the staff, a modern psychiatric library being the only urgent requirement as far as physical facility is concerned.

D.   Facilities utilized in providing constructive diversionary activity for patients. In this respect it must be remembered that patients in a hospital for the emotionally ill are not bedfast most of the time and have relatively large segments of time at their disposal during the course of the day. The exact nature of the diversionary activities must be determined after careful study and consideration, but in my estimation must be kept rigidly free of the atmosphere which is so prevalent in facilities which have existed in most hospitals for the emotionally ill since the advent of psychiatric hospitals.

It goes without saying that in the consideration of physical facilities which will be basic requirements for the establishment of a psychiatric service, provision will need to be made for the application of the most modern forms of psychiatric treatment. As I see it from the point of view of physical facilities, this provides no great problem of cost; it is rather a problem of architectural design.

I have summarized what I feel to be the more or less tangible requirements of an adequate psychiatric service in our community. Important though these tangible requirements are, there are requirements which are not easily definable and measurable; these are to be found in the spirits and efforts of the people in the community, as well as from people outside the community who undoubtedly will be asked or will offer their help.

I picture physical facilities which are modern in construction and design and which can be identified as a concrete symbol of what service we expect to render. The exact size is in need of determination through a careful survey and intelligent weighing of various factors. The exact location also is in need of determination as is the fact of whether it should be located on the grounds of a now-existing general hospital or whether it should stand more alone. However important these physical facilities, their size and location, as well as their general characteristics may be, it must be remembered that bricks and mortar, glass and other material equipment do not constitute a hospital. There needs to be a competent staff who are dedicated to common principles, who are alert, imaginative, and willing to work hard to translate their interests and visions into action and reality. There needs to be a competent, interested and dedicated board of trustees who are at the same time sound in their business judgment and yet not too rigid to fail to have vision and enthusiasm. It goes without saying that among those connected with the hospital, either directly or indirectly, there needs to be cultivated the best and most noble of those ingredients which go into service rendered to our fellowman.

I should like to say just a word about how what I have outlined can be implemented. I am frank to admit that I do not think it will be easy; no worthwhile project ever is. I do, however, have the firm conviction that there is a tremendous need for first-class psychiatric services on a community level. I believe that what we have in mind is somewhat unique, and as the plans are developed, it will arouse the interest as well as the support of a wide variety of people. If we are conscientious and if we are diligent in our efforts, we can have a project which will be thought of as a sort of pilot study for other similar programs in other areas. I have the definite conviction that the community, including the physicians, religious leaders, as well as the average lay person, is eager for such a service and will respond to a degree which will tax our imagination if we are faithful in providing the proper leadership. I am further convinced that once we are organized and have plans that show concretely the reasonableness of our plans, that there will be money available from various foundations. Finally, I am convinced that where there is a need, people will respond in providing what is necessary to meet the need. I believe that a project of this kind cannot be done half way. I should like to find it possible to spend most of my time in the next six months, with the help of a very competent assistant, in drawing up plans on the basis of careful investigation and thorough consultation with competent people. At the same time, I would hope that there would be efforts in the direction of forming a permanent organization of a non-profit corporation type through which our program would be administered.

Organizing principals

Dr. Loux's proposal was eagerly received by Dr. Peters and the handful of Bux-Mont laymen at the forefront of the organizing movement. Here, finally, was tangible evidence that a community-based psychiatric program might get off the ground with Dr. Loux at the controls. Prospective trustees discussed the proposal at a series of informal meetings, some of which were held over coffee and homemade pastries at Charles Hoeflich's Elderberry Farm in Bedminster Township, Bucks County. "Obviously, the first and most important thing [discussed at the earliest of these gatherings] was the need to put together a larger group," Charles would write in 1983. "Four men accustomed to the world of business 'out there' needed the company of others with similar qualifications and interest and commitment.

Fortunately each man knew a name or two of persons who could be counted on to bring an added dimension to the possible effort and who would be equally dedicated to the project."

During a recruitment period that spanned the remainder of 1954 and the first months of 1955, the number of "organizing principals" swelled to nearly a dozen. Souderton attorney Elvin E. Souder volunteered his considerable legal expertise. Hatfield Township dairyman Raymond H. Rosenberger offered his extensive business connections, as did Perkasie oil merchant Russell M. Moyer and Quakertown hosiery manufacturer and real estate manager Marcus A. Clemens. Union National Bank President Russell M. Hillegass joined the effort, along with Lloyd R. ("Poppy") Yoder, the legendary Bucks County educator, athletic coach, and director of Pearl S. Buck's "Welcome House" for orphaned children. Except for Russell Moyer, who belonged to the United Church of Christ, and the Lutheran Russell Hillegass, all of these men were active and influential members of local Mennonite congregations.

As the organizational groundwork was being laid on the "the use side," a couple of important developments occurred on "the supply side." According to Ruby Horwood, it was around this time that "[Butler's] Board decided to close the hospital for financial reasons. It was a very sad occasion, because the hospital had such a long tradition. It was a difficult time, very hard on the staff, very upsetting. Everybody was talking about 'What do we do next?'" This turn of events coincided with an offer of $6,000 in start-up funds or "seed money" from Nelson Moyer, owner of North Penn Hide Company, a rendering business located a few miles outside Souderton. "Nels" Moyer indicated the funds could be used to cover Dr. Loux's salary and expenses during the months it took him to establish a psychiatric practice in Souderton—the first phase in what Nels and other supporters hoped would be the organization of a community mental health center.

Ruby Horwood contemplated an invitation from Dr. Zilboorg to continue in his employ after Butler Hospital closed, assisting him with research projects in America and Europe. Then Dr. Loux posed another intriguing possibility. Would Ruby be interested in moving with him and his family to southeastern Pennsylvania, where she would be invaluable as an administrator of a private psychiatric practice, and then—if everything worked out—of a pioneering mental health center? "I didn't really know specifically what I'd be doing," Ruby recalls, and she recognized she had virtually no experience with the Pennsylvania Dutch culture she would be immersed in, but she enjoyed such a "friendly situation" with Dr. Loux and his family in Providence, and she felt such "enthusiasm for his dream," that she agreed to accompany the Louxes to a new home in the Souderton area. The decision to embark on this venture together appears to have been confirmed around the time Dr. Loux turned thirty-six, on July 27, 1955.

Return to Souderton

By the following September, the Loux family and Ruby were unpacking in temporary quarters outside Souderton, on a farm owned by "seed money" provider Nels Moyer ("Nels was Penn Foundation's first 'angel,' Charles Hoeflich has remarked). Here the Louxes would stay until renovations could be completed on their new home: the farmhouse where Dr. Loux had been born and raised. Dr. Loux remembers planning to "spend the first six months [in the Souderton area] evaluating, looking

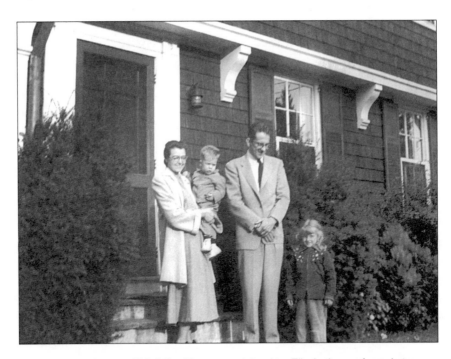

Mother Esther, son Phil, father Norman, and daughter Elizabeth pose for a photograph in front of the Loux family residence in Providence, Rhode Island in the spring of 1955. The family was a few months away from moving back to the Souderton area, where a cadre of concerned doctors and businessmen were eager to help Dr. Loux establish the first psychiatric practice in the Bux-Mont region.

around, seeing what the best approach would be" to addressing the community's mental health needs. Now that he was back among friends and family, however, much of his time was devoted to seeing a backlog of patients, some of whom he had been serving for years, and others who had been newly referred by relieved local doctors. Several Souderton area physicians offered space in their offices for Dr. Loux to meet with patients. Grand View Hospital Department of Surgery Chief Dr. Leroy Moyer was particularly accommodating. "Can you imagine *that?*" Dr. Loux still asks in wonder. "I was allowed to use a surgeon's office to see psychiatric patients! That really helped me become blended into the community as a physician rather than as a 'shrink' or as a psychiatrist. I think it made a big difference in how I was accepted."

Dr. Loux's dedication to his cause was immediately apparent. "He was really a workaholic," Ruby Horwood recalls. "We had patients day and night. I don't know how many evenings a week he worked. And when he wasn't seeing patients he was scurrying around making speeches and really getting the community interested and helping form a board of directors." While he was working out of Dr. Moyer's office, Dr. Loux's recent commitment to addressing mental health needs in the Bux-Mont area was tested by an invitation he received from representatives of the Mennonite Central Committee's Mennonite Mental Health Association. They wanted him to establish or take charge of a Mennonite Church-sponsored psychiatric hospital elsewhere in the United States. "I remember [MCC founder and Lancaster County businessman] Orie Miller meeting with me in Dr. Moyer's office," Dr. Loux told an interviewer in 1999:

> He brought with him Delmar Stahly, who was secretary of the Mennonite Mental Health Association. Orie said, "Look, you should come to one of the Mennonite hospitals. You can almost have your pick. You could go to one in California.* You could go to one in Kansas.** We are thinking about starting one in Elkhart, Indiana.*** You could go there. That would be a good place for you." And I said, "That won't be possible, Orie. I'm committed here." That's the way we left

---

* King's View Homes, Reedley, California, opened on February 11, 1951 as the second and westernmost of the three Mennonite Mental Health Association in-patient hospitals called for in the 1947 MCC master plan.

** Prairie View opened in Newton, Kansas on March 15, 1954.

*** Oaklawn Psychiatric Center would begin serving the public on September 20, 1963.

it, but Orie was not accustomed to having people not go along with what he expected. A few days later I got a letter from him asking "Now which hospital would you like to go to?" He thought I would have changed my mind. I didn't, though. I have nothing but the highest regard for the hospitals that the Mennonite Mental Health Service [subsequently] started, but they were all in-patient facilities. That wasn't what I wanted. I didn't want a separate mental hospital. I wanted to have a community mental health center that was much more a part of the total medical services in the community.

A temporary home at 19 West Chestnut Street

And then Dr. Loux received yet another remarkable vote of confidence from his Souderton-area supporters. It came to the attention of some of these men that Borough officials were planning to raze several buildings along the north side of West Chestnut Street to make room for an expanded municipal parking lot. One of these buildings—located at 19 West Chestnut Street—was a vacant house owned by a group of Souderton merchants, including Paul K. Fisher, founder of Fisher's Furniture Store, and one of the area's wealthiest, most colorful, and most civically active citizens. At the request of Dr. Loux's promoters, Fisher and his colleagues agreed to allow Dr. Loux to use this building as a psychiatric office and as a meeting place for backers of the community mental health initiative. "That was an amazing thing!" Dr. Loux recently remarked about this development. "Where else could something like that have happened? It was truly amazing how things worked out, although it didn't amaze me as much then as it does now."

For her part, Ruby Horwood was astonished to see how the organizers and their wives—middle-aged pillars of the community—rolled up their sleeves and dove into the task of readying the house on West Chestnut Street for service as a psychiatric facility. "I remember all these people, the Miningers and the Souders, coming to the house, cleaning and working, getting all dirty," she told an interviewer recently. "Mrs. [Mahlon] Souder was a real great worker, in particular. I can still see her out on the porch roof, cleaning windows. As a cultural thing, that was a great surprise to me. I mean, I couldn't see this kind of involvement happening in other communities." Ruby was particularly appreciative of cleaning efforts on the building's second floor, which would serve as her living quarters for the foreseeable future.

As noted in the prologue to this narrative, the first organizational meeting of the future Penn Foundation for Mental Health for which minutes were recorded took place in the West Chestnut Street building on Thursday, October 20, 1955 (Dr. Loux probably began seeing patients in this facility around this time). On hand for the "informal and exploratory" session was a self-described "nucleus group" comprising Dr. Loux, Roland Detweiler, Charles Hoeflich, Elvin Souder, Mahlon Souder, and Ruby Horwood, with Ruby serving as secretary (she was still so new to this scene that she spelled the banker's name "Charles Hoflick"). According to Ruby's minutes, "the following topics were brought up for discussion: 1) The legal requirements for the establishment of a non-profit organization which would be recognized as eligible to receive tax-deductible gifts. . . ; 2) The procedures to be followed in the registration and incorporation of an organization formed to promote the establishment of a psychiatric facility. . . ; 3) Choice of a name for the organization. . . ; 4) Selection of members of the Board of Trustees. . .; 5) Publicity. . . ; and 6) Dr. Loux's relationship to the organization." Attorney Elvin Souder provided most of the input on the legal issues, and Charles Hoeflich took the lead in matters of publicity. Among other things, the organizers quickly agreed that two principles should guide the selection of Trustees: "(a) The Board should include only those who are genuinely interested in the promotion of the proposed program, [and] (b) Various denominational groups, business and professional groups and different localities within the community should be represented." Dr. Loux opined "that it would be desirable to have an advisory board of physicians representing the various specialties and the hospitals in the community," and that "it [was] of utmost importance that the physicians on the advisory board meet regularly and have an intimate acquaintanceship with the policies of the hospital."

A "North Penn Foundation for Mental Health"?

The task of adopting a corporate title proved a little more difficult, according to the October 20 meeting minutes:

> Dr. Loux thought that it might be possible to select a name which could be used during the organizational period but

which might not necessarily be the name of the institution. It was decided, however, that it would be preferable to select a name which would be permanently associated with the entire program. It was suggested that a name associated with a geographical location would be preferable to one honoring an individual. It was felt that "Souderton Foundation for Mental Health" might limit its appeal. "North Penn Foundation for Mental Health, Inc." was accepted, though there was some misgiving because of its wide use for business concerns, etc.

This "misgiving" would lead to the adoption of a different corporate title a few weeks down the road. In the meantime, the "nucleus group" resolved that "the community should be made aware of the fact that this project [is] to be a community effort and not a personal project on the part of Dr. Loux," and that "at the time Dr. Loux announces the opening of his office some indication could be given of tentative plans that have already been discussed for the establishment of a psychiatric facility." This strategy was implemented almost immediately, as Charles Hoeflich generated the organization's first press release (he would churn out scores

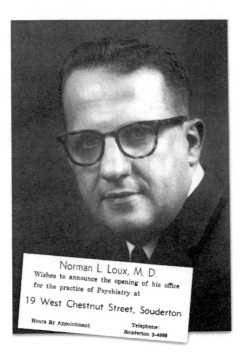

Norman L. Loux, M. D.
Wishes to announce the opening of his office for the practice of Psychiatry at

19 West Chestnut Street, Souderton

Hours By Appointment   Telephone:
                              Souderton 3-4989

Having opened an office in a temporarily vacated house on Souderton's West Chestnut Street, thirty-six-year-old psychiatrist Norman Loux began advertising his services in October 1955 issues of the *Souderton Independent*.

more in the coming years). Charles' write-up was published verbatim in the next issue of the *Souderton Independent*, which hit newsstands on October 27:

Psychiatry Office Opened in Souderton

Dr. Norman L. Loux has recently announced the opening of his office for the practice of Psychiatry at 19 West Chestnut St., Souderton.

Dr. Loux is a native of Souderton. He is a graduate of Goshen College, Goshen, Indiana and Hahnemann Medical College, Philadelphia. After his internship he practiced general medicine in Souderton for several years until he and his family moved to Providence, Rhode Island where he began his psychiatric training. In the meantime he has done postgraduate work in Psychiatry at Yale University School of Medicine. Before returning to this community he was associated with Butler Hospital in Providence, Rhode Island, serving in the capacity of Assistant Superintendent and Clinical Director. While in Providence he participated in many community activities including Parent-Teacher Association programs, group discussions sponsored by ministerial associations, and seminars for teachers of the Rhode Island Department of Education. He was consultant to various community agencies and a director of the Providence Child Guidance Clinic.

In making the decision to return to his home community, he was strongly influenced by the generous encouragement given to him by physicians as well as other citizens of the community who are interested in the establishment of a psychiatric facility on the community level. Dr. Loux feels that the wholesome interest in mental health shown by physicians and lay people alike in a fast developing and progressive community presents a unique challenge for rendering service in this branch of medicine.

Dr. Loux is married and has two children, Elizabeth Ann, age 7 and Philip Michael, age 2. They plan to live south of Souderton on the Cowpath Road.

3

A NEW HOME
WITH A GRAND VIEW

No one in the "nucleus group" of organizers meeting in Souderton's first psychiatric office in the fall of 1955 expected the work of establishing a community mental health center to be quickly or easily accomplished. A portent of the challenging road ahead presented itself almost immediately, as Roland Detweiler, Charles Hoeflich, Elvin Souder, Mahlon Souder, Ruby Horwood, and Norman Loux struggled with what purported to be a relatively simple task: choosing a name for their organization. Of the titles suggested during the first gathering of these pioneers, "North Penn Foundation for Mental Health, Inc." had met with the broadest approval. But a couple of the parties to the discussion worried that adopting such a geographically distinctive appellation might "limit [the organization's] appeal." So the organizers gave themselves a few more days to stew in their creative juices.

At the second meeting of the "nucleus group," held on Saturday afternoon, October 29, name-choosing topped the agenda. The task was deemed "most urgent," according to Ruby Horwood's minutes, because "no application for incorporation could be filed until [a name] was decided upon." A host of corporate titles—all of them ending in "Foundation for Mental Health, Inc."—were proposed, probed, and pondered over the course of the next hour. Despite the growing sense of urgency, no consensus was reached. "It was decided that the matter should be tabled for consideration at the next meeting," Ruby Horwood noted, which meant that filing for incorporation would have to wait at least a few more days. The organizers got better traction when they "agreed unanimously that Dr. Loux would be retained as Medical Director on a salary basis," after which "Dr. Loux stated that he could guarantee a considerable portion of the administrative expense for one year so that a minimum amount of the money solicited for the building fund would have to be used for current administrative expenses." Souderton's first professional psychiatrist was able to make this guarantee because of the seed money provided by Nels Moyer.

The meeting concluded with all parties agreeing that the number of pro tem Directors should be doubled, and that invitations to join the still-unchartered Penn Foundation Board should be extended to six locally prominent businessmen who had been instrumental in enticing Dr. Loux back to Pennsylvania, and who had been helping promote the concept of a community mental health center in the North Penn region. Three of these men—Harold Mininger, Marcus Clemens, and Paul Souder—immediately agreed to serve as Directors; the others expressed "definite interest," but asked for time to consider the implications. Harold and Marcus were so eager to participate in the venture that they managed to attend the very next gathering of organizers, held on the morning of Saturday, November 5. They thus had an opportunity to add their two cents to what turned out to be the final go-round in the "corporate title" deliberations. The list of worthy options had been winnowed to twelve, with each of the names concluding with the universally acceptable "Foundation for Mental Health, Inc." The candidates were "North Penn"; "Penn Valley"; "Penn Hill"; "Penn Dale"; "Penn Ridge"; "Upper Montgomery"; "Montgomery Bucks"; "Souderton"; "Franconia"; "Penn Montgomery"; "William Penn"; and simply "Penn." One-by-one, the prospective titles were considered. Then, as Ruby Horwood related in the meeting minutes:

> The [pro tem] Chairman, Dr. Loux summed up the discussion of previous meetings concerning the selection of a name and reported on the opinions of various people he had consulted. He felt it to be the consensus of opinion that the word Penn should be used to designate the locality and stated that he would be satisfied with any of the aforementioned names that the Board would agree upon. After further discussion, it was proposed by Mr. Hoeflich and seconded by Mr. Clemens that the organization be named The Penn Foundation for Mental Health, Inc. This name was adopted by unanimous consent. The application form to be forwarded to the State Department at Harrisburg was signed by all members present.

Organizing "The Penn Foundation for Mental Health, Inc."

After taking a collective breath, the Directors waded into the choppy seas of organizational structure at their November 5 meeting. With the pro tem Board having grown by three men, and with two more excellent candidates on the cusp of joining, "it was considered desirable to make no further appointments until a more definite program had been formulated." Then the need for advisory boards was discussed. All agreed that Dr. Loux should take the lead in pulling together a "Medical Advisory Board" comprising "representatives of the various medical specialties and hospitals in the area." A "Community Advisory Board" would also be valuable, but "it was agreed that it was a little too early for this to be feasible." Dr. Loux and Elvin Souder were appointed to draft a constitution to be presented at the next meeting, and then Charles Hoeflich set the stage for a discussion of a "Public Relations Program." It quickly became apparent that all parties recognized the critical importance of making a good first impression:

> Mr. Hoeflich stated that it was essential to have a well thought out public relations program set up and that the promotional aspects should be worked out carefully from the beginning. Mr. Mahlon Souder suggested that there should be a good deal of thought given to this matter so that the program should not be over-sold before definite plans had been formulated. Mr. Mininger pointed out the importance of making the right decisions at this time because once an impression has been formed it is apt to be a lasting one. He thought that a well-integrated program had to be presented although it was necessary to estimate in advance what support would be available for such a program. In this connection Dr. Loux summed up the aims and purposes of the Board in this way:
>
> (a) To provide hospital care for the mentally ill.
>
> (b) To provide an out-patient service for those who do not require hospitalization.
>
> (c) To provide a consultation service to ministers and teachers in the community.
>
> (d) To promote an educational program within the community to foster a better understanding of mental illness.

After two-and-a-half very productive hours, the organizers of the Penn Foundation for Mental Health, Inc. adjourned their November 5 meeting, agreeing to meet again in a week, and then to gather on the first Tuesday of each month thereafter, while allowing for the possibility that time-sensitive developments could necessitate the occasional "special meeting." And meet they did, as four more proponents of the local mental health care initiative—Russell Moyer, "Poppy" Yoder, Russell Hillegass, and Raymond Rosenberger—joined the group. By February 1956, Penn Foundation's charter Board comprised a dozen of the area's most well-connected businessmen, with Ruby Horwood serving as a kind of super administrative assistant.

Each of the founding fathers brought at least one form of expertise to the venture. It was attorney Elvin Souder, for instance, who filled out and filed the Application for Articles of Incorporation on February 14. Roland Detweiler, Harold Mininger, and Paul Souder, meanwhile, took responsibility for investigating potential sites for a permanent home. And even though all of the psychiatric laymen on the Board added their responsibilities to demanding day jobs, none of the Directors were busier during this critical period than Medical Director Norman Loux. As he noted in a report submitted to fellow Board members and Grand View Hospital personnel on April 10, 1956, Dr. Loux saw 148 patients during his first twenty weeks on the job, most of them at least several times. Patients visited his office 558 times over five months, a pace that worked out to five visits per day, six days per week. Most of these office visits were conducted in the late morning or afternoon, after Dr. Loux had made his rounds at Grand View Hospital. "All of the doctors at the Hospital made their rounds in the morning," he has explained. "That was the most convenient time. It was important to be there when the other doctors were there, so we could consult with each other. That gave me a chance to talk with the doctors who had referred my patients."

Beyond his treatment of patients, Dr. Loux found time to respond to what he described as the "genuine and intelligent interest in a psychiatric service . . . evidenced by the number of requests that I have had to talk to various groups on the subject." By his count, Dr. Loux had made twenty-six presentations to local professional associations, service organizations, parent-teacher associations, student-faculty groups, church groups, and student nurses at Grand View Hospital during his first five months in Souderton. He had also advised "ministers, teachers, lawyers, and members of the Police department [who] frequently requested help in solving problems that have arisen." In each of his public forays he was keenly aware of the implications his contributions might have on the future of the Penn Foundation for Mental Health.

Dr. Loux's April 1956 report to Penn Foundation Directors and Grand View Hospital personnel was chock-full of statistics he had gleaned from a variety of sources: his own experience as a practitioner; the responses he received to a questionnaire submitted to a hundred local doctors; and his analysis of a regional health survey conducted in 1950. All of these data, examined in light of countless discussions he had had with both laymen and professionals, led him to the following conclusions:

1. There is a definite need for facilities to care for the emotionally ill in our community.

2. Up to the present time, the emotionally ill have not been adequately cared for because of the unavailability of facilities. Many of those cared for outside of the community could have been treated to the greater satisfaction of the patient, his family and the referring physician, had adequate care been available within the community.

3. There exists an unusually wholesome and intelligent interest on the part of the people of the community.

4. On the basis of actual experience to date, the majority of patients have been referred by their family physicians, which indicates the physician's support of the program. Personal communications with many physicians indicate their intelligent support and willingness to participate in a psychiatric service.

5. There is a need and a great desire for a counseling service for individuals as well as for those whose work brings them in contact with the problems of others, for example, ministers, teachers, etc. Even though the present-day emphasis is on out-patient care, it is reasonable to assume that there is need for facilities for patients who need to be hospitalized.

So there was no question in Dr. Loux's mind that the Penn Foundation for Mental Health had a future. But what shape would this future take? And where, exactly, would this future take place? The house on Souderton's West Chestnut Street would soon be razed in order to expand the municipal parking lot. Where should the Directors look for a permanent home?

Overtures to Grand View Hospital

It had been clear to Dr. Loux for some time that the Foundation's services should be tightly integrated with those of Grand View Hospital, and that (as Hospital historian Walter J. Hendricks would write in 1966) "no inpatient beds should be developed [for the Foundation] apart from the hospital." Initially, at least, Dr. Loux's fellow Directors had another model in mind. "The Board thought of developing an inpatient facility in a quiet place where emotionally ill people could rest and where the community could rest from the disturbed people," Walter Hendricks recalled. "This was the pattern of existing psychiatric facilities everywhere," including the inpatient hospitals lately established by the Mennonite Health Association in Virginia, California, and Kansas. Director Harold Mininger already had his eye on a vacant tract south of Souderton. "It was down at the end of Hunsicker Lane," he remembered recently, "in back of Hunsicker's ice house. There was about an eighteen-acre spot in there, and a woods below. It was pretty isolated. I thought that would be a good place to start a mental hospital."

But Dr. Loux, after exhaustive research and consultation, was envisioning a compelling new paradigm: a community mental health center working in concert with a neighboring general hospital. This vision was encapsulated in the final section of his April 1956 report, under the heading "Suggested Plan for Meeting the Psychiatric Needs of the Community." Here Dr, Loux strongly recommended that the Foundation's headquarters be situated next-door to Grand View Hospital. Great care should be taken to ensure that the Foundation's services did not compete with those of the Hospital, which meant arranging for the Hospital to provide all inpatient services. To further enable the close collaboration of the two institutions, the Foundation's medical staff should—where possible and appropriate—also be part of the Hospital's staff.

The collaboration envisioned by Dr. Loux already had a fervent supporter on the Grand View Hospital staff in the person of Chief of Medicine Dr. Michael Peters. In fact, Dr. Peters had helped convince Dr. Loux this was the way to go, as Dr. Loux recalled recently:

> Soon after I opened my Souderton office, they brought to the hospital a little old lady, quite harmless, but she was very psychotic. She was having hallucinations and delusions. I said to Dr. Peters, "Goodness! We can't have someone so psychotic

in a general hospital here. We'll have to send her down to Abington [Memorial Hospital's psychiatric facility], or somewhere." He said, "What are you talking about? That's why we brought you here! We didn't send people away before you came. We're certainly not going to start now." And so we cared for her right there at Grand View, and it worked out very well. For a long time we cared for mentally ill patients on the medical floor, because Mike Peters was very willing to be helpful. He often ran interference for us.

Dr. Loux also went out on a limb to make this unusual arrangement work. Trustee Harold Mininger remembers hearing from Dr. Loux how the admission of the first psychotic patient to Grand View Hospital had transpired:

Norman told me he had a delusional patient who needed to stay overnight in the hospital so he could supervise her treatment. "I went over to the hospital," he says, "and I told them 'I'd like to have this person have a room over here.' And the nurse said, 'But we don't have any way of locking the doors. There's no way we can keep her here.' And Norm said, 'You don't need to lock her in. I'll be available. If anything should happen, I'll take care of it.' And that was our first experience with having a psychiatric patient in the hospital. It worked. That helped everyone see that the world was not going to come to an end, and you wouldn't have [psychotic] people running up and down the halls.

Dr. Peters has remarked that through the first admissions of emotionally disturbed patients to the Hospital "we wanted to take the stigma away from psychiatric illness by treating these patients the same as we did the patients who had pneumonia or appendicitis or gallbladders and so on. We wanted to show the other physicians and the nurses and the other patients that psychiatric patients could be mixed in. And I think we accomplished our mission."

There were other issues that made some Hospital authorities leery of linking up with an independently-run mental health center, particularly one that could be operating in the Hospital's literal shadow. Even if the two institutions managed to avoid offering overlapping services, they would still have to compete for grants and private donations. Dr. Peters reminisced late in life about a pointed exchange he had early in 1956 with William M. ("Hospital Bill") Moyer, the long-time president of Grand View's Board of Directors, frequently credited with pulling the Hospital back from the verge of financial collapse during the Great Depression. As Dr. Peters told an interviewer in 1990:

> Bill was "Mr. Grand View Hospital." He had a lot to do with getting the funds every year for programs and buildings. I remember, he came over to me one day, and he had me in a corner, and he said, "Now, look! We can't have people from a mental health center going and taking money from the same people we go to [for contributions]." And I said, "Look, if the community and the hospital needs this [mental health] program, then the money has to be raised. If the hospital was running the program, then you would have to go get that money. You ought to be glad [that the Penn Foundation Directors] are going to do it for you!" And I never heard another word about it from Bill after that. That was the end of it.

A farm on Sellersville's "Hospital Heights"

Just how amenable the other members of Grand View's Board were to the prospect of partnering with Penn Foundation would soon be divined. "One day I was walking up on the second floor of the hospital," Dr. Peters would later report, "and the head nurse up there says to me, 'Hey, I hear you're interested in getting that mental health thing set up near the hospital. Did you know the farm across the street is for sale?" Well, I promptly got on the phone and called Dr. Loux. I said, 'Dr. Loux, the farm across the street from the hospital is for sale! Fifteen acres and a house.' He said, 'Okay!' And right away he called Harold Mininger and the other trustees. They soon found out that Dr. Winn already had an option on the property."

This development was the principal topic at the February 14, 1956 meeting of Penn Foundation's organizers. Dr. Loux had quickly made some phone calls and learned that surgeon Charles L. Winn, having just moved into the area, was indeed negotiating with a real estate agent to purchase the small farm across Lawn Avenue (a.k.a. Almont Road) from Grand View Hospital, on the ridge overlooking Sellersville Borough, in

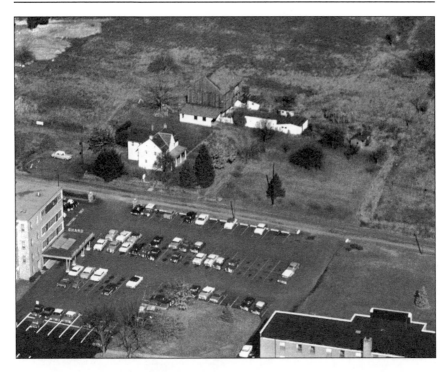

Shortly after Dr. Loux persuaded his fellow organizers to embrace the new paradigm of a community mental health clinic working in concert with a general hospital, word arrived from Grand View Hospital's Chief of Medicine that a fifteen-acre farm across Lawn Avenue from the Hospital was up for sale. Foundation Directors quickly made an offer on the property, and secured an option in March 1956. The farmhouse seen in this northward-looking aerial photograph (taken in 1961) would become Penn Foundation's new home following an August 1956 settlement.

Buck's County's West Rockhill Township. The doctor was, however, only interested in acquiring enough land upon which to construct a medical arts building, so he might be willing to let Penn Foundation's Directors purchase the property if they agreed to then sell him a suitable building lot. The Directors decided that their three-man Building Committee should hasten to "contact the real estate agent and take whatever steps they deemed advisable in securing an option on the property." Naturally, the Committee members also took it upon themselves to visit the farm on "Hospital Heights" and see exactly what it had to offer.

Three days later, Building Committee members Harold Mininger and Paul Souder reported back to their colleagues at a special meeting called for this purpose. The men happily related:

[that] they had looked over the property very carefully and thought it most desirable both from a practical point of view for building purposes and because of its attractive location. Mr. Mininger reported that the house was in fairly good condition and could be made useable for office space without too much expenditure. He felt that the building was a definite asset in that it provided a permanent office address without delay and also a place for business meetings of the Foundation. The committee felt that if it was the consensus of opinion that proximity to Grand View Hospital was an important factor that it would be unwise to defer the matter longer. After some discussion, it was moved by Mr. Mahlon Souder and seconded by Mr. Raymond Rosenberger that the committee be authorized to negotiate for the purchase of the property for a sum of $19,000. The motion was carried unanimously.

How did this informally-constituted Board, still without a corporate charter, propose to finance this acquisition? "Harold Mininger agreed to purchase the property in his name and make the initial down-payment on the basis of a loan to the Foundation," the meeting minutes recorded. "Mr. Paul Souder stated that the wording of the agreement of sale was such that the property could be transferred to the Foundation on the date of settlement. In this way the transaction would come under the tax laws governing non-profit organizations."

The Directors quickly contacted Grand View Hospital officials to let them know what was in the works. "We wanted to make sure they found out about it before the talk was on the street," Charles Hoeflich recalls. "That could have been very threatening to them." The Building Committee also conferred with Dr. Winn, acknowledging that Penn Foundation was now "morally bound to sell [him] a piece of land for a medical office building." Dr. Winn agreed to release his option on the property so long as he was assured of a building lot. The parties shook hands on the deal, and Harold Mininger went off with his checkbook to make the down payment.

All systems were "go" when the Directors gathered for their next regularly-scheduled meeting on March 13. The view of Penn Foundation's future had grown much clearer in recent days, particularly in Dr. Loux's mind. He was asked to comment on "developments he foresaw in the use of [the Lawn Avenue] property during the next few years." As Charles Hoeflich noted in the minutes:

> Dr. Loux thought that for the present the building would be used in the same way as the Souderton building. He thought that we should first plan a building for offices and a day care program and later have buildings for complete hospital facilities added. As for staff, he suggested that one social worker and one clinical psychologist be employed as soon as feasible. . . . As far as finances were concerned Dr. Loux felt that the professional staff might nearly pay for themselves in fees collected for services. He thought that a day hospital might be operated so as to nearly pay for itself. However, complete hospital facilities would lead to high operational costs which might not be covered by fees. He emphasized that the real need was to get personnel with an understanding and feeling for the job that has to be done.

An even more pressing need was money—first to reimburse Harold Mininger for his down payment on the property, and then to cover the remainder of the purchase price at settlement, scheduled for June 19. In discussing "the ways and means of meeting the problem of financing," the Directors concluded that "there should be a well-worked out program before there was general solicitation," and that a Finance Committee should be created to oversee the program. This conclusion, and the recent progress of their venture, inspired the Board to adopt a more formal organization, with elected officers, an Executive Committee, and several subcommittees. A round of voting resulted in the election of Marcus Clemens as President of the Board, Mahlon Souder as Vice-President, Charles Hoeflich as Secretary, and Harold Mininger as Treasurer. Shortly afterward, the officers huddled as an Executive Committee to name a Finance Committee as well as a Publicity Committee. Though these elections and appointments were not yet official—*nothing* would be official until Penn Foundation received its corporate charter—the framework of a community mental health center was taking shape.

A key piece of this framework was installed on the afternoon of Tuesday, April 10, as Dr. Loux officially presented to the Grand View Hospital Board of Directors Penn Foundation's plan to set up shop in the farmhouse across Lawn Avenue from the Hospital. Mahlon Souder, who also served on the Grand View Board, reported later that day at a meeting of Penn Foundation Directors "that he felt this Board was unanimous in its approval of the plans of the Foundation, and . . . that Dr. Loux's explanation had dispelled any doubts that might have been held in regard to the probability of our work competing in any way with the services offered by Grand View" (as Secretary Hoeflich noted in the April 10 meeting minutes).

With this hurdle cleared, Penn Foundation's Directors focused their energies on "the creation of income for the following two purposes: (a) To meet current operating expenses; (b) To make the financial settlement for the property in West Rockhill Township." Charles Hoeflich would later recall how the Foundation's first general solicitation was prosecuted. "The whole Board raised money," he reported. "We didn't just leave it to the Finance Committee. The Directors formed themselves into six teams. Each of us paired up and sat down with three-by-five notecards of where we knew the money was. Then we went out in the evenings [and solicited]. That Board was a fundraising committee *in toto*." During their first two months of soliciting, the Directors raised $9,000, a total that included their own contributions. They had set their initial fund-raising goal at $50,000, half of which would be needed shortly to cover the negotiated cost of the Lawn Avenue farm ($18,000), as well as the anticipated renovations and equipment purchases (another $7,000).

Charles Hoeflich has characterized Penn Foundation's charter Board as "unique." "One of the criteria" for being selected to join this Board, he told an interviewer in 1999, "was that the individual must be interested in psychiatry as a medical discipline. He also had to have certain other commitments, including a commitment to making the psychiatric unit a strong testimony. The universal admiration of the Board for Norman and our complete understanding of [Dr. Peters'] fine hand behind all of this made that Board into a unique board. It was not your typical board where you have one person from the Rotary and one from the Chamber of Commerce and one from the Board of Education and one from something else. It was a group of men who were dedicated to psychiatry, who were sold on the leadership, and as a result they themselves worked. That Board of Directors was a speaker's bureau. We would go out and speak to service organizations, to Sunday school classes, to anywhere we could get from ten to a hundred people together. We talked about the Penn Foundation and what was going on."

"One of the most progressive concepts in the treatment of mental illness"

Charles Hoeflich found time between soliciting donations and speaking to civic groups to draft the first press release bearing the "Penn Foundation for Mental Health" imprimatur. He mailed the communiqué to local papers early in May, along with a photographic portrait of the Foundation's "Officers" taken by Souderton photographer Arnold Moser (only ten of the twelve Directors were on hand for the photographic occasion). The *Souderton Independent* published the historic release and accompanying photo in its May 17, 1956 edition, under the heading: "Penn Foundation For Mental Health Meeting At Souderton—Dr. Norman L. Loux, Souderton, Appointed Director of New Progressive Community Project—Sanctioned By Medical Profession." The article read:

> A new facility for dealing with problems of mental health was announced today. Primarily devoted to the communities of Upper Bucks and Montgomery counties, it will be known as Penn Foundation for Mental Health. Simultaneously it was announced that negotiations have been entered into for the acquisition of a fifteen acre tract of land, together with the existing buildings located directly across from Grand View Hospital, at Sellersville, Pennsylvania. Dr. Norman L. Loux, of Souderton, has been appointed Medical Director of the Foundation and a board of trustees has been created by Marcus A. Clemens, hosiery manufacturer from Quakertown. Pa. Other officers of the Foundation include Mahlon A. Souder, of Blooming Glen, Vice-chairman, Charles H. Hoeflich, of Keller's Church, Secretary and Harold M. Mininger, of Souderton, Treasurer.
>
> It was announced that this would be a non-profit organization dedicated to the establishment of a psychiatric service for the area and would seek to render service to all those in the community who need such help without regard to race, creed or ability to pay. Clemens speaking for the Foundation stated, "For some time it has been obvious to many thoughtful citizens that there is a need within the community to help those suffering from emotional illness and to provide counseling for

those with problems concerning family relationships, child rearing, etc. . . ."

Dr. Loux, in commenting, said "It is a well known fact that the problem of emotional illness is the nation's number one health problem. There are more people in mental hospitals in the United States than in all other types of hospitals combined. On the basis of experience it is reasonable to assume that many who in the past have been hospitalized can be helped without hospitalization if facilities are available for early treatment. . . ."

Considerable enthusiasm for this entire project has been indicated by a number of medical, civic and religious leaders who likewise have voiced the need for mental health facilities.

It is expected that considerable interest will be shown also by psychiatrists elsewhere in what is believed to be one of the most progressive concepts in the treatment of mental illness at a community level.

There was no summer vacation for Penn Foundation's Board in 1956. Indeed, the Directors added some crucial components to the organizational framework during June, July, and August of that year. Elvin Souder reported at a special Board meeting held on June 19 that "the Articles of Incorporation had been approved by the Pennsylvania Department of Welfare. These articles are to be filed in [the Bucks County] Court on July 6 and the Charter should be granted shortly thereafter." In fact, the charter was granted on the same day the articles were filed. The Board was finally authorized to conduct a "formal organizational meeting," which it did on July 25. The Penn Foundation for Mental Health, Inc. was—as of that date—an official Pennsylvania non-profit agency.

Having helped Penn Foundation get its administrative feet on the ground, Ruby Horwood resigned as Dr. Loux's full-time assistant-receptionist in order to take a job at the Eastern Pennsylvania Psychiatric Institute, a research-oriented hospital established on the Philadelphia campus of the Medical College of Pennsylvania in 1949. "I was invited to come and set up the library in a building that was just being built," Ruby would later report. "It was a rather difficult decision for me to make, because I had come to work so closely with Dr. Loux. Eventually we worked it out that I would continue to work on a part-time basis with Dr. Loux [at Penn Foundation], several evenings a week on different projects."

The vacancy left by Ruby was partly filled when a receptionist was hired on July 24. But Dr. Loux still needed a proper secretary, and he was pressing the Board even harder to hire a social worker. At the August 9 meeting of the Board, Dr. Loux was "asked to elaborate on the role of a social worker in the program of a psychiatric clinic," Secretary Hoeflich noted. "He pointed out that one of the most important contributions of a social worker was to act as a liaison between the patient, the patient's family, and the physician. In a treatment program it is essential that the patient's family have some understanding of the problem so that they are better able to deal with situations that arise. Because of time limitations, it is impossible for the psychiatrist to see all those concerned very often and the work of the social worker in this respect is invaluable." A few weeks later, Dr. Loux presented to the Board yet "another good reason to hire a social worker: any application for State funds would be considered on

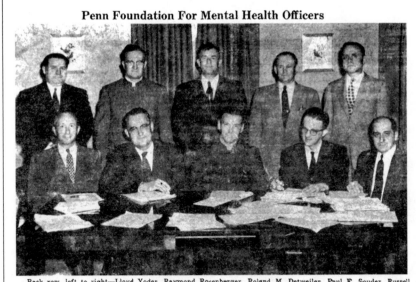

Penn Foundation For Mental Health Officers

Back row, left to right—Lloyd Yoder, Raymond Rosenberger, Roland M. Detweiler, Paul F. Souder, Russell Moyer. Seated, left to right—Charles Hoeflick, Harold M. Mininger, Marcus A. Clemens, Norman Loux, Elvin E. Souder. Two members not present—Russell M. Hillegas and Mahlon A. Souder.

—Moser Studio Photo

The first press release issued by the Penn Foundation for Mental Health made the front page of the May 17, 1956 edition of the *Souderton Independent*. The communiqué was accompanied by this portrait of the new organization's "Officers" engaged in a meeting. The pictured men were ten of the twelve charter members of the Foundation's Board of Directors, all but two of whom were active and influential members of local Mennonite congregations.

the basis of staff. A social worker is considered essential to the program of a psychiatric clinic and this might be a determining factor in the allocation of grants."

Dr. Loux already had someone in mind for this important position at Penn Foundation. Early in July he had conducted a promising interview with Louise DiGiorgio, a Catholic senior case worker at Philadelphia's Friends Hospital, and the holder of a Master of Social Work degree. When the Board finally agreed at its September 11, 1956 meeting to hire a social worker, Dr. Loux was ready to recommend Miss DiGiorgio. The Directors deferred to Dr. Loux's experience, and offered Louise a one-year position at a salary of $5,500. She accepted, even though taking the job would mean commuting daily from her home in south Philadelphia, where she lived with—and looked after—her aging mother. Louise's term of employment was scheduled to begin on December 1.

From Souderton to Sellersville

Perhaps the most dramatic development of the summer was the relocation of Penn Foundation's headquarters from Souderton to Sellersville. The Board made settlement on the Lawn Avenue property on the afternoon of Wednesday, August 1, a month ahead of the scheduled demolition of the West Chestnut Street house. Charles Hoeflich remembers that on "the morning of the signing, we didn't quite have the money" to make the settlement in full. The Directors' faith in their mission was rewarded when "enough money arrived in the mail that very morning to make the settlement."

When the Board next assembled—on August 9, for its monthly meeting—the location was "the new home of the Foundation in Sellersville," as Secretary Hoeflich delightedly entered into the minutes. Among the subjects discussed at this gathering was the need to test the property's "sufficiency of water supply" (this test would reveal the need for a new well), the division of plumbing and heating upgrades between contractors Norman Good and Frank Myers, and the awarding of a painting contract. Renovations would need to proceed quickly so staff and clients could concentrate on the work of the Foundation. Beyond that, the Directors were eager to orchestrate a dedication ceremony that would generate some much-needed publicity. Local papers such as the *Souderton Independent*, Perkasie's *News-Herald*, and Allentown's *Morning Call* were proving able allies in spreading the news of the region's first community mental health center. The *Morning Call* pulled out the most stops on September 16 when it published in its Sunday edition a feature article on Penn Foundation, under the headline: "Souderton Has Unique Agency—One Community Trying to Help Mentally Ill." The author made clear in this piece that, as "one of the first non-profit corporations in the nation designed to fill the psychiatric needs of what is primarily a rural community," Penn Foundation was "Centered In Community":

> The foundation's plans are in keeping with a current nation-wide interest in bringing psychiatric facilities to the community rather than having a large, central facility, according to Dr. Norman L. Loux, medical director of the foundation and chief psychiatrist at Grandview Hospital, Sellersville.
>
> "Taking mental patients out of a community militates against community understanding and participation," he adds. "And since educational programs are being emphasized, the most effective process educationwise seems to take place in situations where families, ministers, teachers and the patient's community are involved."
>
> Penn Foundation's program for the emotionally ill will be related to the medical program at Grandview Hospital in line with a trend to integrate psychiatry with regular medicine. But its administration will be self-governing, although some members will probably serve on both boards.

A "crossroads day"

Penn Foundation's gestation period was initially slated to climax in an outdoor dedication ceremony at the Lawn Avenue farm on the afternoon of Sunday, October 28. But when organizers learned of a scheduling conflict with the man hand-picked by Dr. Loux to present the keynote address at the dedication—old friend Dr. Kenneth Appel, Chairman of the Department of Psychiatry at the University of Pennsylvania Medical School—the event was put off until Sunday, November 11. In the end, the extra days of preparation came in handy. The challenge wasn't so much in arranging for a large tent and refreshments as it was in preparing and mailing out "approximately 1,500 invitations . . . to County & State officials, physicians, teachers, ministers, and officers of service clubs."

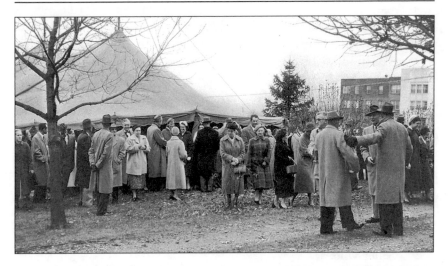

An overflow crowd of well-wishers attended the outdoor Dedication of Penn Foundation's new Lawn Avenue headquarters on the chilly, overcast, but otherwise glorious afternoon of Sunday, October 28, 1956.

Dedication Day dawned chilly and gray. The tent laboriously erected by the trustees ("I can remember yet the Directors out there holding the poles and the ropes and taking so long to put up that great big tent," says Charles Hoeflich) proved indispensable, as organizers quickly imported space heaters to cut the chill. No one was really sure what kind of turn-out to expect. Dr. Loux lunched in his Souderton home with Dr. Appel and another special guest, Dr. Lauren Smith, Physician-in-Chief of Pennsylvania Hospital's Department for Nervous and Mental Diseases. A half-hour before the dedication ceremony was scheduled to begin, the party climbed into a car for the short drive to Sellersville. "We came up Route 309," Dr. Loux recalls, "and we got into a traffic jam." The congestion, they discovered, was caused by traffic funneling toward Penn Foundation's new home. "There were so many people there for the Dedication when we arrived, the tent was overflowing. And I knew then that [this venture] would succeed. I didn't really understand it, though. I couldn't imagine why so many people would come out. They didn't come to hear Dr. Appel, really. They didn't know him from Adam. They came because they were interested. I remember Dr. [Arthur] Noyes, the famous superintendent of Norristown State Hospital [and the former President of the American Psychiatric Association], he attended the Dedication with his aide. Years later the aide told me that Dr. Noyes had told him he was eager to go to that Dedication because 'Something *important* is happening up there in that community!'"

Charles Hoeflich, who served as the event's master of ceremonies, was thrilled that Dr. Appel's keynote address "struck just the right note of concern, as he held forth on the deep inner longing each person has for help as he or she passes through the turbulent emotional crises almost everyone faces at one time or another. It was a crossroads day, and the Foundation knew it was truly moving forward." Also impressed was one of the youngest attendees, ten-year-old Henry L. Rosenberger, son of Board member Raymond Rosenberger. "I remember the occasion very well," Henry would tell an interviewer in 1999. "It was solemn and wonderful, because it was addressing a need that was very pressing. And here was my dad and these other local guys, all in their prime. They were *doing* something about it!"

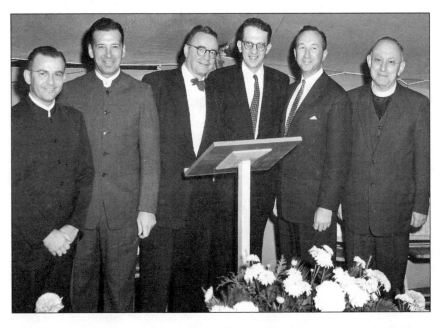

Inside a tent raised the previous day by the Directors themselves and warmed by some hastily-imported space heaters, the throng thrilled to a Dedicatory address delivered by Dr. Kenneth Appel, Chairman of the Department of Psychiatry at the University of Pennsylvania Medical School. Dr. Appel (third from left in this newspaper photo) was joined at the podium after the proceedings by (from left) David Derstine, pastor of Blooming Glen Mennonite Church; Marcus Clemens, President of the Foundation's Board of Directors; Dr. Loux, Medical Director; Charles Hoeflich, Secretary of the Board; and Dr. William Seaman, pastor of Emanuel Lutheran Church in Souderton.

4

A DEDICATED
"DAY CARE CENTER"

Two days after the November 11 Dedication, Penn Foundation's Directors gathered for their monthly meeting. Excitement still hung in the air as Vice-President Mahlon Souder led the men first in opening devotions, then in an exchange of congratulations. Spirits high, the trustees turned to confront some prickly fiscal realities in the form of Treasurer Harold Mininger's financial reports from September and October. There were glints of red ink in the documents, and they warned of an eventual hemorrhage. Mahlon reminded his colleagues that "continuous operating deficits would create serious problems in the near future, and that it was essential to place the work of the Foundation on a sound financial basis without delay" (according to meeting minutes). "[He] urged that a determined effort be made by every Board member to obtain financial contributions."

The Directors did indeed redouble their fundraising efforts in the ensuing weeks. They quickly compiled a list of local business firms and divvied up responsibility for pitching each of them in person. They drew up a letter of financial appeal and mailed copies to a thousand area residents. More importantly, they broadened their base of support by fostering the formation of two important affiliates: a Ladies Auxiliary and the "Friends of Penn Foundation." The seed of an Auxiliary had been planted earlier that fall when several Directors' wives volunteered to provide furniture for the Foundation's new headquarters. The women wound up purchasing some of the new gear with books of trading stamps. Then they offered to lend a much-needed feminine touch to the Dedication. A few days after that event, Board President Marcus Clemens mailed a letter to Grace Souder (wife of Director Paul Souder), thanking her and her colleagues for their assistance. He concluded by suggesting the women "give some serious thought to the organization of a ladies auxiliary for the foundation."

This was all the encouragement the wives needed. By January 1957 they had a rudimentary Auxiliary up and running (its formal organization and adoption of by-laws lay several months in the future). Membership in the sorority—described in a December 1957 magazine article as "probably the first such group ever attached to a psychiatric out-patient facility" in America—quickly swelled to ninety. Under President Viola Yoder (wife of Director "Poppy" Yoder), the women set their sights on "developing among the membership a deep interest in and a loyal support of the Penn Foundation for Mental Health." Charles Hoeflich would recall that this

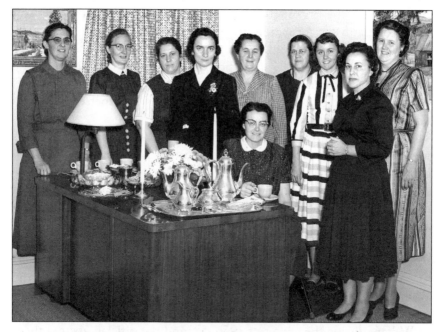

Board members' wives pitched in from the start—cleaning, baking, sewing, decorating, hosting, and even providing furniture for the Foundation's new headquarters. This photo was taken at a reception held for new social worker Louise DiGiorgio (second from right) on December 20, 1956. Standing with Miss DiGiorgio were (from left) Helen (Mrs. Marcus) Clemens, Myrtle (Mrs. Harold) Mininger, Grace (Mrs. Paul) Souder, Patty (Mrs. Elvin) Souder, Miriam (Mrs. Mahlon) Souder, Sallie (Mrs. Raymond) Rosenberger, Sonya Derstine, and Evelyn (Mrs. Russell) Moyer. Esther (Mrs. Norman) Loux was seated behind the tea service. Within weeks of this occasion, most of these ladies would begin formalizing their association with Penn Foundation through the organizing of a Women's Auxiliary.

interest was cultivated through "meetings held in the conference room in the old Nurses' Home over in Grand View Hospital, where the ladies listened to mental health and medical speakers." In the coming years, enthusiasm generated by these information sessions would be manifested most prominently in the Auxiliary's hosting and catering of such Foundation-related events as Educational Teas, Board of Directors Luncheons, Annual Meeting Buffets, and Christmas Teas.

The Auxiliary's fraternal twin—the Friends of Penn Foundation—was also conceived in the winter of 1956–57. Taking its first steps without the benefit of a ready-made core of functionaries (like that enjoyed by the Auxiliary), this alliance of supportive citizens needed more time to gather momentum. Most if its energy in the first half of 1957 was expended in planning Penn Foundation's first annual dinner meeting, scheduled to coincide with the organization's second anniversary in September (on which occasion the formation of the Friends would finally be formally announced). Organizers of this group hoped it would serve as a hot-bed of private support for the Foundation, as well as a vehicle for educating the community in matters of mental health. By the close of 1957, scores of Friends would be receiving quarterly bulletins interspersed with invitations to forums, lectures, and special meetings.

While welcoming every donated dollar, Penn Foundation's Directors were aware that the gap between patient-insurer payments and operating expenses (not to mention the cost of physical improvements and expansion) could hardly be bridged by individual and corporate contributions alone. Their organization would only be able to realize its potential through a steady infusion of federal, state, and county funds. Now that a community program staffed by a licensed social worker (Louise DiGiorgio) was officially underway, Penn Foundation was eligible to pursue some forms of tax-based funding (and even more would be available if and when the Foundation hired a clinical psychologist). Dr. Loux and a Board member or two met several times with officials of the Pennsylvania Department of Welfare during the winter of 1956–57, and the officials assured them "that financial aid was available and that the necessary application forms and endorsements were in process" (as noted in Board minutes). Russell Hillegass, in his capacity as Chairman of the Board's Finance Committee, briefed two Bucks County Commissioners on the Foundation's program and ambitious goals. As soon as schedules permitted, he would sit down for a similar session with one or more Montgomery County Commissioners. In the spring of 1957, Dr. Loux heard through the grapevine that the Grant Foundation of New York—the charitable arm of the W.T. Grant store chain—was interested in supporting community mental health initiatives. He wasted no time in making an appointment to meet with the Grant Foundation's Director.

As it turned out, the first major infusion of funding came by way of Pennsylvania's Department of Welfare. Marcus Clemens learned in April 1957 that the Commonwealth would be providing Penn Foundation with approximately $4,600 in public money for the quarter ending on June 30. If the current conditions continued, Penn Foundation could expect similar amounts from the State in each of the remaining quarters, adding up to about $18,000 per fiscal year (which was $2,000 more than Dr. Loux's annual salary). Then, in May 1957, the Grant Foundation came through with an offer of $2,500, contingent on Penn Foundation's elimination of its $8,604.26 debt by the following October 31. The Directors girded themselves for another round of solicitations, buoyed by the prospect of debt-free operation.

Though Dr. Loux resigned his position on the Board at the end of 1956—pointing out that "standard practice [dictated] that the Medical Director of an institution should not be a member of the Governing Body"—he continued to attend Board meetings, often with Louise Di-Giorgio in tow. He usually presented his "Report of the Medical Director" right after the minutes of the prior meeting were reviewed and approved. If Louise was in attendance, she followed Dr. Loux with a "Report of the Psychiatric Social Worker." These updates allowed the Directors to keep their fingers on the pulse of the Foundation, which they generally found to be beating resolutely despite a nearly suffocating case load and an endless succession of public speaking engagements for both Dr. Loux and Louise. In January 1957, Dr. Loux added a new component to his reporting: a quarterly accounting of "clinical activities of the Foundation." Through these periodic presentations of statistical analyses and anecdotes, he hoped to keep the Directors conversant in the language of psychiatric services, while helping them appreciate the staff's day-to-day challenges and achievements.

Obliged to expand

A snapshot of the Foundation's achievements during its first twenty-two months of operation was presented by Dr. Loux in an historic "plan for action" he helped draft in August 1957 (a few months after he had

been appointed to the new Board of Mennonite Mental Health Services).
The "recapitulation of accomplishments" read:

> Since [September 1955] there have been approximately 30
> new patients accepted each month, with a total of 629 dif-
> ferent individuals having been seen through July, 1957. Of this
> total, 249 were from Bucks County, 331 were from Mont-
> gomery County, 49 were from outside either Bucks or Mont-
> gomery County. Of the total number of patients seen, 55 were
> hospitalized because of their emotional illness. The great
> majority of those hospitalized could profitably have been hos-
> pitalized in the type of facility that the Foundation conceives
> as part of its expansion program. It is also true that a num-
> ber more of those seen who were not hospitalized could have
> been more satisfactorily helped with the facility which the
> Foundation conceives.
>
> What have been the apparent results of our program thus
> far? Trying to be as realistic and intellectually honest as pos-
> sible, it is our feeling that the psychiatric results have been
> more than gratifying. There have been a number of notable
> results. For example there have been instances where people
> have been ill over a period of years and have been treated in
> various hospitals who seem well on the way to recovery at the
> present time, at least partially in response to the efforts of the
> Foundation. There have been numerous folks who have been
> severely ill who have been carried and treated successfully
> without hospitalization through working closely with the fam-
> ily and other responsible people in the community.
>
> In psychiatry, as a general rule, results are not as spectac-
> ular as in some other branches of medicine, but they are often
> dramatic as experienced by those working with patients as we
> do through the Foundation. The results are dramatic in that
> we can often see the transformation of a person with almost
> unbearable mental anguish and complete incapacity, into a
> person who is free to live a life with feeling and purposeful-
> ness. The fact that there have been not more numerous dra-
> matic results must be assumed to a large extent to be due to
> our own inaptitudes and to a lesser extent to lack of facilities
> for utilizing treatments which would be helpful. However, the

fact that there have been so many good results leads us to believe that there can be many more good and dramatic results as we accumulate more knowledge and become wiser in applying the knowledge that we have and improve the facilities with which we work. There obviously have been enough failures in treatment to keep us humble, but the good results challenge us to work diligently. . . .

What facts stand out from our previous experience?

1. The community continues to be intelligently receptive to a psychiatric program to a degree that is beyond our expectations and beyond anything that experienced people have observed previously.

2. The community is not only receptive in a passive way but is willing to participate on all levels.

3. Emotionally ill folks can be cared for in most instances in their own communities and frequently without prolonged hospitalization, providing help is available for helping families and other people in the community meet the patient's needs.

4. There continues to be and probably always shall continue to be a number of emotionally ill patients who will require a period of hospitalization and types of treatment which require hospitalization.

Dr. Loux and his colleagues on the Board cited these facts as evidence that Penn Foundation dearly needed to expand its facilities and services. As they noted later in their August 1957 "Outline of a Suggested Plan for Action for Expanding Psychiatric Facilities of the Penn Foundation for Mental Health, Inc.," "the results have been challenging enough so that it leads us to believe that the expansion of Penn Foundation . . . is an obligation which we have to the community as well as to the psychiatric profession." The Board identified four overarching "needs" in the section of its "Plan for Action" labeled "What Do We Concretely Propose?":

A. Since the backbone of our psychiatric program is our outpatient facility, the first need is to construct office space which will enable us to render service to our out-patients. The principles governing the construction of out-patient facilities would seem to be as follows:

a. The facilities should be easily and unobtrusively accessible.

b. They should give due consideration to the privacy of the individual patient.

c. Adequate waiting area facilities should be constructed where a sense of privacy is possible for those occupying the waiting area.

B. The next most important aspect of our program is the need for facilities for day-care patients. Day-care patients would be those who would profit by being removed from their environment for a period of time during each day for three reasons;

1. For diagnostic study in a way that is not possible on out-patient visits.

2. Because the environment is a serious deterrent to the processes of recovery.

Thanks to furnishings and decorating touches applied by Directors' wives, the reception area of the newly-dedicated Penn Foundation headquarters had a home-like warmth, as this publicity photo taken in November 1956 attests. The "patient" on the left is actually trustee Russell Moyer. The other two "patients" have not been identified.

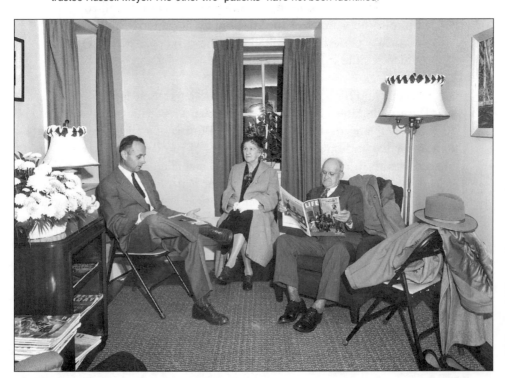

3. Because special therapies need to be administered which can only be administered while the patient is in our care for longer than an out-patient visit, for example:

    a. Electro-convulsive therapy.

    b. Drug therapy under closer supervision than would be possible at home.

    c. Occupational and recreational activity.

It is true that our aim must be to help members of families or other significant people in the patient's environment, to help the patient to become well, but at times especially trained people are necessary during a part of the patient's recovery process.

C. The third need is for a limited facility for in-patients. This includes the actual rooms where patients live while in the hospital. These should be, in my estimation, semi-private rooms including a total space for 12 in-patients.

D. The next and final aspect of our need centers around our general educational responsibility. The physical needs for this aspect are chiefly those of a meeting place for groups perhaps up to 100 in number where public meetings in the general interest of Mental Health could be held. Also needed is a conference room, especially where physicians and other professional people in the community such as teachers and ministers could meet for conferences centering around cases and problems in which they are interested.

The facilities must form a functioning unit and in reality one cannot exist without the other. However, in structural design and layout, consideration need be given to the privacy of the individual groups if desired by them.

It is our feeling that the overall principles reflecting the needs of the community and the general manner in which these needs can be met is clearly in mind.

The next step is the translation of these principles into concrete facilities.

"Marking Two Progressive Years"

The Board of Directors unveiled its vision of a new multi-purpose mental health care facility to 425 supporters at the first annual Penn

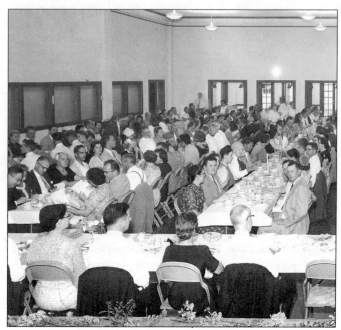

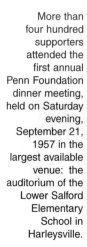

More than four hundred supporters attended the first annual Penn Foundation dinner meeting, held on Saturday evening, September 21, 1957 in the largest available venue: the auditorium of the Lower Salford Elementary School in Harleysville.

Foundation dinner meeting, held on Saturday evening, September 21, 1957. Organized by the fledgling Friends of Penn Foundation, the banquet and program of music and addresses was staged in the largest available venue: the auditorium of the Lower Salford Elementary School in Harleysville. "An overflow crowd of enthused friends heard the Penn Foundation for Mental Health lauded by government officials and leaders in the psychiatric field," a local newspaper reported of the red-letter event:

> Dr. Robert Matthews, Commissioner for Mental Health, Department of Welfare of the State termed the Foundation's progress "one of the most exciting developments in the field of mental health I have ever seen." Warm words of commendation were read from Governor [George M.] Leader who wrote that only absence from the State prevented him from expressing in person his gratitude for the part that they have played in bettering community mental health.
>
> One of the evening's high points was reached when the Foundation's Chairman, Marcus A. Clemens, announced that "now for eleven days we have been debt-free"—a notable

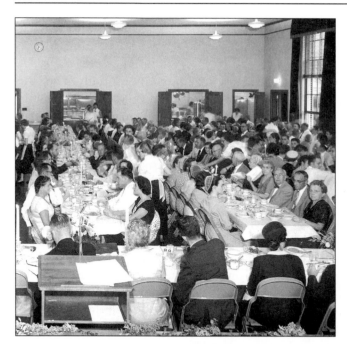

At this gathering, which marked "Two Progressive Years" of providing mental health services in the Bux-Mont region, the Foundation's Directors announced their intention to build a multi-purpose mental health care facility beside the converted farmhouse on Lawn Avenue.

achievement considering the work that has been accomplished in two short years. He went on to say that in view of the demand for additional facilities this would probably be a "temporary situation."

Dr. Stanley Moyer, president of the medical staff of Grand View Hospital and representing the Bucks County Medical Association reviewed the accomplishments which led the Association to name the Foundation the recipient of its Annual Benjamin Rush Award, presented in recognition of "an outstanding contribution to community mental health."

Certainly the atmosphere of the affair was an ebullient one and as Dr. Norman Loux, Medical Director remarked was "full of thanksgiving for the many benefits which we have received." Dr. Loux stressed the fact that such progress as has been made is only "because we have enjoyed such a wonderful measure of understanding and cooperation from physicians, as well as each and every segment and person in our community. Without this whole-hearted response from everyone we should never be able to reach the goal we envision."

A photograph accompanying this article (page 214)—with the lead caption "Marking Two Progressive Years"—showed a beaming Marcus Clemens shaking hands with one of the evening's guest speakers: Dr. Lauren Smith, the Pennsylvania Hospital Chief Administrative Physician who had placed his stamp of approval on the Dedication ten months earlier. Looking on were Dr. Loux (holding the Benjamin Rush Award for 1957) and State Commissioner for Mental Health Dr. Robert Matthews. Charles Hoeflich recalls that Dr. Matthews was highly impressed with the display of public support at Penn Foundation's first annual banquet:

> This was in the days when all Mennonite ladies wore their coverings. Dr. Matthews and I were seated side-by-side at the speakers' table during the meal, looking out over this sea of white caps. He turned to me and said, "You sure have a marvelous turnout! I've been to the State Mental Health organization's annual meeting, and they're lucky if they have thirty-five people attend. You must have over four hundred here. Do you have a particular religious group behind you?" He was clearly intrigued by all those white caps. I said, "No, *everybody* is behind us!" Then I added, "It's true that Mennonites have been taking a little bit of a lead with this, maybe because of their experiences in the war. But, really, all of the local churches have been supportive."

On this ebullient occasion, the Directors managed to squeeze in a special Board meeting to tend to some important business: lifting some of the administrative load from Dr. Loux's shoulders. Ever since Ruby Horwood's resignation, the Foundation's Medical Director had been prodding the Board to round out the clinical staff through the hiring of an Executive Secretary. In the ensuing year Dr. Loux had been doing double-duty as both doctor and administrator. This could not continue—not with the "clinic carrying a maximum patient load," and "no decrease in the number of referrals" through the spring and summer of 1957. Now that Penn Foundation was debt-free (at least for the time being), the Directors could see their way to hiring a new "Ruby." Their September 21 special meeting was devoted to discussing the prospect of engaging a women who had earned Russell Moyer's endorsement. This was Marjorie Alexander, a forty-year-old Perkasie resident employed as a supervisor at the Harleysville

Insurance Company, which is where Russell (Chair of the Board's Personnel Committee) got to know her. On his hearty recommendation, the Directors agreed to invite Marge in for an interview, and she became Penn Foundation's third full-time employee as 1957 drew to a close. She would be a fixture with the organization for the next quarter-century.

A few months after Marge joined Penn Foundation, Dr. Loux added a fourth employee to the payroll. Swiss-born Dr. Lily Brunschwig, author of the 1936 monograph A *Study of Some Personality Aspects of Deaf Children*, was engaged as a clinical psychologist "on a one-day-per-week basis" in February 1958 (a year later her work schedule would be expanded to three days per fortnight). The hiring of a psychologist relieved Dr. Loux of some duties, but just as importantly, it allowed Penn Foundation to apply for additional State funds. This consideration was also behind Dr. Loux's stepped-up search for an assistant psychiatrist. Despite efforts that included placing an advertisement in the American Psychiatric Association's newsletter and conducting interviews with Pennsylvania Hospital's Associate Clinical Director, Dr. Loux was not able to find a suitable second psychiatrist throughout the remainder of 1958, and well into 1959.

Beyond the day-to-day operations of the clinic, Penn Foundation's primary focus during this period was on building a new home. Board meeting minutes chronicled the Directors' slow-but-steady progress in "translating principles into concrete reality":

> **October 8, 1957:** Building Committee Chairman Harold Mininger "presented a revised set of plans for the new building. There was considerable discussion on the direction that the Board should take in the initial planning. It was the consensus of opinion that an approximate [construction cost] should be set so that the plans can be made in accordance with the funds available. It was proposed that the plans made by Mr. Mininger be discussed with Dr. [Daniel] Blain [Medical Director of the American Psychiatric Association] and other experts in the field."

> **November 11, 1957:** Mahlon Souder "expressed his deep concern over the fact that the building plans were not being finalized. He felt that a determined effort should be made to coordinate plans without delay."

December 10, 1957: "Dr. Loux reported that the visit of Dr. Blain had been most worthwhile. Mssrs. Hoeflich, Rosenberger, and Paul Souder reported briefly on their meeting with Dr. Blain. It was the consensus of opinion that their discussions with him had proved most reassuring and they felt that the future plans for the work of the Foundation were being made in accordance with current trends in patient care and treatment."

January 14, 1958: Harold Mininger "reported for the Building Committee on the visit of Dr. [Charles] Goshen, Architectural Consultant of the American Psychiatric Association. It was proposed that final drawings be done to be submitted to State authorities for approval." Charles Hoeflich suggested that "solicitations from individuals be done before May, and that business firms be contacted during the latter half of the year. A figure of $140,000 was suggested as a goal. It was proposed that half of this amount be raised before the building program is begun."

February 11, 1958: Harold Mininger was authorized "to have detailed plans drawn up, and that these building plans be submitted to the American Psychiatric Association as soon as possible."

March 18, 1958: Harold Mininger "presented plans for the proposed building and invited comments and suggestions from members of the Board."

May 13, 1958: "The members of the Board visited the proposed site of the new building and discussed location, landscaping, parking facilities, etc. It was the consensus of opinion that the building location had been well chosen. It was emphasized that the building should be placed in such a way that space would be available for an expanded program which might include Research and Custodial buildings in the future."

At some point in this process, Dr. Loux and the Directors decided to omit costly in-patient accommodations from the construction plans. It had never been their mission, after all, to run even a small hospital, especially with a large and cooperative hospital right across the street. Indeed, Grand

View officials would eventually offer "to reserve a number of [the Hospital's] beds for psychiatric patients."

An artist's rendering of the proposed day care center (page 215)—a long, rectangular, perfectly symmetrical one-story structure now expected to cost upwards of $150,000—was unveiled to the public at Penn Foundation's "Third Anniversary Dinner" (the second annual fund-raising dinner), held a couple of weeks before Thanksgiving 1958 with the participation of another overflow crowd of supporters at the Lower Salford Elementary School. Among the evening's speakers was Dr. Gilbert L. Guffin, President of Eastern Baptist Theological Seminary and of Eastern Baptist College. Also addressing the audience was the Foundation's old friend Dr. Arthur Noyes. Both men "lauded the dramatic work done at Penn Foundation" and applauded the Directors' resolve to construct what Mahlon Souder described for the audience as "a building designed to bring to our area the best for a modern program of recreational and occupational activities as well as housing [for] the newest forms of psychiatric treatment" (as reported in a local newspaper). The facility would "also relieve a physical situation which is now so overloaded as to be almost unbearable," Mahlon noted. If everything went according to plan, construction of the day care center would begin early the following year.

In fact, everything did *not* go according to plan, and work on the building did not commence in early 1959. Nor was ground broken later that year, or even in 1960. More than two years would pass before construction got underway. Moreover, when Penn Foundation's new home finally opened it doors in the summer of 1962, the building would look nothing like the artist's rendering unveiled at the Third Anniversary Dinner in 1958. What happened?

A "crossroad" demands a "heady decision"

Funding the construction project turned out to be much more difficult than anticipated, and this in turn slowed progress in retaining an architect, nailing down the final design, and choosing a general contractor. For more than a year following their decision to proceed with expansion, the Directors assumed that a significant portion of the amount needed to underwrite this venture would be provided by the Federal government through the 1946 Hospital Survey and Construction Act. Widely known as "the Hill-Burton Act" (having been sponsored by Senators Lister Hill and Harold Burton), this legislation was originally designed to provide Federal grants for the modernization of hospitals rendered obsolete during the Great Depression and World War II. As early as May 1956, Dr. Loux had conveyed to Penn Foundation's Board assurances he had received from such experts as Dr. Kenneth Appel that "Hill-Burton funds for building purposes would be made available" after a community fund-raising effort had begun. These assurances were recalled in January 1959 as the Directors worked out the last details of their upcoming solicitation, and approved what they hoped would be the final revisions to their "Day Care Center" construction plan.

Through his contacts at Pennsylvania's Department of Welfare, Dr. Loux learned that the administrator of the Hill-Burton program for Bucks County was a man named Ira Mills, and that Mr. Mills had already indicated to a State official he "was most optimistic regarding the availability of funds for the Foundation" (according to March 10, 1959 Board meeting minutes). This so encouraged the Directors that they quickly appointed a committee to "call on Mr. Mills [in Harrisburg] and explore fully the matter of financial aid so that all necessary formalities could be completed at the next meeting." In their excitement, they even discussed the possibility of scheduling a groundbreaking ceremony. They concluded, however (wisely, it turned out) that further talk of groundbreaking exercises should wait until "the availability of funds has been fully explored."

Meetings and correspondence with Ira Mills during the spring, summer, and·fall of 1959 did nothing to dampen the Directors' spirits. They were further encouraged by a visit in mid-October 1959 from Dr. John A. Davis Jr., the new Commissioner of Mental Health for Pennsylvania's Department of Welfare. Dr. Davis reviewed the plans for the day care center and consulted with each of the staff members. As reported in a local newspaper, the visitor "was enthusiastic in his praise of the work which is being done and indicated that the program of the local Foundation is 'very much in keeping with the most advanced thinking and planning in the field of psychiatry today.'"

The Directors' painstaking completion and submission of Hill-Burton applications in September and October 1959 was rewarded with news in December that the nation's Secretary of Welfare had responded to the applications (and Mr. Mills' attendant recommendation) by approving the granting of $108,000 in Hill-Burton funds to Penn Foundation for construction purposes, pending approval of the Foundation's construction plans. This amount would be added to community contributions, plus at least $150,000 the Directors were preparing to raise through the sale of a bond issue to meet a projected cost now approaching a quarter-million dollars. The Building Committee was poised with recently-retained architect Willard Van Ommeren of Stanley Horn Associates of Perkasie to begin soliciting bids from contractors.

Then, one evening in early spring 1960, Dr. Loux received an unexpected and disheartening phone call from Ira Mills:

> [Ira] said, "I didn't realize it, but there's a stipulation in the Hill-Burton [regulations] that the funding has to be for beds [i.e. in-patient accommodations]," Dr. Loux would later recall. "Construction has to revolve around beds, and you don't have any beds in your plans. That's an obstacle we will have to overcome, but I'm not sure quite how we can do that." He said, "Let's set up a meeting [with Department of Welfare officials] in Harrisburg."
>
> I can still remember that meeting. We went all through the regulations. They said, "Why don't you just put a few beds in your center? You can always use a few beds. Emergencies come up. We can work around that." I remember on the way home [from this meeting] there was a lot of serious thought and talk. Then the Executive Committee met, and we had a Board meeting. We decided that it just wasn't right for us. If we really were committed to avoiding beds as a matter of principle, then to make a change in order to receive federal funding was ridiculous.

Charles Hoeflich recounted this pivotal sequence of events in his 1983 retrospective as follows:

> Another crossroad had been reached and another heady decision must be made. The Foundation had developed a program involving outpatient care with family, employer, and community involvement. Bulwarked by group therapy, day treatment, marital counseling, and other methods of treatment, the program was showing positive, measurable results. Should the Foundation surrender this concept and become a twenty-bed mental hospital or give up the money which was unquestionably important in the scheme of things at the time?

The answer took a special meeting and deep discussion.

Choosing a name had been child's play compared to this, for the entire future of Penn Foundation could be at stake. There was an added option—the Foundation could keep the grant if it would become an integral part of [Grand View] general hospital. But its unique identity and reputation, which by now had been recognized through being the recipient of the Benjamin Rush Award, several cash awards and numerous feature articles in magazines and professional journals, would all be lost.

After an all-morning session [on May 26, 1960], the decision was made to scrap the plans, graciously decline the government funds, and start all over. The community's needs—not bureaucratic standards—must be the criteria for action.

The significance of this "heady decision" can hardly be overstated. In the decades since they made their choice, the Directors and Dr. Loux have come to view the "Hill-Burton affair" as one of only several occasions when the soul of Penn Foundation hung in the balance. "The money the government was holding out to us was *such* a juicy plum," Dr. Loux reflected recently. "We *really* wanted those funds so we could continue with our building project. But we suspected, and it is all the more clear in hindsight, that taking the money with the strings attached would have meant we were partly owned by the government. And when you're *partly* owned by the government, you're *totally* owned by the government. I'm sure that if we had taken the Hill-Burton funds, Penn Foundation would be an entirely different organization today."

So the Building Committee went back to the drawing board in June 1960, and began devising plans for a smaller day care center that would cost less than a half the amount projected for the Hill-Burton-funded facility. In consultation with a new architect—George Hay of Media, Chester County—planners exchanged the single-story design with a split-level configuration. Exteriors walls would be constructed not of brick but of more economical cinder block and stucco. The roofing material would be asbestos shingles rather than slate. Halls would be slightly narrower. "The new plans turned out to be more acceptable to the staff and others involved, anyway" Charles Hoeflich later observed. Dr. Loux noted that it was easier to design a suitable facility—and projected construction costs dropped dramatically—once the many stipulations attending Hill-Burton eligibility were removed from the equation. "We ended up getting more built for less money than if we had utilized Hill-Burton funds," he commented recently. "That was another one of those 'very interesting' developments along the way."

Human resource developments

There were several lower-profile developments on the human resources front as Penn Foundation turned the corner from the Fifties to the Sixties. The clinical staff of three full-time employees (Loux, DiGiorgio, and Alexander) and one part-time contributor (Brunschwig) was expanded in July 1959 when Dr. Loux was finally able to hire a full-time assistant psychiatrist after "many months of diligent searching for the right man who would combine the qualifications and sense of dedication we have been seeking" (as reported in a local newspaper). This appointment was followed closely by the hiring in September 1959 of secretary-receptionist Patricia Clay. Pat had her work cut out for her. Between scheduled clinical activities and the growing number of emergency situations the Foundation was asked to handle, telephone calls were coming in at the rate of twenty-to-thirty a day, six days per week.

With growth came the potential for growing pains, and that potential was realized in October 1959 as Dr. Loux concluded—after evaluating a series of "not entirely satisfactory" performance reports concerning his new assistant psychiatrist—that "many months of diligent searching" had not resulted in the hiring of the "right man" for Penn Foundation after all. The junior psychiatrist was asked to resign only three months into his tenure, and November 1959 found Dr. Loux back in the hunt for an assistant. He had remarkably more success this time around. His interview with child psychiatrist John M. Dunn in January 1960 was as promising as the new decade. Dr. Dunn—known to friends as "Mike"—was hired at the end of February to work one day per week (Saturdays). In making the part-time appointment for a "trial period," Dr. Loux was mindful of the recent experience with his first assistant psychiatrist. Penn Foundation's Medical Director noted in his March 1960 report to the Board, however, that "the hiring of professional staff on a part-time basis was impractical unless it was done with a long-range plan, that is . . . with a view to a permanent full-time staff position." Any view toward hiring Dr. Dunn on a full-time basis proved to be fully justified. He immediately began "making a real and greatly appreciated contribution in his work with school children," according to Dr. Loux. In August 1961 Dr. Dunn's position was expanded to three-quarter time, and he would continue his valuable affiliation with Penn Foundation at least on a part-time basis for another thirty-one years.

The policy of hiring professional staff on an initial part-time basis was applied again in August 1961 when clinical psychologist Dr. James T. Barbash was brought in to replace the recently departed Dr. Brunschwig. Most of Dr. Barbash's time (as little as three hours per week) was devoted to psychological testing. Like his colleague Dr. Dunn, Dr. Barbash proved to have staying power. He would be made a full-time employee in 1968, and go on to log another dozen years with the Foundation.

Doctors Barbash and Dunn had tied themselves to a rising star. The future was looking bright for Penn Foundation on the evening of Friday, June 23, 1961 as the Directors, staff members, and Auxiliary representatives welcomed local doctors, dignitaries, and Grand View Hospital employees to a field overlooking the Foundation's headquarters. There the group conducted a brief groundbreaking ceremony for the new day care center. After pastor Elwood Reitz of St. Michael's Lutheran Church in Sellersville offered a prayer of dedication, Grand View Hospital President Arthur Alderfer stepped forward and "accented the value of the cooperative effort of the hospital and the foundation" (as reported in a local newspaper). "He stressed the importance of the contribution of a mental health facility to the well-being of a community and the desirability of a rounded medical center able to provide the maximum in medical care to our brothers whose keepers we are."

New Board President (as of October 1960) Harold Mininger then announced that the construction contract—worth approximately $150,000 —had been awarded on the basis of competitive bidding to Lawrence M. Knaefler of Telford. "We have come a long way in a short time," Harold continued. "While there have been hurdles, they have been remarkably few, and the response of the people in our entire area has been a constant challenge to each of us. This new building is in reality the fulfillment of our original purpose—to create a climate for the best in mental health here."

During the year that it took Lawrence Knaefler and his subcontractors to erect Penn Foundation's new quarters, the Directors concentrated on raising money for the building program. The centerpiece of this effort was the fifth annual fund-raising dinner, held on November 4, with mental health care lobbyist, author, and lecturer Thomas Francis ("Mike") Gorman serving as featured speaker. Nearly five hundred supporters turned out for the affair in what one reporter characterized as "an unusual display of enthusiasm." Though the Directors ultimately covered out of their own pockets the $121.45 difference in receipts versus expenses for this event, they were rewarded when donations of "sizable amounts" began rolling in shortly thereafter.

Attention then turned to an alarming shortage of operating funds resulting from a combination of uncollected fees and smaller appropriations of public funds. In recent years both Bucks and Montgomery Counties had significantly reduced their annual "grants-in-aid"—Bucks from $9,000 to $5,000, and Montgomery all the way down to $3,000. This was hard to swallow considering that ninety-three percent of Penn Foundation's patients lived in one of these two counties. Dr. Loux and Russell Moyer traveled to Norristown in October 1961, and there they received assurances from Montgomery County officials that the appropriation for Penn Foundation would be "considerably increased" in 1962. A visit with Bucks County's Commissioners the following November offered equal promise. But in mid-January 1962, the Directors learned that Montgomery County's contribution for the new year would be no more than $3,000 after all. A month later they received Bucks County's contribution—an un-increased $5,000. Fortunately, the operating budget had grown a little fatter by that time through an increase in fees for service. With the rate increase to $15 per hour, an "all-time high in fees collected" was achieved in January 1962. Dr. Loux reported a month later that "there had been no resistance" to the increase, and that "the fees were [still] conservative when compared to other private agencies."

There was certainly no shortage of billable hours. Dr. Loux's patient load was so heavy in the spring of 1962 that new non-emergency patients were having to wait at least a month for an appointment. The need for a second psychiatrist was painfully acute, and it was now combined with a wont of several professionals—a full-time clinical psychologist, a registered nurse, and a "maintenance man"—to fill out the staff for the new day care center. Once the hiring of staff representing an additional $40,000 in annual salaries was approved by the Board at its April 10 meeting, Dr. Loux and the Directors conducted a flurry of interviews. By mid-May, Dr. Loux was ready to recommend the employment of Ruth Lefever (a "capable and energetic Graduate Nurse with post-graduate training in psychiatry") as Day Care Coordinator, and Dr. Wilbert A. Lyons, a general practitioner in Sellersville for the previous decade, as staff psychiatrist.

These recommendations were affirmed by the Directors in a landmark gathering on May 15, noteworthy in that it was the first Board meeting conducted in the new facility's snug, bookshelf-lined conference room. Elsewhere in and around the building—which a local reporter described as having "the look of a lovely, oversized split-level ranch house"— carpenters, painters, electricians, and plumbers hastened to meet their approaching deadline. They were close enough to done that the Directors confidently scheduled a Dedication program only eight weeks down the road. It appeared that the finishing touch to the center's interior could be the hanging of nine large impressionistic paintings of local scenes rendered by Sellersville's renowned artist, writer, and educator Walter

A groundbreaking ceremony for Penn Foundation's new day care center was conducted in a field just north of the Foundation's headquarters on the evening of Friday evening, June 23, 1961. On hand for the occasion were Grand View Hospital representatives Arthur Alderfer (Board President, fifth from right) and Dr. Michael Peters (Chief of Medicine, 13th from right,

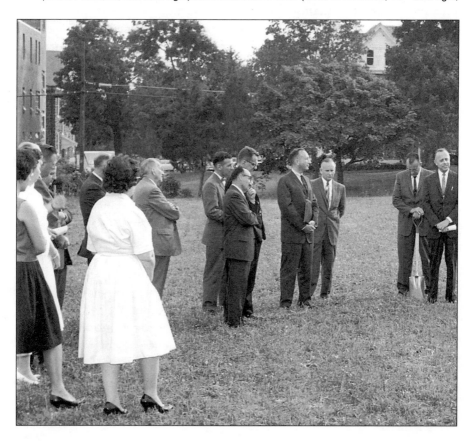

Emerson Baum, who offered to sell the artwork to the Foundation for a modest $810.

"Fulfillment of a dream"

Five years of planning, fundraising, constructing, and hurdling obstacles culminated in a joyous Dedication service for the new day care center on the sun-drenched afternoon of Sunday, June 17, 1962. Among the dignitaries rising to the podium to address the crowd of five-hundred visitors seated on folding chairs on a patch of bare earth between the new 7,194-square-foot facility and Lawn Avenue were Congressman Willard

standing in front of Chief of Psychiatry Dr. Norman Loux), as well as Penn Foundation's Directors. The trustees visible in this photo were (from right) Roland Detweiler, Mahlon Souder, Lloyd "Poppy" Yoder, Raymond Rosenberger, Russell Moyer (8th from right), Harold Mininger, Paul Souder, Charles Hoeflich, and Marcus Clemens (14th from right).

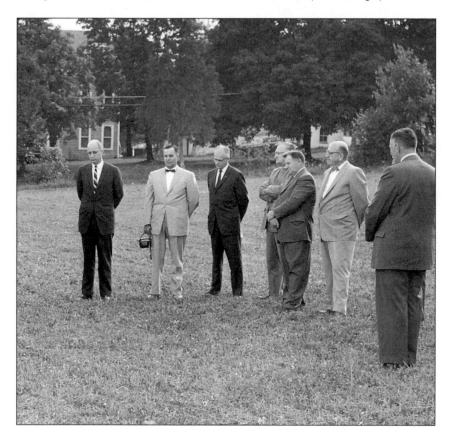

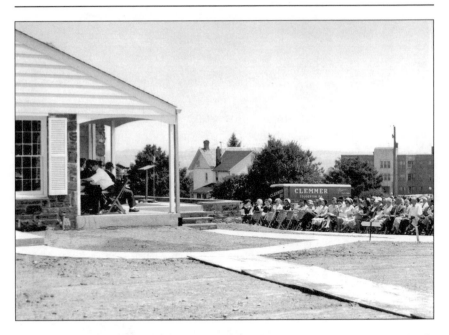

On the sun-drenched afternoon of Sunday, June 17, 1962, more than five hundred well-wishers assembled on a patch of bare earth across Lawn Avenue from the Grand View Hospital to join in the Dedication of Penn Foundation's new 7,194-square-foot, $125,000 multi-purpose mental health facility. The homily of keynote speaker Richard Detweiler—

Curtin, Dr. Kenneth Appel, and Dr. Daniel Blain, the latter now serving as Commissioner of Mental Health for the State of California. Having traveled to Sellersville several times over the years to advise Foundation officials on their expansion project, Dr. Blain characterized the Dedication as "the fulfillment of a dream with which I am proud to say I was identified at the very outset."

The keynote speaker was Richard Detweiler, pastor of the Perkasie Mennonite congregation, bishop in the Franconia Mennonite Conference, and Principal of Christopher Dock Mennonite School. In selecting the Souderton-born churchman-educator to deliver the afternoon's main address, organizers hoped to highlight the connection between Penn Foundation's medical mission and the Christian call to "love your neighbor." Richard did not disappoint. His homily on the theme of "recovering the lost" perfectly fit the occasion (one of the five hundred supporters in attendance spoke for many when he remarked after the Dedication that "seldom, if ever, has the aim of the Penn Foundation been described as well").

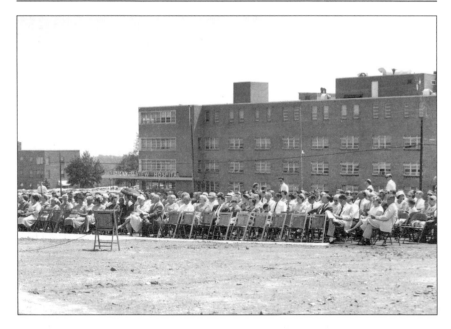

pastor of the Perkasie Mennonite congregation, bishop in the Franconia Mennonite Conference, and Principal of Christopher Dock Mennonite School—made an indelible impression on many in attendance. One supporter remarked that "seldom, if ever, has the aim of the Penn Foundation been described as well."

Richard began his sermon by noting that "upon occasion our Lord Jesus Christ sought to explain His ministry among men," and that "in the Gospel of Luke, Chapter 15, His words in story form have marked out for us three concerns that should characterize the dedication of these facilities." Penn Foundation's first objective, he continued, should be "finding the one who is lost." He recalled Jesus' rhetorical question: "What man of you, having a hundred sheep, if he lose one of them, doth not leave the ninety and nine in the wilderness, and go after that which is lost, until he find it?" So should we seek out and reclaim our neighbors who have "lost touch with reality" or are "emotionally at sea."

The second "concern" of the Foundation should be helping persons find "faith in the revealed Word of the living God." A man may be rich in many things, but if he loses his faith—an increasing likelihood in an ever-more impersonal, automated, and convictionless world—Penn Foundation should be ready to help him be as "the woman with ten pieces of silver who loses one, then lights a candle and sweeps the house seeking diligently to find it." "We look to the staff of this center not only to neutralize inner conflicts and expose hidden fears and remove false guilt," Richard declared, "but to assure persons that even in the twentieth century . . . there are trustworthy absolutes to live by. This does not mean we are suggesting naive and superficial answers to the deep-seated problems of the mentally and emotionally ill. Neither are we recommending that those who minister here should tear apart the personal fabric of every man's creed and exploit the sacred right of a man to his religion. But we do expect that this center will function on the promise that there are universal laws by which man has been ordained to live and that those laws have their being in the wisdom and love of a personal God who can be known."

As the basis for his final point—that "we must find and share forgiveness and restore to man the healing of his broken relationships"—Richard recalled the exclamation of the Prodigal Son's forbearing father: "This, my son, was dead, and is alive again; he was lost and is found!" "We dedicate this center," Richard remarked in conclusion, "to helping persons with broken relationships to be forgiven and to forgive, for therein lies the healing of human society. This is the highest calling on earth—to the art of healing. It is the divine approach to the restoring of the brokenness of man. We can dedicate ourselves and the work of Penn Foundation to nothing less and nothing greater than the healing of forgiveness."

The bishop's words struck a chord in his listeners, opening hearts and—as was soon demonstrated—checkbooks. Harold Mininger remembers an old friend approaching him after the service and without explanation thrusting into his hand a check for a sizable donation. Harold passed the word along to his fellow Directors, and together the men resolved to broadcast Pastor Detweiler's message to a wider audience. They hit the jackpot when the editor of Perkasie's *News-Herald* agreed to publish the Dedication address in the next issue of his newspaper.*

---

*The text of Richard Detweiler's Dedication speech, as printed in the July 5, 1962 edition of the *News-Herald*, is reproduced in Appendix 1.

5

"A MODEL FOR THE COUNTRY & THE WORLD"

Many in the throng attending the Dedication service for Penn Foundation's new $125,000 community mental health center lingered after the speeches and the benediction to inspect the facility. According to a Foundation press release, the building's "look of a lovely, large split-level home is carried into its interior. When one enters the reception room, one senses the warmth of welcome in the colors, the mixture of Early American and modern furniture, the curtains, the fireplace, and most of all the smile of [secretary-receptionist] Mrs. Marjorie Alexander, whose living room this might well be." A newspaper reporter also likened the reception area to "a handsome living room," but offered no assessment of the other interior components, identified as "five offices for the staff

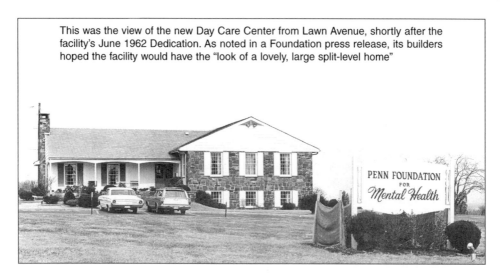

This was the view of the new Day Care Center from Lawn Avenue, shortly after the facility's June 1962 Dedication. As noted in a Foundation press release, its builders hoped the facility would have the "look of a lovely, large split-level home"

Penn Foundation's primary publicist, Board Secretary Charles Hoeflich, opined in a June 1962 press release that "when one enters the reception room [of the new Day Care Center], one senses the warmth of welcome in the colors, the mixture of Early American and modern furniture, the curtains, the fireplace, and most of all the smile of [secretary-receptionist] Mrs. Marjorie Alexander, whose living room this might well be." Perhaps the most noteworthy of the room's appointments were several large impressionistic paintings of local scenes rendered by Sellersville's renowned artist, writer, and educator Walter Emerson Baum.

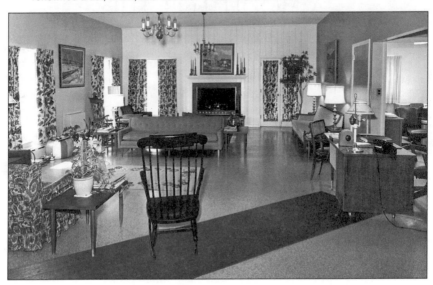

to receive patients, a library-board room, and a child's playroom on the first floor, a kitchen, a group-therapy room, a fully equipped occupational therapy room, a sitting room, and lavatories on the ground-level room." A third visitor recorded a mix of facts and impressions concerning the center: "An exceptionally pleasant split-level building, residential in feeling, it consists of a large and attractive reception room with open fireplace, a series of spacious and pleasantly decorated offices for the professional staff, a multipurpose room where the day hospital is held, a kitchen, two patient sitting rooms, which are used for group therapy, an employees sitting room, a quiet room, and appropriate storage area."

Of the four overarching needs spelled out in the August 1957 "Outline of a Suggested Plan for Action for Expanding Psychiatric Facilities," the new day care center fully addressed the first two: offices and a reception area arranged with "due consideration to privacy" for the treatment of out-patients; and facilities "to accommodate the delivery of day care services." Not part of the new building were bedrooms for in-patients (Grand View

Hospital had agreed to make those available), nor was there "a meeting place for groups perhaps up to 100 in number where public meetings in the general interest of Mental Health could be held." Addressing this final need would have to wait until the next round of expansion.

Monday, July 2, 1962 was the first day on the job for Day Care Coordinator Ruth Lefever and staff psychiatrist Wilbur Lyons. The Directors hoped the new employees could have the day treatment program up and running in about a month. As Nurse Lefever and Dr. Lyons dove into their work, however, they discovered that preparations would take much longer. The task proved so complex that they were obliged to make research trips to psychiatric day care centers in Pennsylvania, Maryland, and New York (it would later be reported that "all of these services were much more heavily staffed, more elaborately equipped, and had more complicated programs than anyone at Penn Foundation had in mind, but the visits provided a starting point for planning"). Back home, Nurse Lefever and Dr. Lyons spent their days ordering supplies, devising legal forms, negotiating payment plans with Blue Cross, and generally trying to keep their heads above the surface of a sea of administrative details.

The summer had all but elapsed before the program was ready to admit its first patients. When it did, the many weeks of preparing—and years of dreaming—quickly began paying dividends. At the October 1962 Board meeting, Dr. Lyons and Nurse Lefever reported on "the opening of the Penn Foundation Day Care Program" and "presented two cases" for the enlightenment of the Directors. The medical teammates noted in conclusion that they "were most encouraged by the fact that both patients had responded dramatically to this type of treatment, and they are convinced that both patients have been spared long hospitalizations because of the availability of day care" (as recorded in meeting minutes). These charter patients, and all other patients admitted to the Day Care Program during its first eighteen months of operation, were female. "The Program originally appeared more suitable for women than for men," the authors of an organizational profile would note several years later. "For the first eighteen months, only women were admitted."

A layman's view of the Day Care Program shortly after its inception was provided by a staff writer for Doylestown's *Daily Intelligencer*, who visited Penn Foundation in November 1962 and filed the following report:

> Day patients arrive early in the morning and spend their
> time in a variety of ways, perhaps an hour with the doctor,

perhaps partly in group therapy, with time to read, or work at ceramics, woodworking, or weaving.

It's a unique and progressive approach to treating emotionally disturbed people in that while they are under proper psychiatric care, they spend most of their lives with their families. This eliminates an often difficult adjustment of getting back into the community life.

Most patients are referred to the Foundation by their pastors, doctors, or they come on their own. Some 2,500 persons have availed themselves of the Foundation's services; 447 are now under treatment. . . . The Foundation turns down no one who seeks aid. Persons who cannot pay full rates are charged according to their ability to pay. Some cannot pay at all. Consultant fees are, says [Medical Director Norman] Loux, "all the way from $15 per hour down to nothing."

A reporter from a competing newspaper was most impressed by the ambience he perceived while touring the new facility:

It is truly well named. Day Care Center. And the accent is on the word "care." Whether visiting with Louise DiGiorgio, the social worker, Dr. "Mike" Dunn, the child psychiatrist, Dr. Wilbert A. Lyons, staff psychiatrist, Dr. James Barbash, clinical psychologist, or Dr. Loux himself, the atmosphere of prevailing peace and of technical competence go hand in hand.

This is undoubtedly true because the group which has come together reflect the original purpose for which the Foundation was founded—to provide the best in the medical specialty of mental health to all who need it in its area of activity. And the word "all" is meant to reflect the concern of the founders, which is the same as the Good Samaritan had for his neighbor.

"Fine spirit of unification"

The newest method of treatment available to the Foundation's psychiatrists in the fall of 1962—electroconvulsive therapy (ECT), or "shock treatment"—was practiced not in the day care center but across the street in Grand View Hospital. Administered almost exclusively to patients diagnosed with clinical depression, this not-entirely-understood but undeniably effective technique had not been an option at Penn Foundation prior to the hiring of a second psychiatrist (Dr. Lyons) several months earlier. The nature of ECT was such that (as Dr. Loux explained to the Directors at the time) "it is essential to have a team of two psychiatrists and a nurse in attendance."

The close association of Penn Foundation and Grand View Hospital, epitomized by Dr. Loux's service as Medical Director of the former and Chief of the Neuropsychiatry Department of the latter, was demonstrated again in September 1962 when officials of the two organizations worked out an arrangement whereby Foundation personnel would perform ECT using the Hospital's facilities, and all related billing would be handled by Foundation administrators. This new collaboration was soon lauded in a local newspaper editorial as "another milestone in the fine medical care that is available to the area." Under the headline "Another Step Forward," the editorialist continued:

> Last week's announcement said that shock treatment will become available and 24 hour emergency service for those requiring mental health care will be instituted.
>
> The introduction of shock treatments at Grand View means that people requiring such service will no longer be required to travel as distant as Abington or Allentown which had been the closest hospitals offering such aid.
>
> It emphasizes other things, too. People responsible for directing the hospital and foundation program are not content to sit back and rest on their record which has for years provided more than the normal services and care of a general hospital.
>
> Rather they have continued to make available more services and in return better care. This latest move emphasizes as well the fine spirit of unification that exists between the hospital and the foundation which while run independently are closely associated through the every day demands of patients.
>
> It's nice to know that while the area already enjoys the advantage of an excellent hospital and mental health clinic, officials of both continue to work hard to incorporate new services to meet the medical needs of the community.

The institution of "24-hour emergency service" for psychiatric cases alluded to by the editorial writer was another manifestation of "the fine spirit of unification" between Penn Foundation and the Hospital. This service had become available when a Foundation telephone line was wired into the Hospital's switchboard. After-hours calls to the mental health center, formerly diverted to an answering service, would now be received and promptly acted upon by Hospital personnel. It was the most tangible gesture of cooperation since the Hospital had allowed Penn Foundation to tie into its sewer line when the Day Care Center was constructed. The parties had entered into a contractual agreement regarding their usage of the sewer line, but "all other matters pertaining to patient care and provisional services were, and remain, a gentleman's agreement [between Hospital and Foundation personnel], maintained by mutual respect and personal integrity" (according to the author of a 1968 study of Penn Foundation).

Within ten weeks of the ECT apparatus's deployment in Grand View Hospital, 115 shock treatments were administered to Penn Foundation patients. The delivery of day care and after-care to these patients was the principal factor in the dramatic increase—from two to thirty-four—in the number of persons treated in Penn Foundation's day care program from late-September 1962 through the first week of December. The rapid growth put tremendous pressure on the program's limited human resources, prompting Dr. Loux to recommend to the Directors that "the use of volunteer help be fully explored," with the stipulation that "volunteers be supervised by trained staff."

Yet another avenue of program expansion was opened in November 1962 when Dr. Loux met with the Superintendent of Bucks County Schools to discuss the possibility of Penn Foundation "providing psychiatric services to the school system." The Medical Director came away from this meeting impressed by the opportunity, but mindful too of the potential pitfalls. Before Penn Foundation took on such a challenge, he advised the Directors, "the problem of long-term financing and administrative responsibility would have to be carefully worked out."

Major administrative issues would be "worked out" a bit differently after the Board's adoption of a streamlined meeting schedule in January 1963. The full Board would meet in the Foundation's library/board room once every two months, while the Executive Committee—comprising the four officers of the Board—would meet with Dr. Loux at the Union National Bank in Souderton on the first and third Thursday of each month. The site of Executive Meetings was chosen in deference to Board Secretary Charles Hoeflich, just completing his first year as President of Union National, and Treasurer Russell Moyer, the former oil merchant whom Charles had recently brought to the Bank to serve as Assistant Trust Officer.

A Presidential appeal

The Directors' first brush with Federal legislation—the unrequited Hill-Burton Funds affair of the late 1950s—had convinced them that Penn Foundation should remain as free as possible of financial assistance with strings attached, especially strings emanating from Washington, D.C. A second brush in the mid-1960s yielded much more positive results. Indeed, activities in the nation's capitol helped raise Penn Foundation's profile from backwater community mental health center to "a model for the country and the world."

The curtain of the national stage onto which Penn Foundation would be ushered was raised by President John F. Kennedy, whose sensitivity to issues of mental health had been sharpened through childhood experiences with his mentally retarded sister, Rosemary. In his first year in office (1961), President Kennedy appointed a cabinet-level committee to review a new report submitted to Congress by the Joint Commission on Mental Illness and Health following a five-year study. Entitled *Action for Mental Health*, the report called for federally-funded programs of training, treatment, and research in the field of mental health. The call had been picked up and amplified by the American Medical Association, the American Psychiatric Association, and the National Association of Mental Health by the time President Kennedy established his "President's Panel on Mental Retardation" and charged it with investigating the services available for persons with mental retardation and other forms of developmental disability. The paucity of services confirmed by this Panel, and the general inattention to issues of mental health revealed by the Joint Commission's studies, prompted President Kennedy to address Congress on the urgent need for action. As he noted in the opening passages of his "Special Message to the Congress on Mental Illness and Mental Retardation," submitted on February 5, 1963:

> . . . Mental illness and mental retardation are among our most critical health problems. They occur more frequently, affect

more people, require more prolonged treatment, cause more suffering by the families of the afflicted, waste more of our human resources, and constitute more financial drain upon both the public treasury and the personal finances of the individual families than any other single [health] condition.

There are now about 800,000 such patients in this Nation's institutions—600,000 for mental illness and over 200,000 for mental retardation. Every year nearly 1,500,000 people receive treatment in institutions for the mentally ill and mentally retarded. Most of them are confined and compressed within an antiquated, vastly overcrowded, chain of custodial State institutions. The average amount expended on their care is only $4 a day—too little to do much good for the individual, but too much if measured in terms of efficient use of our mental health dollars. In some States the average is less than $2 a day.

The total cost to the taxpayers is over $2.4 billion a year in direct public outlays for services—about $ 1.8 billion for mental illness and $600 million for mental retardation. Indirect public outlays—in welfare costs and in the waste of human resources—are even higher. But the anguish suffered both by those afflicted and by their families transcends financial statistics—particularly in view of the fact that both mental illness and mental retardation strike so often in childhood, leading in most cases to a lifetime of disablement for the patient and a lifetime of hardship for his family.

This situation has been tolerated far too long. It has troubled our national conscience—but only as a problem unpleasant to mention, easy to postpone, and despairing of solution. The Federal Government, despite the nation-wide impact of the problem, has largely left the solutions up to the States. The States have depended on custodial hospitals and homes. Many such hospitals and homes have been shamefully understaffed, overcrowded, unpleasant institutions from which death too often provided the only firm hope of release.

The time has come for a bold new approach. . . .

The President went on to describe the goals he envisioned for this "bold new approach." They included "seeking out the causes of mental illness and of mental retardation and eradicating them," as well as "strengthening the underlying resources of knowledge and, above all, of skilled manpower which are necessary to mount and sustain our attack on mental disability for many years to come." It was President Kennedy's third assertion that held the key to Penn Foundation's elevation to national notoriety: "We must strengthen and improve the programs and facilities serving the mentally ill and the mentally retarded. The emphasis should be upon timely and intensive diagnosis, treatment, training, and rehabilitation so that the mentally afflicted can be cured or their functions restored to the extent possible. Services to both the mentally ill and to the mentally retarded must be community based and provide a range of services to meet community needs."

If the ears of Penn Foundation officials were not yet tingling at this point in the President's Message, surely a tingle commenced when they read the following words from the leader of the free world:

> Central to a new mental health program is comprehensive community care. Merely pouring Federal funds into a continuation of the outmoded type of institutional care which now prevails would make little difference. We need a new type of health facility, one which will return mental health care to the main stream of American medicine, and at the same time upgrade mental health services. I recommend, therefore, that the Congress (1) authorize grants to the States for the construction of comprehensive community mental health centers, beginning in fiscal year 1965, with the Federal Government providing 45 to 75 percent of the project cost; (2) authorize short-term project grants for the initial staffing costs of comprehensive community mental health centers, with the Federal Government providing up to 75 percent of the cost in the early months, on a gradually declining basis, terminating such support for a project within slightly over four years; and (3), to facilitate the preparation of community plans for these new facilities as a necessary preliminary to any construction or staffing assistance, appropriate $4.2 million for planning grants under the National Institute of Mental Health. These planning funds, which would be in addition to a similar amount appropriated for fiscal year 1963, have been included in my proposed 1964 budget.

Penn Foundation supporters responded to these recommendations with a collective "Would you look at that! The President of the United States is calling for the establishment of community mental health centers like Penn Foundation all across the country!" It was entirely possible, however, that the President and his advisors—including National Institute of Mental Health founder and Director Robert H. Felix—were unaware of Penn Foundation and its pioneering program. As chairman of the Foundation's Publicity Committee, Charles Hoeflich quickly drafted a letter of introduction to Dr. Felix, and mailed it off with the Board's approval. The Foundation's original supporter, Dr. Michael Peters, took it upon himself to write President Kennedy directly. "I told him we had been [operating a comprehensive community mental health center] like he described since 1955," Grand View Hospital's Chief of Medicine later recalled. "I told him we felt this was *really* a good program. And he wrote back, saying 'I'm glad to hear it. Keep up the good work and you'll hear from us.'" This was not, as Foundation officials soon learned, an empty promise.

Congress responded to President Kennedy's appeal by passing two pieces of legislation in October 1963 (less than a month, it turned out, before the President's assassination in Dallas). Public Law 88-156, known as "The Maternal and Child Health Mental Retardation Planning Amendments of 1963," provided funds for research into links between maternal health and mental retardation in children. A week later, Congress enacted Public Law 88-164, "The Mental Retardation Facilities and Community Mental Health Centers Construction Act of 1963." This legislation would provide matching funds of $150 million over a three-year period for states to use in constructing "comprehensive community health centers." It also stipulated that regulations be formulated concerning the types of services which would together constitute "comprehensive care." In the coming years, persons responsible for establishing community clinics under Public Law 88-164 would seek out "model" programs for study and consultation. More than a few of these clinic builders would find their way to Penn Foundation's door.

Community outreach through education

One of the program components for which Penn Foundation would receive particular attention in the mid-1960s was community outreach. This facet of the Foundation's mission was lifted to a new level in March

1963 with the initiation of twice-monthly classes for local clergy, organized in collaboration with the Upper Bucks County Ministerial Association and the Grand View Hospital chaplains. "We are attempting not only to help ministers learn something of our techniques and knowledge of psychiatry," Dr. Loux explained in a press release, "but of equal importance, we feel we also need to learn from them. Group study with persons of similar interest and with a group the proper size can be very meaningful. This particular course has been designed to broaden the understanding of the ministers in the matter of problems which face the individual today." At the March 19 gathering of pastors and chaplains at Penn Foundation, Drs. Loux and Lyons lectured on the topic of "Defense Mechanisms" before the dozen participants divided up for group discussions.

Encouraged by the response to these pastoral classes, Dr. Loux and the Directors began planning a series of day-long seminars geared for doctors, school superintendents, and law enforcement officers, in addition to clergy. Dr. Loux's reputation and professional connections enabled him to recruit some eminent authorities for the inaugural sequence of four seminars. He was also able to persuade Lemmon Pharmacal Company of Sellersville to underwrite the sessions, conducted once every few weeks beginning on October 31, 1963. Nearly one hundred doctors and ministers turned out for the first seminar in which the Reverend Seward Hiltner, Professor of Theology and Personality at Princeton Theological Seminary, held forth on "the meaning and place of the various professional groups in the community in the care of the total person." The guest lecturer for the second seminar was Dr. Loux's old friend from Yale University and the Yale Child Study Team, Dr. Milton Senn. The final two sessions featured addresses by Dr. Edward T. Auer, Professor and Director of the Department of Psychiatry and Neurology at St. Louis University, and the new President of the American Psychiatric Association (who needed little introduction to Penn Foundation audiences), Dr. Daniel Blain.

Other high-profile visitors to Penn Foundation in the latter months of 1963 came to learn rather than lecture. Among them was the Foundation's long-time ally, Dr. Lauren Smith of the Pennsylvania Hospital. He was conducting a nation-wide study of community mental health centers in preparation for an American Medical Association-sponsored Congress on Mental Illness and Health, scheduled for November 1964. After spending "considerable time" in Sellersville in the fall of 1963, Dr. Smith departed having assured Dr. Loux and the Directors that they would "undoubtedly be asked to participate in a substantial way in the conference next November in Chicago" (according to Board meeting minutes). Two other estimable visitors arrived together as representatives of a committee appointed by the National Institute of Mental Health (NIMH) while Congress was deliberating over what turned out to be Public Laws 88-156 and 88-164. Dr. Robert Strauss of the University of Kentucky's Medical Center and Dr. William Soskin of the U.S. Department of Health, Education and Welfare were dispatched to Sellersville to find out if Penn

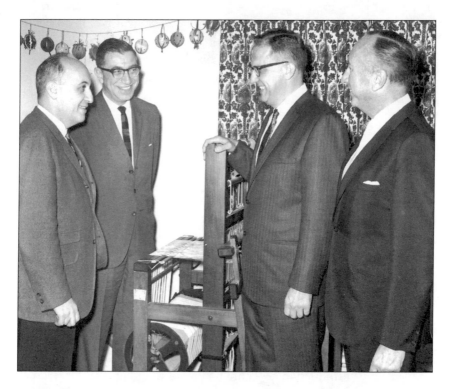

Penn Foundation brought scores of psychiatric luminaries to Sellersville. Some came to observe and take notes, others to dispense wisdom. Included in the latter group were dozens of experts imported through the Foundation's public education program, which took a major step forward in October 1963 with the inauguration of an annual Seminar Series funded by the Perkasie-based Lemmon Pharmacal Company. Generally comprising four public lectures spaced about a month apart and commencing in November, the Series was entering its fifth season on November 28, 1967 when this photo was taken of guest lecturer Dr. Stanley F. Yolles, Executive Director of the National Institute of Mental Health (second from left) conferring with Pennsylvania's Commissioner of Mental Health Dr. Joseph Adlestein (far left), Dr. Loux, and Penn Foundation President Charles Hoeflich beside a hand loom in the Foundation's occupational and recreational therapy area.

Foundation had any particularly valuable advice, insight, or experience to offer organizers or operators of community mental health centers. The answer was "Yes" on all counts, and Drs. Strauss and Soskin returned to Washington to file their enthusiastic report. Once again, the Foundation's officers were told they'd be hearing soon from federal officials, and once again the promise was kept.

The report filed by Drs. Strauss and Soskin was reviewed by personnel of the newly-formed Joint Information Service (JIS) of the American Psychiatric Association (APA) and the National Association for Mental Health (NAMH). Dr. Loux learned late in 1963 that Penn Foundation had been one of 234 psychiatric facilities across the country evaluated by the JIS in an attempt to identify *truly comprehensive* mental health centers for further study. Sellersville's entry not only made the initial cut of 65, it was among the handful of programs selected by the JIS for in-depth examination. Interestingly, the chosen eleven—three located in New York, and one each in California, Colorado, Kansas, Massachusetts, Missouri, Nebraska, Pennsylvania, and Saskatchewan—included Prairie View Hospital, the institution founded ten years earlier by the Mennonite Central Committee's Mennonite Mental Health Association in Newton, Kansas.

Penn Foundation's staff and Directors scrambled during the winter of 1963-64 to compile data for use by an investigative team of JIS-appointed doctors and administrators scheduled to visit the Foundation in mid-March 1964. Most of the data reflected clinical activities recorded during the previous year, categorized as either "Outpatient Service," "Part-time Hospitalization," "Inpatient Service," or "Services for Children." These activities were ultimately summarized in the JIS report as follows:

> OUTPATIENT SERVICE. In 1963 [Penn] Foundation saw 450 new outpatients, for an average of 15 visits each. Most of the patients are seen in one-hour sessions, some in half-hour sessions. About 75 per cent of the patients are seen either once or twice a week at the beginning of therapy, the others less frequently. A number of them have been treated in the inpatient or day programs, to and from which they are readily shifted as needs indicate. In addition to individual psychotherapy, the program includes group therapy, family therapy, and, for some depressed patients, electroshock. About 50 per

cent of outpatients receive psychotropic drugs at any given time, and about 75 per cent receive such drugs at one time or another during their outpatient experience. In 1963, 60 per cent of outpatients were women, 40 per cent men; 8 per cent were under 20 years old, 84 per cent were between 20 and 59, and 8 per cent were 60 or older. They represented the following diagnoses:

Psychoneurotic depressive reactions:	30%
Schizophrenic reactions:	22%
Psychotic disorders other than schizophrenic reactions:	18%
Psychoneurotic disorders other than depressive reactions:	10%
Transient situational personality disorders:	9%
Other personality disorders:	8%
Other diagnoses:	3%

PART-TIME HOSPITALIZATION. For the occasional patient who can work during the day but needs to sleep at Grand View Hospital at night or who needs to spend only the weekend in the hospital, the program is sufficiently flexible that he can do so. The need arises very rarely.

There is a formally organized day care program, held on Mondays, Wednesdays, and Fridays. Inpatients at Grand View who can benefit from the day program come across the street to the Foundation, where the day program takes place in a large, cheerful room. During 1963 a total of 31 patients were treated on the day program. The average attendance was 9. Of these, an average of 8 came from their homes and one from Grand View Hospital. There were 26 new admissions during the year, and a total of 16 discharges. All members of the professional staff devote some of their time to the day care program, which includes individual psychotherapy, a group therapy session each day, a variety of occupational and recreational therapy activities, a variety of interesting and entertaining field trips, and an emphasis on total milieu therapy, including, for example, discussion groups, preparing lunch for fellow patients and staff members, and group singing. The social service staff maintains regular contact with the families of patients on the day program. . . .

INPATIENT SERVICE. During 1963 there were 150 psychiatric patients admitted to Grand View Hospital. Of these 72 per cent were women, 28 per cent men. Five per cent were under 20 years old, 82 per cent were between 20 and 59, and 13 per cent were 60 and older. Sixty per cent were given psychotropic drugs, another 38 per cent were given such drugs plus electroshock, and 2 per cent were given neither. They represented the following diagnoses:

> Schizophrenic reactions: 40%
> Other psychotic disorders: 36%
> Psychoneurotic disorders: 17%
> Other diagnoses: 7%

The average length of hospitalization for these patients was 15 days. Following the inpatient episode, 76 per cent were referred to the outpatient or day care services at Penn Foundation. Another 14 per cent were referred to their family physicians. The remaining 10 per cent were transferred to private psychiatrists, state and private psychiatric hospitals, and elsewhere.

SERVICES FOR CHILDREN. Of the 70 children seen in 1963, 30 were between 10 and 19 years old and in the data furnished us are included in the statistics presented above. Physicians and parents were the source of referral for about one-third each of these 70 children. The schools referred 19 per cent, and the remaining 8 per cent came from the courts, attorneys, and other sources. Two-thirds of them were boys, one-third girls. Sixteen per cent were under 7 years old, 47 per cent were from 7 through 12 years old, and 37 per cent were between 13 and 19 years old. They represented the following diagnoses:

> Transient situational personality disorders: 33%
> Other personality disorders: 27%

Psychoneurotic disorders: 16%
Psychotic disorders: 9%
Chronic brain syndromes: 0%
Psychophysiologic reactions: 16%
Mental deficiency: 0%

As of the end of 1963, 20 per cent continued in treatment at the Foundation, 4 per cent had been referred elsewhere, 43 per cent had been terminated as improved, and 21 per cent had been terminated as not improved. As for the form of treatment, in 40 per cent of cases the mother and child were both seen, in 35 per cent of cases only the parents were seen, and in 24 per cent there was no treatment.

The mental health experts charged with evaluating these data and getting a first-hand look at Penn Foundation in action arrived at the center on March 10, 1964. Led by JIS Chief Raymond M. Glasscote, the team of professors and psychiatrists spent several days in Sellersville, shuttling back and forth between the Foundation and Grand View Hospital, observing, interviewing employees and patients, taking copious notes. When they finally moved on to their next destination, Dr. Loux declared to a local reporter, "There is no doubt in my mind but that the results of what they are doing will serve as an invaluable reference for other areas which might need and want to establish a mental health unit." The prediction would prove spot on.

Expanding personnel

Among the Penn Foundation staff members observed by the JIS team in March 1964 was a relatively recent hire: psychiatric social worker G. Lawrence Landes. Larry had come "highly recommended by his teachers and former employers" when he was brought in for an interview a year earlier. When he "favorably impressed" Dr. Loux and the Directors in a series of interviews, he was invited to become the Foundation's second social worker. Two weeks after his first day on the job (May 1, 1963), Dr. Loux reported to the Directors that Larry "is proving to be a most worthwhile addition to the staff."

Had the JIS observers visited Penn Foundation a couple of months later, they would have found two additional employees at work. Thirty-six-year-old Arthur C. Isaak was hired on a part-time basis in April 1964 to set up and direct a recreational and occupational therapy program. A native of Idaho and a member of the West Swamp Mennonite congregation in Quakertown, Art had served the previous six years as assistant minister at Zion Mennonite Church in Souderton. Because he would be spending some of his time with patients across the street at Grand View Hospital, the Hospital administration agreed to pick up a portion of his salary once he became a full-time employee in July 1964. It was the beginning of another long and fruitful employee-employer relationship

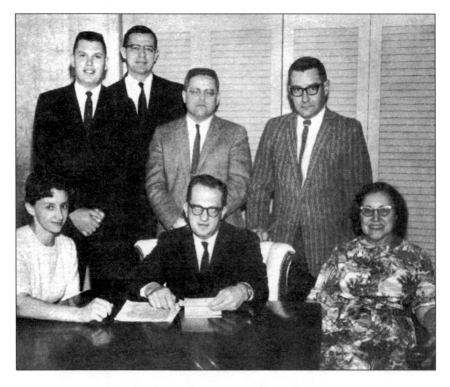

This publicity photo of Penn Foundation's professional staff was published in local newspapers in the spring of 1964, shortly after Art Isaak (standing, far right) was hired to set up and direct a recreational and occupational therapy program. Art's new colleagues comprised (seated, from left) Day Care Coordinator Ruth Lefever, Medical Director Norman Loux, social worker Louise DiGiorgio, (standing) psychiatric social worker Larry Landes, child psychiatrist Dr. John ("Mike") Dunn, and staff psychiatrist Dr. Wilbert Lyons. Not included in the photo was part-time clinical psychologist Dr. James Barbash. A couple of months after this picture was taken, Dr. John Richards joined the Foundation as staff psychiatrist.

along Lawn Avenue. Art would be a valuable player on the Penn Foundation team for the remainder of his life.

The second new hire in July 1964 was former Bucks County general practitioner Dr. John Richards, brought in to serve as a staff psychiatrist alongside Drs. Loux and Lyons. Dr. Loux had begun discussing employment possibilities with Dr. Richards almost a year earlier, but it took months to work out the contractual details and allow Dr. Richards—who had begun his residency in psychiatry at Norristown State Hospital, and had completed it recently at the University of Pennsylvania Hospital—time to tie off his existing responsibilities. One of the sticking points in the lengthy negotiation was the insistence by Dr. Loux and the Directors that any psychiatrist joining Penn Foundation on a full-time basis be totally divested of non-Foundation employment. As Dr. Loux explained to JIS interviewers shortly before Dr. Richards' first day on the job: "A comprehensive psychiatric service cannot succeed in any community if it is staffed by transient professionals, or personnel giving their major energies to other activities, or personnel using their position as a stepping stone to private practice. I believe there needs to be a core of key professional people who have the respect of the community, including the medical community, and who themselves are, or are becoming, a part of the community."

There was yet another new name on the Penn Foundation payroll in July 1964. Kathryn (Mrs. Ernest K.) Landes had begun volunteering her time in the Day Care Program midway through 1963. When her efforts at coordinating the training of additional volunteers proved invaluable (literally "just what the doctor ordered," the "doctor" being Dr. Loux in his December 1962 proposal that the Directors "fully explore" the use of volunteers), Dr. Loux recommended that Kathryn be appointed Director of Volunteer Services on a salary basis. The trustees approached Kathryn with the invitation, which she humbly accepted on the condition that the nominal salary offered—$150 per month—be reduced to an even more modest $100.

The addition of Kathryn Landes, Dr. Richards, and Art Isaak to the Penn Foundation staff was partly offset in July 1964 by the departure of Louise DiGiorgio. Having gamely commuted by train or car to Sellersville every work-day since December 1956, Louise resigned in order to care for her ailing mother in south Philadelphia. Her exit left the Foundation staffed in the summer of 1964 by twelve persons: a medical director and psychiatrist-in-chief, two more full-time psychiatrists, a part-time child psychiatrist, a part-time clinical psychologist, a psychiatric social worker, an occupational and recreation therapist, a registered nurse, a volunteer services coordinator, an executive secretary, a full-time secretary, and a part-time secretary.

The additional manpower made it a little easier for Dr. Loux to take on professional speaking and consulting engagements being offered at a rate rising along with Penn Foundation's reputation. He was also able to continue serving as the Foundation's eyes and ears at numerous regional and national mental health conferences. As even a partial list demonstrates, his résumé was lengthening impressively:

- March 1963: Presentation of paper, "Comprehensive Psychiatric Services in a Semi-Rural Community with special emphasis on Day Care," in New York City.
- April 1963: "Discussant" in "Goals of Healing" session in "Academy of Religion and Mental Health, Fourth Annual Meeting," in Philadelphia.
- March 1964: Attendance at New England Hospital Assembly; attendance at "Catholic Hospital Association's conference on psychiatric hospitals."
- June 1964: Speaker at staff conference of NIMH conducted by the JIS in Boulder, Colorado.
- November 1964: Chairman of panel at AMA Congress on Mental Illness and Health in Chicago

In his travels, Dr. Loux made many professional connections while spreading the word of Penn Foundation's "bold new approach." At the April 1963 meeting in Philadelphia, for instance, he talked shop with fellow "discussant" Rev. Seward Hiltner. This encounter set the stage for Dr. Loux to invite Reverend Hiltner to guest lecture at Penn Foundation's inaugural seminar series the following October. Back home, Dr. Loux's standing in the community was further elevated when he was elected President of the Grand View Hospital Medical Staff by his peers at the annual Hospital meeting in January 1964. News of this election was soon followed by two more exciting announcements. The first was that the Grundy Foundation—a philanthropic organization recently established by Bucks County industrialist and State Senator Joseph R. Grundy—had responded positively to a request from Grand View Hospital officials for financial assistance in "developing overnight space for their psychiatric facility, which is provided for Penn Foundation" (as recorded in Executive Committee meeting minutes). The Grundy response took the form of a $35,000 grant to Penn Foundation, "payable one-half in 1964 and one-half in 1965, made . . . with the understanding that as much as needed should be allocated to the proposed improvement to Grand View Hospital to provide improved facilities for in-patient care for by the Penn Foundation. The balance is to be used for the improvement or expansion of the facilities of Penn Foundation."

Prestigious endorsements

The Directors also learned in May 1964 that the Mental Health Association of Southeastern Pennsylvania (MHASP) had chosen Penn Foundation from a pool of twenty-four candidates to receive the first annual Earl D. Bond Award. Established in honor of the oldest living former president of the American Psychiatric Association, and intended to "reward, support, or encourage new and creative approaches to the care of mentally ill persons," the Award was presented to Dr. Loux by MHASP officials and Dr. Bond himself at a ceremony conducted on June 4, 1964 at the Institute of the Pennsylvania Hospital in Philadelphia, where Dr. Bond had served as a psychiatrist for more than fifty years. A lengthy profile of Penn Foundation published in the next issue of MHASP's newsletter, *Lines of Communication*, began by explaining that the Foundation was selected for the Award "for its successful pioneering in the establishment of a comprehensive community mental health center, the only one of its kind in Pennsylvania." After recounting the major steps in Penn Foundation's journey, the article concluded by noting that the "future plans at the Foundation call for expanded children's services and day care, introduction of evening care and, eventually, night care. 'One of the most satisfying aspects of our work has been the harmonious relationship with the family physicians and other medical specialists in our community,' [Dr. Loux remarked to the author]. 'Furthermore, there is an immeasurable difference between participating in a project the community wants and is willing to put forth the effort to have, and introducing an organization primarily from without. Our program has had support from the medical profession, hospital administration, business, industry, private and public agencies, and the community-at-large,' Dr. Loux said. He did not say that his own professional skill, creativity and resourcefulness, personal magnetism and integrity have played a major role. Others in the [mental health] community, however, made it clear when they nominated Penn Foundation for the Earl D. Bond Award."

Penn Foundation received an even more prestigious endorsement later that month when Dr. Loux was informed by JIS officials at the NIMH conference in Colorado that Penn Foundation was "one of four or five services chosen as a model for the most desirable [psychiatric] unit of its type serving a community, and we are to act as a prototype for others to imitate," as Secretary Charles Hoeflich noted in his July 1964 Executive Committee meeting minutes. The Foundation's exalted place in the JIS's estimation was further highlighted when a book compiled by Raymond Glasscote and his team of JIS investigators was released in October 1964. Entitled *The Community Mental Health Center: An Analysis of Existing Models*, the 220-page volume included chapter-length profiles of each of the eleven psychiatric units selected for the study. It was no accident that the chapter on Penn Foundation was placed in the lead-off position, as Charles Hoeflich learned a few weeks later. "I was at a convention for mental health people [probably the AMA Congress of Mental Illness and Health in Chicago]," he recalled recently, "and the head of the National Institute said to me, 'Charlie, I hope you liked our book!' I said I sure *did*. He said, 'Well, we couldn't say who was best and who was not best of the eleven organizations, but I hope you noticed where [the chapter on Penn Foundation] landed up in the order!" I said I sure *did*. That was the closest I ever came to having someone who really knew what he was talking about say Penn Foundation was at the head of the pack." This high standing could no longer go unnoticed after the publication of the JIS study, of which 1,500 copies were distributed at the AMA Congress for use as a source work.

It might have seemed incongruous that even as national acclaim rolled in, there were still occasions when Penn Foundation was hard-pressed to make its payroll. The occasional crises were more understandable when the organization's revenue formula was explained, as it was by a correspondent in the May-June 1965 issue of *SK&F* [Smith Kline & French] *Psychiatric Reporter*: "About 65 per cent of Penn Foundation's operating expenses are paid for by individual fees for service, the rest being made up by money from the state, from Bucks and Montgomery counties, and from foundations. The top charge is $12 for the day-care program and $15 an hour for outpatients, but fees are scaled down so sharply according to ability to pay that the average is only about seven dollars. No one is turned away for lack of money." This policy contributed directly to the "financial emergency" facing the Directors in mid-November 1964. The "primary culprit" in the crisis, everyone agreed, was "overdue accounts" (in other words, tardy patient payments). The short-term solution was to authorize the Treasurer "to borrow funds from the Building Fund account to pay for operating expenses during the emergency." Beyond that, one or more of the trustees would "speak with the Business Manager of Grand View Hospital to see how [Hospital administrators] deal with overdue accounts." The third tack was to fire off another "solicitation letter to a limited mailing list of those who have previously contributed." Year-end contributions amounting to $8,874 ultimately helped stave off what had threatened to be a particularly dicey financial winter. Even so, the Directors had little choice but to "charge off $4,059 uncollectable Clinic Fees and $2,063 uncollectable Day Care Fees for the fiscal period ending December 31, 1964."

Making more news

From the community's perspective, Penn Foundation appeared to be sailing smoothly onward in the winter of 1964-65. A second four-session seminar series bathed the organization in the glow of such psychiatric luminaries as Dr. George C. Anderson, founder and Director of the Academy of Religion and Mental Health; Dr. A.E. Moll, Professor of Psychiatry at McGill University and Psychiatrist-in-Chief of Montreal General Hospital; and Dr. Emily H. Mudd, Director of the Marriage Council of Philadelphia, and Professor of Family Study in Psychiatry at the University of Pennsylvania School of Medicine. Local papers carried stories of other notable visitors to the Foundation, some of international renown. Among them was Belgian psychiatrist Dr. Jan Schrijvers, who spent the work-week of February 1-5, 1965 in Sellersville observing "at close hand an example of how a community psychiatric service can run in a relatively rural area in conjunction with a community hospital" (from Perkasie's *Central News-Herald*). A month later, the red carpet was rolled out for Dr. Klaus Thomas, psychiatrist at St. Elizabeth's Hospital in Washington, D.C., who addressed an audience of "130 persons, including many of Upper Bucks' physicians, psychiatrists, and ministers," on the topic of "suicide: its causes and possible prevention."

A highlight of a busy winter was a visit from Dr. Loux's old friend Frances Braceland, Psychiatrist-in-Chief at the Institute of Living in Hartford, Connecticut. The eminent Dr. Braceland's announced intent on March 16, 1965 was to meet with Penn Foundation staff during the day, and address a gathering of doctors and other professional workers in the evening. His agenda expanded, however, to include a surprise luncheon ceremony in which he helped unveil a portrait of Dr. Loux painted by Grand View Hospital oral surgeon and Medical Staff Secretary-Treasurer Dr. Kermit S. Black. An attending journalist reported that "the portrait of Dr. Loux was hailed by those who saw it as a dramatic likeness 'accenting the tremendous compassion for which he is noted.'"

Penn Foundation was back in the news a week later, as the new psychiatric in-patient wing at Grand View Hospital—built collaboratively using $29,850 in Grundy Foundation grant money—was dedicated in a

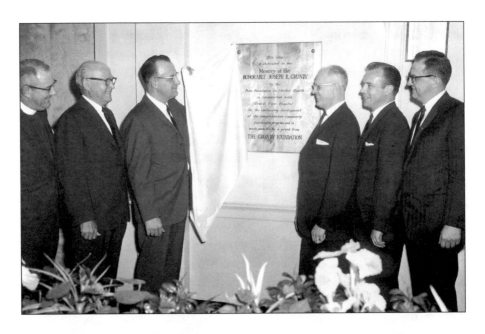

A plaque unveiled at the March 24, 1965 Dedication of the "Grundy Pavilion"—the new psychiatric in-patient wing in Grand View Hospital—was inscribed with these words: "This area is dedicated to the memory of the Honorable Joseph R. Grundy by the Penn Foundation for Mental Health in cooperation with Grand View Hospital for the continuing development of the comprehensive community psychiatric program and is made possible by a grant from the Grundy Foundation." Among the dignitaries on hand for the opening of the seven-room, thirteen-bed facility were (from left) the Rev. Ernest H. Flothmeier, pastor of St. Paul's Lutheran Church in Telford; W. James MacIntosh, Chairman of the Grundy Foundation; Harold Mininger, President of the Penn Foundation Board; Arthur A. Alderfer, President of the Grand View Hospital Board; William H. Waite, Grand View Hospital Administrator; and Penn Foundation Medical Director Dr. Norman Loux.

mid-day ceremony on March 24. Dubbed the "Grundy Pavilion," the new seven-room facility contained thirteen beds and "other facilities to aid the mentally ill." One of the speakers at the dedication, Hospital Board President Arthur A. Alderfer, declared that "this occasion is a testimonial to unselfish benevolence, but further, an example of unselfish community planning. It is evidence that two autonomous agencies can work together collectively for community welfare without costly duplication of identical services, and completely within the spirit of harmony which is so necessary to meet today's pressing problems. Trustees of the Grand View Hospital and the Penn Foundation feel that this gift from the Grundy Foundation has presented us a challenging but rewarding opportunity to demonstrate to the nation the real and only effective answer by which total health problems can be met—namely regional and coordinated planning. We earnestly hope that all in the future (and there will be many who will have occasion to visit our facilities) will be guided and inspired by this functional care unit, its development, and particularly the cooperative atmosphere within which it has been constructed."

The nation did indeed observe and applaud this demonstration of "regional and coordinated planning." The topic of collaboration was front and center in the aforementioned May-June 1965 profile of Penn Foundation in SK&F Psychiatric Reporter, which began:

> "We're here because the family doctors around Sellersville wanted us," said Dr. Norman Loux, medical director of the Penn Foundation for Mental Health. "We couldn't possibly do the job without their cooperation—even though we get lots of help from clergymen, teachers and others. I'd bet many of our patients would drop out of treatment if they didn't have the support of their doctors."
>
> He turned to Dr. Michael Peters, an internist who's medical chief at Grand View, the modern, 147-bed hospital that provides residential care for those of the Foundation's patients who need it. "Would you say I'm exaggerating?" "Not a bit," Dr. Peters said. "You know, if they want to, doctors can easily sabotage a psychiatric service. For one thing, they can simply disregard its existence. Our doctors, however, not only refer patients to the Foundation, they sell them on its value. And they always tell patients what to expect. They keep in touch with the psychiatrists, too—help them out when needed."

We were eating lunch in the staff dining room at Grand View, which also serves the Foundation's staff. Dr. Loux gestured toward the other tables. "A lot of informal counseling between psychiatrists and other doctors goes on every day right here over these tables," he said. "A lot more goes on over the phone. I'd say each of us makes four or five phone calls a day advising general practitioners about patients, or even former patients. There are many emotional problems that the family doctor can handle better than we can."

Celebrating a progressive decade

Penn Foundation rode a wave of local congeniality and national approbation right on through to its twinbill Tenth Anniversary celebration in October 1965. The latter of the two Anniversary events was the more intimate and low-key, as visitors were entertained at an open-house at the Foundation's headquarters on Sunday afternoon, October 10. Dr. Loux was on hand to answer questions, show folks around, and help them appreciate the significance of the day-care patients' work on display. This quiet get-together stood in stark contrast to the main Anniversary event conducted five days earlier, which also served as the first installment of the third annual Penn Foundation Seminar Series. More than five-hundred Foundation supporters had gathered in the Christopher Dock Mennonite School dining hall on Tuesday evening, October 5 to enjoy a banquet and then join a couple hundred more supporters in the adjoining auditorium to hear from no less an authority than NIMH founder and University of St. Louis Medical School Dean Robert Felix. A visiting reporter noted that Dr. Felix spoke passionately that evening of the Foundation's obligation "to push ahead to integrate its work with the community, determining community resources and pin-pointing the need for consultative services. 'Determine the real power structure of the community and use this knowledge to deal with the deeply destructive forces and to protect the community's mental health,' he said. He stressed the urgency of using preventive intervention; of being able to help people meet the stress situations of life which make them more than usually vulnerable to mental and emotional illness, such as entering school, adolescence, marriage, moving, retirement. . . . He praised the center's program as one in which 'the patient can move along as he progresses' and one which keeps him in his community and returns him to his familiar surroundings."

In fact, America's preeminent mental health expert mixed plenty of praise in with his admonitions. His most electrifying comments of the evening could hardly have been more congratulatory:

> If I were to select a half-dozen community mental health centers that nearly approach the dream I dreamed, not only would Penn Foundation be included, it would be one of the top three. Not only is it the only one of its kind in Pennsylvania; it is a model for the country and the world. Go on to bigger dreams; go on and on and on.

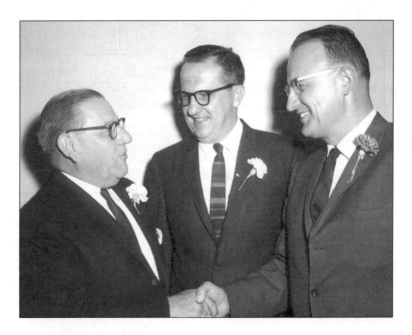

In his address to more than seven hundred supporters gathered in the Christopher Dock Mennonite School auditorium on October 5, 1965 to celebrate Penn Foundation's tenth anniversary, National Institute of Mental Health founder and University of St. Louis Medical School Dean Robert H. Felix lauded the Foundation as "a model for the country and the world." After his stirring speech, Dr. Felix (on left) expressed his appreciation individually to Medical Director Norman Loux (center) and Board President Harold Mininger.

6

"BOLD NEW APPROACH"

In the course of ten years, Penn Foundation had climbed from an obscure birth to the limelit national stage, with the very founder of the National Institute of Mental Health tossing up bouquets. Was the organization's swift ascent about to level off? Not if the first months of the Foundation's second decade were any measure. Indeed, an unusual project already underway at the time of the Tenth Anniversary celebrations would guarantee Dr. Loux and his colleagues at least another couple of years in the spotlight.

In yet another endorsement of Penn Foundation's pioneering program, the NIMH had decided to have half of the footage needed for its next major instructional movie filmed on location in and around Sellersville. With the working title *Bold New Approach* (borrowed from President Kennedy's 1963 Special Message to the Congress), the fifty-five-minute "mood film" was intended "to be used by mental health libraries throughout the United States to stimulate interest in communities where efforts are being made to start community mental health centers," according to a reporter for the *Souderton Independent*. The film would be shot "in black and white because of the technical difficulties of creating 'moods' in color."

The movie-makers hired for the job, Affiliated Film Producers, Inc. of New York, had been turning out short films on psychiatric topics for two decades. Several of these "shorts" were the work of producer-director Irving Jacoby, a founder of the production company in 1946 and a 1959 Oscar nominee in the Live Action Short Subject category. Jacoby took on the job of casting, producing, and directing *Bold New Approach*. His arrival with a film-making entourage in Sellersville in mid-October 1965 created a minor sensation. An article published in Perkasie's *News Herald* under the headline "Area Plays Big Role In Film To Boost Modern Mental Health Work" began with this teaser: "If you've seen camera crews, sound trucks, actors and all of the other paraphernalia reminiscent of Hollywood around the area, there's a good reason. Sellersville and Perkasie are the 'location' for an important motion picture—important, that is, in the field of mental health."

While the handful of actors imported for the shoot had some professional experience, they were hardly Hollywood legends. The female lead was a young actress named Jane Draper, whose short résumé included several roles in live theater productions (her career would peak two years later with a run of five guest appearances on the new television series *Dark Shadows*). Draper played the part of a teenager pushed over the edge by social pressures, but who was lucky enough to live in a community equipped with a mental health center able to deal humanely and effectively with psychotic breaks. Her co-stars in the hospital scenes were none other than Dr. Peters and Dr. Loux, who essentially played themselves (though they were not identified by name). A *Souderton Independent* feature writer witnessed some of the film-making action in a cordoned-off section of Grand View Hospital, and described it as follows:

> Casually dressed in a loose-fitting black sweatshirt, Irving Jacoby leaned back against a low radiator in the little corner room in Grand View Hospital, Sellersville.
>
> "Sound," he called in a firm soft voice, and everyone in the little cluttered room became silent. Everyone seemed to center their attention on the young lady in the hospital gown sitting up in the bed, lulling away time with a jig saw puzzle.
>
> Through the closed door to the corridor came a sharp clear answer.
>
> "Speed."
>
> A moment later Jacoby commanded, "Roll," and there was a faint *whrrr* from the massively padded motion picture camera that seemed to crouch in the corner between the windows on either side of the room.
>
> "Roll 12 . . . take 75," said an assistant as he held a scene board in front of the camera that had the director's name and the title of the film, "A Bold New Approach," painted on it along with space for the roll number and scene number (pieces of adhesive tape numbered in black) to be attached.

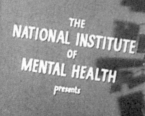

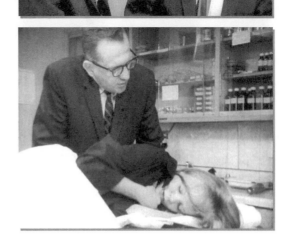

These frame captures from the first half of the National Institute of Mental Health's 1966 "mood film" *Bold New Approach* show Grand View Hospital Chief of Medicine Dr. Michael Peters administering a sedative to a newly-admitted psychiatric "patient" (played by aspiring actress Jane Draper) with help from a nurse and a police officer; Dr. Peters discussing the "patient's" condition with the Hospital's Chief of Psychiatry Dr. Norman Loux; and Dr. Loux addressing the becalmed "patient."

The holder of the scene board sharply snapped the hinged bottom of the board, making both a visible mark on the film and an audible mark on the sound tape that would later be used to synchronize the sound with the picture when both were printed together.

"Come in doctor," Jacoby called a second later.

The door to the hospital room opened and Dr. Norman Loux, medical director of Penn Foundation, entered and carefully closed the door (as rehearsed) and approached the young lady in the bed (Miss Jane Draper, professional actress who played the leading roll).

A few moments of seemingly casual but critically rehearsed dialogue ensued between the doctor and the patient.

"Print that," called Jacoby in a satisfied voice. Everyone began to move about and talk once again.

"Make several silent close-ups of the doctor," Jacoby instructed the "grips" and cameraman. The lighting technicians (grips) moved the "barndoors" on several of the lights to effectively light Doctor Loux's face as he stood by the bed and repeated several of the lines he had used in the dialogue earlier. These silent takes would be worked into the final print of the film to place emphasis on parts of the dialogue and add variety to the film.

A few minutes later, the close-ups completed, everyone in the room began to move about, removing and packing equipment that they had spent several hours setting up, in the room that had been especially chosen because, on this gray but fairly bright day, the windows on two adjoining sides of the room provided the basic light for the scene. Lighting equipment was added to "model and separate" the actors from the background.

During their "extended stay" in Sellersville, Irving Jacoby's film crew also shot scenes across the street in Penn Foundation's reception area, in the day care rooms, and in the library/board room. According to an article published in the *News Herald*, "besides the [Hospital and the] Day Care Center of the Foundation, the home of Tom Hixson and George Spotts, well known growers and florists, on Route 309 south of Sellersville, was selected as the locale for the 'patient's' domicile. The new plant of V&M

Tool Company on 5th St. Perkasie, provided the scene of [another character's] employment, as did the interior of the Electro Mechanical Instruments Company at 8th and Chestnut Sts. Local people lending an assist as actors included Mrs. Ernest K. Landis of Souderton [Kathryn Landis, Director of Volunteer Services for Penn Foundation] and Earl Ludwig, III of Telford. If in the days ahead, the field of mental health gets a boost as a result of this film (which is the reason for its production)—'our communities and our people will have done their part,' a foundation spokesman said."

"Penn Foundation for Mental Health: Ten Years Later"

After several exciting and slightly surreal weeks, the film-makers moved on to shoot in locations as far away as California. There would be little to show for all the hubbub they had created around Sellersville until *Bold New Approach* had its premiere sometime the following year. As the excitement of movie making and anniversary celebrating subsided, Dr. Loux completed a "descriptive paper" he had been working on for months. Entitled "Penn Foundation for Mental Health: Ten Years Later," the report was prepared for presentation at an upcoming NIMH-sponsored Research Seminar on the Evaluation of Community Mental Health Programs, but it wound up also being featured in a collection of Seminar papers published in 1968 under the title *Community Mental Health: An International Perspective* (Richard Hays Williams and Lucy D. Ozarin, editors). The opening paragraphs of Dr. Loux's paper contained the following statistical snapshot of the organization at the close of 1965:

> Penn Foundation for Mental Health, Inc. is a voluntary organization started in 1955 in a semi-rural community in Eastern Pennsylvania, with a primary service area of 75,000 [persons] and a secondary service area of an additional 50,000 people. This population is contained in an area within a 10½ mile radius and is also the area served by Grand View Hospital, the community general hospital. . . . The [Foundation's] staff presently consists of three full-time adult psychiatrists, one part-time child psychiatrist, one psychiatric social worker, a part-time clinical psychologist, a Coordinator of Day Care Activities, a Director of Occupational and Recreational Activities, and a Director of Volunteer Services. . . . Since its beginning through February 21, 1966, there have been nearly

4,000 different patients cared for. In the calendar year 1965 there were a total of 408 new patients seen as outpatients, the majority having been referred by physicians on the staff of Grand View Hospital with which Penn Foundation for Mental Health is intimately identified. There were 50 different patients cared for in the Day Care Program for a total of 1,579 days, with an average patient stay in the Day Care Program of 35 days. There were a total of 193 patients admitted as inpatients to Grand View Hospital for a total of 2,733 days. The average length of hospital inpatient stay was less than 15 days. In addition to the patients admitted to the Inpatient Psychiatric Service, there were 84 formal psychiatric consultations and many informal consultations with physicians concerning psychiatric problems that arose with patients on other services. In addition to the direct clinical services there were many other activities relating to education, project demonstration, and similar activities. . . . As accurately as can be tallied there were approximately 1,500 hours spent by various staff members in activities other than clinical services throughout the year.

In reviewing the achievements of Penn Foundation during its first decade, Dr. Loux identified eleven overlapping "primary factors" in the organization's success:

1. The need for psychiatric services as part of the general medicine of the community was keenly and intelligently appreciated by the physicians of the community. It was they who interested a responsible, creative, and dedicated group of lay people to provide the framework through which such service could be provided.

2. The key lay people who became the Board of Directors of the Foundation were influential and capable leaders, remarkably devoid of self-serving interests in the development of a mental health program. Their primary qualification was a neighborly concern for meeting a relatively unmet need within the community. Their social and economic standing, important though it has been, was secondary to their primary qualification. After careful evaluation, all of these men

literally placed their reputation on the line and gave themselves to developing what they had come to believe was an important need.

3. There was a consistent commitment to the philosophy that psychiatric needs should be discerned, a program to meet the needs developed, and a staff acquired to develop the program. This in contradistinction to introducing a preconceived program from the outside and fitting the community needs into it.

4. The principle of autonomous administrative control did not interfere with the meaningful integration of psychiatric service with the rest of medical services already available This was accomplished largely through constant meaningful communication between interested parties.

5. There was little problem in undoing patterns of caring for emotionally ill people because no previous organized program existed within the community. This enabled us to concentrate on meeting needs without spending great energies in proving that what we were trying to do was better than something already being done.

6. There was and is dedication to the principle of not separating "full pay" patients from "free or low pay" patients. All were treated by the same staff and in the same manner.

7. The principle of full-time professional staff was adhered to from the very beginning. With few exceptions, staff members were required to give full time [to the Foundation,] without holding other positions. We were dedicated from the beginning to the principle that the psychiatric and other professional staff should become a part of the community rather than be thought of as "outsiders" coming in to render a service.

8. It was assumed from the very beginning that members of the community should be wholesomely involved in the activities of the Foundation. It was assumed that the more that was done with helpful community participation, the less stigma would be attached to those receiving treatment.

9. The principle of local responsibility for financial and administrative control was the core of the development of the Foundation.

10. The dedication of the members of the Board, as well as the professional staff, to keep themselves in tune with developing trends in the field of mental health has existed from the beginning. Each staff member is sponsored by the Foundation to annual post-graduate training or experience.

11. It was assumed that community education would need to take place on all levels.

In short, Dr. Loux affirmed that "the present structure of the Foundation is certainly in tune with what was envisioned at the outset in all major areas." This was not to say there was no need for advancement. "We have not [yet] found a way of bringing help to a maximum degree to those people who do not have a solid, stable family or community of friends who will support them in an illness," Dr. Loux confessed. The Foundation also needed to more effectively address "the problems of the alcoholic," the "increasing number of senior citizens with emotional problems," and children who would benefit from a comprehensive diagnostic and evaluative service. More generally, the "belief that with our present facilities we could care for, if need be, all psychiatric problems arising in the community" had been opened to question. Certain manifestations of psychiatric illness had Dr. Loux and his colleagues wondering if "it may be constructive for some patients to be away from their family and the community for given periods of time during some phase of an illness" (which would require the construction of residential accommodations alongside the day care facilities). The coming years would prove that in identifying these avenues of exploration and improvement in the winter of 1965–66, Dr. Loux set out the organization's agenda for program expansion for the next quarter-century.

Penn Foundation's medical director noted in his recap of 1965 that "there were 14 formal on-site visits from groups interested in developing comprehensive community mental health centers in their own communities," and "there were numerous visits from other individuals interested in some phase of the work of the Foundation." None of the time spent by Foundation staff in hosting visitors was remunerated. Employees added these duties to their already-demanding schedules, with no specific increase in salary. Board members frequently paid for visitor entertainment expenses out of their own pockets. This situation could not continue indefinitely, and an important step in providing relief was taken in January 1966 when former executive assistant Ruby Horwood was coaxed back into the picture. Dr. Loux and the Directors invited her back to coordinate and conduct tours of Penn Foundation on a part-time basis. Ruby would keep her job at the Eastern Pennsylvania Psychiatric Institute in Philadelphia while serving as "Demonstration Project Officer" as needed in Sellersville. The position would eventually be funded—it was hoped—by a grant from the NIMH.

Ruby's ability to serve as a spokesperson for Penn Foundation was enhanced by her appointment to a reconfigured Board on January 18, 1966. At the first meeting of the Directors in the new year, Harold Mininger stepped down from the presidency after five years, making way for new President Charles Hoeflich. Ruby took over Charles' former duties as Secretary, and the remaining slate of officers (making up the new Executive Committee with Dr. Loux) comprised Vice President Raymond Rosenberger and Treasurer Russell Moyer. One of the first actions of the new Board was to apply to the NIMH "for a grant to help the Foundation meet with mental health leaders to study and investigate our program and look upon it as a model demonstration project." The grant would come, but only after a long year's wait.

The flow of visitors did not abate while the application for NIMH funding was being processed. Sellersville remained a popular destination for curious psychiatrists, psychologists, and social workers from around the country and the world. Penn Foundation's reputation was further burnished when Bold New Approach was completed in June 1966. It premiered at the national convention of the American Psychiatric Association in Atlantic City, and "was highly praised by those who saw it there," Dr. Loux reported. Three months would pass before a copy of the film finally arrived in Sellersville. Foundation personnel and other local folks who had participated in the filming enjoyed a "private preview" of the movie in the day care center on October 18. Dr. Loux described the film to a local reporter as "stark at times, but always realistic. One thing is certain," he added, "one cannot view it without a warm feeling of appreciation that ours is truly a community effort, successful because of the involvement of so many people." The general public got a chance to experience this for themselves when Bold New Approach premiered locally in the Christopher Dock Mennonite School auditorium on October 20. In its local angle, "moody" atmospherics, and educational orientation, it contrasted sharply with the competing cinematic offerings of the day, including recently released Alfie and Georgy Girl.

"'Snake pits' give way to the new clinics"

Three weeks later, another laurel landed on Penn Foundation's doorstep. This one arrived in the form of a three-page feature article published in the November 5, 1966 issue of *Business Week*. Entitled "'Snake pits' give way to the new clinics," and subheaded "At the Penn Foundation, the old style of mental institution has been pushed aside completely," the unattributed profile was illustrated with eight whimsical ink sketches of day care and out-patient activities at the Foundation, drawn during a recent visit to Sellersville by freelance artist and illustrator Joseph W. Papin of New York City. Like many other feature articles designed to introduce Penn Foundation to a wider audience, the *Business Week* profile began with a recap of the organization's community-based birth and growth, followed by a recitation of statistics relating to patient services and budget. Then, pushing beyond the numbers, the author attempted to put a human face on the life-changing work of the Foundation:

> Penn Foundation concentrates on day-time care of patients who have the usual variety of mental disturbances. Among them, there are:
> ● Alice, a compulsive talker. When she can't dominate the conversation, she withdraws into a psychotic state.
> ● A successful businessman and his younger, attractive wife. They have a marriage that won't work.
> ● A teenager, with an IQ of 140, who is the product of a broken home. He has adjustment problems.
> ● An older teenager, an unmarried girl who is pregnant. Her minister brought her to the Penn Foundation for help.
> The foundation recorded over 8,000 visits by patients last year. Their problems are handled in an atmosphere vastly different from that prevailing in older mental institutions. They are met with warmth and friendliness, not isolation. Since they come from their own homes by day, they wear their own clothes, not drab hospital gowns. They are encouraged to maintain their independence and individuality, not to adapt to the abnormal atmosphere of a state mental asylum. . . .
> "Historically," [Dr.] Loux told a session of the American Medical Assn., "when psychiatric treatment was thought of, it was not automatic to associate it with the existing medical

services in the community, especially in rural areas. It was much more natural to think of a locked ward hospital, state or private, outside the community with very little meaningful communication between the hospital and the community. In a hospital, all responsibilities for living are given up," he continues, "and this encourages regression. We emphasize the forces within a person that cultivate wellness. We let the post-partum mother care for her baby a little, or the businessman go to his office for half-an-hour or half a day. Even the big industries are adapting themselves to this."

Loux believes that "the inter-personal relationships of an individual play a significant part not [only] in the development of a mental illness, but also in the recovery process. In a sense," he says, "we are saying that the communities which have helped produce mental illnesses in the first place are areas of key importance in treatment, as well as in prevention

---

Ink sketches by freelance artist Joseph W. Papin of New York City served as illustrations for a feature article on Penn Foundation published under the heading "'Snake pits' give way to the new clinics" in the November 5, 1966 issue of *BusinessWeek*. Papin captioned the images as follows:

"In Penn Foundation's relaxed surroundings, Dr. Richards (left) counsels husband and wife whose marriage is coming apart."

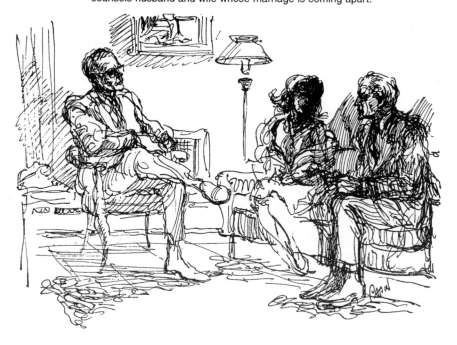

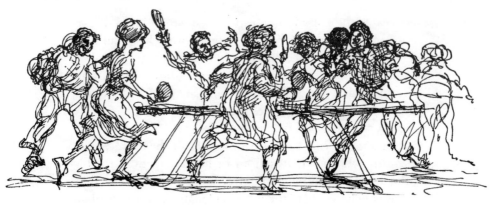

"Group therapy plays a big role—here in the form of run-around Ping Pong."

of mental illness. The patient must live with responsibilities," he adds, "rather than remove them. He must live with as much as he can safely take. At Sellersville, community psychiatry carries no stigma. Mental health is accepted as a medical problem that can be brought under control. Emotional problems are being treated in the community—where they begin."

Like every other writer charged with telling Penn Foundation's story (and explaining why "Federal officials call Penn Foundation one of the models of a community approach to psychiatry that is needed across the U.S."), the *BusinessWeek* reporter faced the challenge of understanding and conveying to readers the significance of intensely private communications between mental health workers and their clients. A standard tool for measuring the success of service providers—customer satisfaction—was hardly in

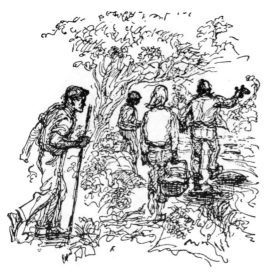

"Off to the hills for birdwatching and a picnic is part of the recreational therapy for Penn Foundation patients"

play when it came to evaluating a community mental health center. Most of Penn Foundation's services were provided behind closed doors, in utter confidentiality, and their healing effects were generally not broadcast beyond a patient's inner circle. It was thus as surprising as it was heartwarming when Directors learned from clients or their relatives how Penn Foundation was helping individuals deal with troubling facets of

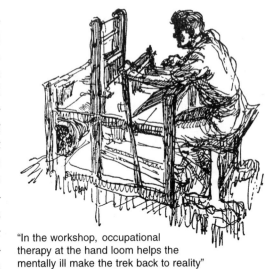

"In the workshop, occupational therapy at the hand loom helps the mentally ill make the trek back to reality"

their lives. Board President Charles Hoeflich would often tell the story of how "a lady came into the bank one day, and she said, 'Oh, Charles, I can't thank you enough!' I said, 'What for?' 'Oh, for what you did for my husband!' I said, 'I didn't do *anything* for Sam.' I tried to think of a loan I'd made to her husband, but I couldn't recall any. She said, 'No, what you did for Sam *at the Foundation*.' I said, 'Oh, has he been a patient at the Foundation?' 'Didn't you know that?' she asked. I said, 'No. We don't have access to patient files. They're confidential." And she replied, 'Well, that's just wonderful! Keep up the good work!' The element of confidentiality was uppermost in everything we did. I think that really encouraged people to participate."

Fellow trustee Harold Mininger remembers similar exchanges. "I'd meet relatives of patients, and they would say 'It's been wonderful, the last six months, how so-and-so has improved!'" he recalled recently. "They would just be elated that Penn Foundation was doing such a good job." Harold cites this kind of feedback as one reason he and his colleagues did not always insist on a "pay-as-you-go" business approach. "We would hear all this gratitude and think, 'What's happening here really seems to be hitting the mark. I'm not going to be that tough as a board member and watch every penny or tell the staff they can't start up a new kind of program if it's really going to help people. We'll just have to do something to make it work financially. You might have an auditor or accountant who says, 'Two and two is four, and that's it!' But you can't let it stop there.

You have to find a way to make two and two add up to five, and then have a little bit left over."

In this spirit, the Directors gave the green light early in 1967 to "Dr. Dunn and other staff members [to] work out plans for an expansion of services to children." They also authorized the Building Committee to set up "a meeting with [architect George] Hay to discuss plans for an additional building," a section of which would be devoted to providing children's services (according to Board meeting minutes). A few weeks later came word that the NIMH had finally awarded Penn Foundation a grant of $10,762 to cover the part-time salary of a Demonstration Project Officer for one year. This wouldn't change anything for Ruby Horwood, who had already been busily serving in that capacity for fifteen months, but it meant that money used to pay her could now be directed toward addressing what Dr. Loux described in March 1967 as "an urgent need for an additional social worker and a psychologist." One-half of this need was met in August with the hiring of psychiatric social worker William Swartzendruber. His primary responsibility would be working with parents of children being seen by Dr. Dunn, and his engagement meant Chief Psychiatric Social Worker Larry Landes could take a partial leave of absence to receive training and certification in marriage counseling. The hiring of William Swartzendruber represented only the second substantial increase in the Foundation's payroll in three years, the first being the engagement of secretary-receptionist Margaret ("Peggy") Emerick in March 1966.

The growing Penn Foundation family suffered its first major loss in the fall of 1967. While traveling to watch his son play football at the Franklin and Marshall College stadium in Lancaster on Saturday, November 11, charter trustee Lloyd ("Poppy") Yoder suffered a fatal heart attack. The sudden passing of this vigorous, beloved, and inspiring figure at the relatively young age of sixty-two stunned a wide circle of friends and colleagues. The outpouring of grief that followed was a testament to Poppy's influence across the Bux-Mont region. Local sportswriters and columnists paid their final respects in glowing testimonials, such as the following, offered by Buzz Cressman of Perkasie's *Central News-Herald*:

> Here was a man of general simplicity, of uncomplicated thinking. He established his life around spiritual convictions, developed and practiced in the Mennonite Church, around his family and around sports. He approached and spoke on all these subjects in such simple natural terms, it seemed

almost unreal in today's complex society. But the points he always made—on clean living, courage and conviction, rubbed off on everyone he knew. His mark of greatness was not the standings of his team, but in the character of the men he coached. And in those he educated in the classroom. The fact he started with limited capacity in almost everything, and eventually touched upon so many was a sign of human greatness in itself.

He was actually a self-taught athlete and coach. He was a teacher who educated high school students although in the start he began his teaching career with but one semester of post high school education at Millersville. He became a Christian layman of tremendous intelligence with no formal education on the subject.

Yoder molded all of these things into a philosophy that made men of boys. The fact that Pearl Buck chose Poppy to guide and train her Asian-American children in his home was perhaps the supreme compliment to the great traits of this man. Miss Buck, an extremely wealthy woman, could have sought specialists, foster homes anywhere in our great land for her needs. She chose Poppy Yoder. For here was warmth, friendship, a Christian home atmosphere, things only character, not money can develop among others.

It was not by accident that Yoder developed men, rather than great teams. He said the score would soon be forgotten. But the character of his men would never disappear

Poppy Yoder was renowned more for his contributions as a coach, teacher, and father than for his thirteen years of quiet service as a Penn Foundation Director. But those who worked with him in launching one of the nation's first community mental health centers knew that his sincerity, his enthusiasm, and his belief in human dignity and decency had served to propel as well as ballast the Board on its voyage. He would be dearly missed.

"Fresh blood"

It was ironic, if not prescient, that during what turned out to be Poppy Yoder's last Board meeting, he and his colleagues had "discussed the desirability of adding one or two members to the board," the consensus being "that the addition of 'new blood' would have great advantages." Now Poppy's vacated chair would have to be filled, and an expansion of the Board would require at least a second new trustee. Two likely candidates were quickly identified, both of them local Mennonite businessmen with demonstrated interests in community mental health care. One was Hatfield Township resident Vernon L. Derstine, a vice president and co-owner of the V.&J., Inc. trucking company. Vernon was already serving as a Director of Brook Lane Psychiatric Center in Maryland (known upon its establishment by the Mennonite Central Committee in 1949 as "Brook Lane Farm," this first-ever "rest home for Mennonites needing mental care" had recently been steered by new leadership away from the "community mental health center" model toward a general hospital model, with its formerly-salaried psychiatrists now permitted to work on a private or fee-for-service basis after two years of employment—a practice Dr. Loux and his colleagues at Penn Foundation vigorously eschewed). Vernon Derstine was also a colleague of Directors Charles Hoeflich and Russell Moyer through his service on the Souderton Regional Board of the Union National Bank and Trust Company.

The other candidate for the Foundation's Board in the winter of 1967–68 was Curtis Moyer, younger brother of seed-money provider Nels Moyer. Curt was busy expanding his family's beef packing and rendering businesses in Franconia Township, but his sensitivity to mental health issues—heightened through his relationship with Nels (who had died a decade earlier in only his fifty-third year), as well as his experience managing a growing family of employees—led him to accept the Foundation's invitation to leadership. Both he and Vernon Derstine began injecting their "fresh blood" into the Board mid-way through 1968. They quickly learned why this body had been repeatedly cited for its "unusually active involvement" in Foundation affairs. A local newspaper reporter treating this very topic in a November 1968 article titled "Penn Mental Health Foundation Directors Actively Involved" included a telling anecdote with his commentary:

> Boards of directors often give the impression they are aloof from all but the general aspects of the operation they direct. Such is not the case with the board of directors of the Penn Foundation for Mental Health in Sellersville. The foundation is in the process of expanding its physical plant and the

directors are deeply committed to seeing all the details are just right.

Staff psychiatrist Dr. John C. Richards believes, as do other staff members, that the involvement of the directors is among the reasons for the foundation's success. . . . [He] said he recently visited an area business to inspect a new type of radiant heating system the building committee was contemplating using in the foundation's new wing. When he arrived, he discovered the three board members who were on the committee with him were already there, having taken time off from the operation of their businesses.

Along with their willingness to pitch in wherever needed, Foundation Directors were unusual in their commitment to a decision-making process inspired by Mennonite Church practice. As Charles Hoeflich explained recently, "the Board always acted by consensus. That was our policy. If there was a question, it was discussed back and forth, back and forth, until everybody agreed. There was never a case of needing a two-thirds vote or a majority vote to make something happen. It was always 'decision by consensus,' whether we were deciding to hire someone or begin a building project."

Expansion Phase 2

The building project demanding attention in 1968 had been kick-started early that year when the Grundy Foundation poured a $50,000 gift into the Penn Foundation building fund. Dr. Loux and his fellow staffers already had a clear sense of what they wanted in the next phase of expansion. Topping their wish list was a "Child Development Center" where a "Comprehensive Diagnostic and Evaluative Service" could be offered to children through the age of eight. As proposed by Dr. Dunn, this service would "combine the skills of a pediatrician and clinical psychologist with those of specialists in hearing and vision, or in identifying reading difficulties. [Children enrolled in the Penn Foundation program] would present a wide range of problems, primarily in the psycho-social area of development. Some of the children will have underlying physical defects; i.e. in the central nervous system, but this will not be a program for the primarily physically handicapped. The emphasis will be on a total evaluation, using a multiple discipline approach."

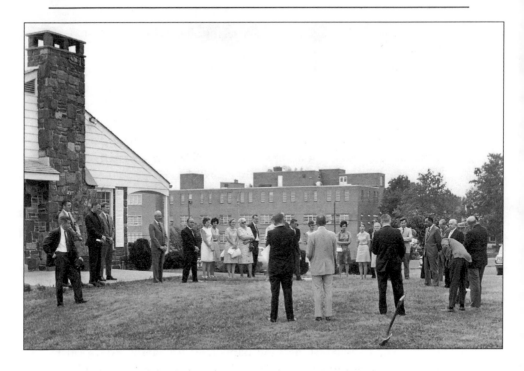

In addition to a "child psychiatric wing," the building project initiated in February 1968 was expected to equip the Foundation with an auditorium-gymnasium—the long-awaited "meeting place where public meetings in the general interest of Mental Health can be held." The Grundy grant would be applied to the construction of this particular facility. In the six months between the conception of the building project and its formal announcement, the Foundation's staff and trustees developed plans with architect George Hay that would more than double the organization's 7,194 square feet under roof along Lawn Avenue. An estimated $350,000 would be needed to cover the cost of building and equipping the children's wing, group therapy rooms, more consultation offices, occupational therapy workshop areas, and a greenhouse. In announcing that Andrichyn & Schnabel, Inc. had been awarded the $204,000 construction contract in July 1968, the Directors also noted that a local corporation—Sylvan Pools, Inc.—had offered to install a swimming pool valued at $8,700 as its special contribution to the new recreational area.

The second groundbreaking ceremony in Penn Foundation's history was conducted with the participation of "community leaders and those prominent in the field of medicine" on Thursday, August 8, 1968 (a few hours before Richard Nixon accepted the Republican Party's nomination for President of the United States in Miami Beach). Like the Foundation's first building project, the next phase of expansion would be undertaken without any federal subsidies. "All funds will be raised from private sources," Charles Hoeflich declared in both the "local" and "national" versions of his latest news release. "We believe those who have a dedicated interest in the field of mental health, particularly in the work which we have been doing, will support us again as they have in the past. Our constituency has been wonderfully loyal and the splendid staff of the Penn Foundation has repaid them with solid results."

The second groundbreaking exercise in Penn Foundation's history was conducted on the north side of the 1962 building on August 8, 1968. The building project would double the Foundation's square footage through the addition of clinical offices, a Children's Unit, occupational therapy space, and a gymnasium-auditorium. One of several groups photographed wielding a ceremonial shovel at the groundbreaking ceremony was this collection of "Foundation officers": (from left) Board President Charles Hoeflich; Board and Building Committee members Roland Detweiler, Raymond Rosenberger, and Harold Mininger; and Medical Director Norman Loux.

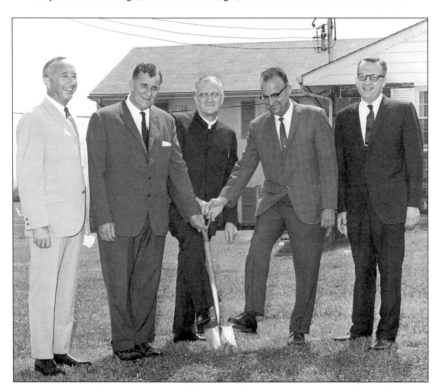

Anticipating a significantly expanded program, Penn Foundation's enlarged Board retained the accounting firm of Detweiler and Landis in August 1968 "to take care of Foundation accounts under the general supervision of the treasurer." At the same time the Directors approved the promotion of part-time clinical psychologist Dr. Barbash—in his eighth year with the Foundation—to a full-time position. He quickly "became more involved in psychotherapy than in testing" (according to a corporate report), "and divided his time between patients, serving as a consultant to social agencies and schools, and planning the new children's services, of which he is to be the Administrator. A young psychologist [David Clayton of Worcester, Montgomery County] was engaged on a part-time basis to do most of the testing" (Dr. Clayton would be serving as a psychologist in the Foundation's Outpatient Program thirty-six years later).

These staffing changes were documented in a 130-page "comprehensive study" of Penn Foundation completed early in 1969 through a contract with the Commonwealth of Pennsylvania's Office of Mental Health. The purpose of the study—organized and overseen by psychiatrist Catherine M. Fales—was to furnish State officials with data they could use in establishing county-based programs for the provision of mental health and mental retardation services, as mandated in Pennsylvania's "Mental Health and Mental Retardation Act of 1966." Penn Foundation was among the few community mental health centers in the East deemed worthy of a $25,000 "research study" and possible emulation by the Office of Mental Health. The product of the year-long examination, entitled *A Comprehensive Study of the Services Provided by the Penn Foundation for Mental Health, Inc: 1955–1968*, presented a highly-detailed picture of the Foundation on the cusp of a major expansion. Most of the information was statistical in nature, geared toward helping authorities project staffing, facilities, and financial needs for the new generation of community mental health centers. But some sections of the report were more descriptive than statistical, and in those passages the reader was offered a window into the setting and day-to-day activities of the Foundation circa 1968. Among the descriptive passages was the following "tour" of "the buildings and grounds":

> The Penn Foundation occupies an attractive, split-level, wood and stone building (with a floor space of approximately 7, 194 square feet) which is located on the side of a hill directly across the road from Grand View Hospital.

Windows facing south look out over the valley below in which lies the Borough of Sellersville, its homes, churches and industries, and the surrounding rolling countryside on either side of the East Branch of Perkiomen Creek. The Foundation grounds, approximately fifteen acres, which stretch to the east and south of the buildings are nicely landscaped, and building and grounds create for the newcomer, as well as for those who know it well, the impression that the Foundation is informal and welcoming.

Once inside the front door this impression grows. The large waiting room is light and cheerful, flowered cretonne curtains frame the windows, three fine landscape paintings by a local artist hang on the walls, and, in winter, a wood fire burns all day in the large stone fireplace. A rocking chair and children's corner with inviting toys make the young feel welcome, while comfortable chairs and couches are thoughtfully arranged so that persons waiting may choose whether to talk with others or read quietly alone, almost unnoticed. In an alcove at one side of the waiting room and facing the front door is the receptionist's desk, and behind this a secretarial office. On the other side of the desk the office of the Executive Secretary opens into the waiting room.

At the end of the waiting room, opposite the fireplace, three steps lead up to the offices of the Clinical Staff. These are seven in number and include a playroom for play-therapy with children. On this floor there are also a library-conference room with a kitchenette concealed behind folding doors at one end, a small record and mail room and wash-rooms for men and women.

The space beneath these offices is the location of the Day Care Program. Two medium-sized rooms, furnished as living rooms, are used by patients to rest and read and for the daily group therapy sessions. Next to these is the nurse's office, a drug room, and a large recreation room with an adjoining fully equipped kitchen. In the recreation room is a grand piano, ping-pong table, two large tables that can be used for crafts or eating luncheons, a loom for weaving, a sewing machine, an aquarium, and whatever equipment is necessary for the current project. Behind the kitchen there are locker

rooms for men and women and a storage room. In the furnace
room beyond is a small kiln for ceramics.

The recreation room opens out-of-doors onto a ball court
where either volleyball or basketball can be played. Further
to the east, a large garden is planted and tended each summer.

A description of the Day Care Program included in the *Comprehensive Study* accounted for the sharp increase in activity in and around the
Foundation on certain days of the week:

> The Day Care Program is in session . . . Monday,
> Wednesday and Friday from 9:00 a.m. to 3:30 p.m. on the
> ground floor of the Penn Foundation. Although the present
> facilities are in many ways too small for the size of the group,
> the atmosphere is warm and friendly.
>
> The program for each day is flexible and to some extent
> is chosen by the participating patients. The day is divided
> informally between a variety of activities, (1) social or total
> milieu therapy, (2) recreational therapy, (3) occupational ther-
> apy, (4) field trips or excursions, (5) individual psychother-
> apy, (6) group psychotherapy. The social activities or therapy
> include such occupations as group singing, piano playing,
> informal discussions over a cup of coffee, planning the week's
> menu and preparing and serving luncheon to the group.
>
> As for occupational therapy, equipment for woodworking,
> ceramics, weaving, sewing, leather work, basketry and other
> handicrafts is available and the staff is always on the lookout
> for a new idea. Recreational therapy includes indoor-outdoor
> activities, volleyball, croquet, bowling, etc. Gardening should
> be included under one or perhaps all of the above mentioned
> types of therapy, for the Day Care Staff and patients plant and
> tend two large gardens.
>
> Almost every week, the group leaves the Foundation for a
> field trip or excursion, a picnic by the river, a visit to Philadel-
> phia to the Aquarama or Independence Mall or an afternoon
> of bowling. Many times these excursions have been requested
> by the patients, and the staff makes the necessary arrange-
> ments. If the group is large, volunteers are found to supply
> and drive cars.

A great deal of credit goes to the two full-time staff members, the Nurse [Ruth Lefever] and Occupational Therapist [Art Isaak], for maintaining an interesting and varied program. Their success in this endeavor is due in part to the fact that they are sensitive to and aware of the needs of both individual patients and the group as a whole, and they vary the program to keep step with needs. Another reason that the program remains alive and interesting is that both staff members participate enthusiastically in all activities. No one stands aloof in a supervisory capacity. This participation by staff members in daily activities helps to prevent the program from becoming an artificial experience. In fact, the continual encouragement to remain involved with the community, and the positive response of the community to this involvement, is a manifestation of the beliefs and convictions which were largely responsible for developing the Foundation.

Because of the emphasis on communication and group participation, one to one-and-a-half hours of group therapy are planned for each day; the sessions are held at 11:00 a. m. so that discussions can continue into luncheon if need be. Three different therapists are involved, and each directs the group for one of the three days each week. The Friday Group is continuously supervised by the Psychiatrist in charge of the Day Care Program [Dr. Lyons]. Leadership of the Monday session is divided among staff members. The Wednesday group is directed by the Psychiatric Social Worker [William Swartzendruber] who is acquainted with families of the patients. Since the group on Wednesday includes patients who are planning to leave the program in the near future, the leadership of the Social Worker who has been acquainted with the family situation throughout the patient's illness is particularly helpful, as he tends to direct attention toward consideration of community resources. Continuity from session to session is provided by the presence of the Nurse who is co-therapist with each leader. She is also responsible for keeping a record of each session.

A determined effort is made to involve relatives in the care of each Day Care participant. One member of a family, usually parent or spouse, is asked to come in and talk with the Psychiatric Social Worker associated with the program and is encouraged to return on a regular weekly basis. In cases where families have become successfully involved, a patient can be carried through a severe illness while living at home and attending the Day Care Program, for the family can be given some knowledge of the medication to be taken and the types of behavior that might be expected from the patient, as well as assurance that a member of the Foundation staff will be available if help is needed.

Another method of involving families with the Foundation is through the "evening social" that takes place about every two months. These are planned and organized by the Day Care Staff for the patients and their families and may consist of a square dance, a Halloween party, a covered dish supper, a card party or possibly a lecture with slides that describe a trip someone in the community has recently taken. A quantity of good food and a well-planned but informal program is the formula for parties that are greatly enjoyed. In addition, the Nurse, Occupational Therapist, Director of the Volunteer Services, the Psychiatrist-Director of the program and Social Worker regularly attend, and other members of the staff frequently come for a short time.

Patients stay in Day Care long enough to become thoroughly familiar with the Foundation and the Staff. However, prolonged dependence on the program to fulfill one's needs is discouraged and discharge to home and normal activities is always the goal. A procedure for encouraging progress and recognizing its occurrence is the informal division of the group into three sub-groups based on improvement. A patient on admission attends all three sessions— Monday, Wednesday, and Friday. With improvement, he omits the Wednesday group and comes only on Monday and Friday; when discharge is planned, he attends only on Wednesday, and, as mentioned earlier, the group session on Wednesday, supervised by the Social Worker, is geared to the needs and problems of a person contemplating return to full activity in the community.

The Day Care Program originally [in the fall of 1962] appeared more suitable for women than for men, and for the first eighteen months, only women were admitted. After a good deal of discussion, men were included, and everyone soon agreed that the mixed group was a great improvement since it provided patients with a less artificial environment in which to work out their problems. Since then, men and women from 15 years of age up have been admitted, if, in the opinion of the staff, the program would help them to recover. There have always been more women than men, but that is because a greater number of women with illnesses that would benefit from this type of treatment come to the Foundation.

The program started with four persons. During the 5½ years of operation, there have been as many as 23 persons in attendance on one day. As presently staffed and housed, the optimum number for the program is 12 to 14 persons. If there are more persons than this, it is difficult to have effective group therapy, and activities lose the combination of informal organization and participatory supervision that is characteristic of the program at present. With the additional space that the new building [will provide], at least twice that number can be treated.

The *Comprehensive Study* was completed as Penn Foundation's "new building" was in its final phase of construction. The *Study* authors were therefore able to include a description of the various spaces soon to be occupied:

> The new addition, which will have a floor space of approximately 10,086 square feet, has three distinct sections. The front part of the building, which is reached from the waiting room, contains four clinical offices, a room for group therapy with a one-way viewing window and additional offices for Secretarial and Administrative Staff.
>
> As in the original building, the floor beneath the clinical offices is the location of the Day Care Program. A new doorway leads from the previously described recreation room onto a wide hallway and further into a spacious occupational therapy room and woodworking shop. A small greenhouse is located on the southern side of the occupational therapy room.

The most easterly part of the building is the children's unit. This can be entered by a door from the main building or by its own outside entrance which leads into a waiting and reception room. Upstairs, the unit includes a secretary's office, a doctor's examining room, two clinical offices, one of which has a connecting play room for play-therapy with a one-way viewing screen. On the ground floor are a classroom for a special education class, a play room, large kitchenette and small conference room. The play room opens by wide sliding glass doors onto the lawn recreation area.

Between the children's unit and the clinical offices, and opening into both of them, is a fine auditorium with an attractive stage at the far end. This room will be the center for a great deal of activity as it will function both as a gymnasium and recreation area and as an auditorium with a seating capacity of 200. As a recreation area it will he shared by the Day Care Program and the children's unit. It will also become a community center for lectures, meetings, seminars, and discussions concerning mental health.

The two-hundred-person seating capacity of the new auditorium was exceeded by fifty percent when Penn Foundation's new wing was finally dedicated on Sunday afternoon, September 7, 1969. A standing-room-only crowd spent most of the dedication service listening to the President of the American Psychiatric Association, Dr. Raymond J. Waggoner, deliver a sober keynote address on "the role mental health agencies must play in helping to solve the many social problems of our time—the campus disorders, draft dodging, and the generation gap in general" (shockwaves from Woodstock, the weekend-long anti-establishment binge attended by more than half-a-million Baby Boomers a couple of weeks earlier, were still rocking the nation). The challenge of living in such a "deeply troubled and profoundly unsettled time," Dr. Waggoner asserted, was developing "some special alchemy to ensure that the dialogue between the young and the old is not stopped precipitously, since it must be sustained if the common interest of facilitating an orderly transition to a better, more humane, more rational and improved society is to be realized without the violence that destroys the human values for which man has fought so long and so hard."

The good doctor fully expected community mental health centers to be part of that "special alchemy." His faith in Penn Foundation in particular was strengthened by "the remarkable support from this community, [which] indicates that there is public understanding that mental illness is not something of which to be ashamed, but which is to be dealt with by appropriate treatment as one would deal with other health problems." Like many visiting dignitaries before him, Dr. Waggoner concluded his address to Foundation staff and supporters with a memorable blessing:

> With the completion of this very functional, comfortable, and attractive addition, one must recognize that the soul of the unit, the very essence of it, is what goes on inside as a result of the efforts of those who work there. It is made up of people skilled, knowledgeable, and capable, dedicated to the task of making life more comfortable for those who are unfortunate enough to have an illness. . . . May I suggest that you here in Sellersville, and at the Penn Foundation for Mental Health, have made a most positive and aggressive approach toward the solution of many of these problems. By your coordination of effort, by your amazing community drive, by the devotion of the hard-working people in this community, by your initiative, creativeness, determination, and altruism in the commitment and motivation to help one another has come the ability to do this with the maintenance of man's dignity, for those who have unfortunately developed mental illness. May I also plead for your continuing support of this magnificent development, for only by continuing support can Dr. Loux and his associates provide the greatest degree of care for those in need.

7

CATCHMENT AREAS
091 AND 462

The dedication of a new wing in September 1969 marked the dawn of a new era at Penn Foundation. The 1970s would pose unique challenges to the pioneering community mental health center on Sellersville Heights, and Foundation officers and employees would rise to these challenges with a combination of conviction, time-tested techniques, newly-acquired expertise, and creativity. The sailing wasn't always smooth. Results were occasionally mixed, particularly when institutional well-being was measured in terms of fiscal fitness. Like a lot of organizations and individuals coming of age amid the aftershocks of the social, economic, and political earthquakes of the 1960s, Penn Foundation sometimes struggled to find its footing in a shifting world order.

Looming over the new order for psychiatric institutions in Pennsylvania was the Commonwealth's "Mental Health and Mental Retardation Act of 1966," which took effect in 1967 but needed a few years to begin producing widespread results. The legislation mandated that programs for the provision of mental health and mental retardation services be established in every county and first-class city of the Commonwealth, and that appropriations and regulatory oversight for these community programs be provided by the State Mental Health/Mental Retardation Department through county-based Departments with Administrators and Advisory Boards. The smaller and least populated counties could be served by a single "base service unit." Larger and/or more populous counties had to be divided into two or more "catchment areas," with one unit serving each area. Where catchment areas were not yet equipped with a State-approved provider, the County was obligated to get one up and running.

Dr. Loux and his colleagues learned in the spring of 1969 that—to no one's surprise—Penn Foundation had been approved as a base service unit under the Mental Health and Mental Retardation Act of 1966. Among other things, the new regulatory regime would reshape the catchment area Foundation officials had delineated more than a decade earlier, described as follows in the 1964 Joint Information Service profile:

> The express purpose of establishing the Foundation [in 1955] was to provide psychiatric service to essentially the same clients served by physicians on the staff of the Grand View Hospital. Because of the scarcity of psychiatric facilities in the vicinity, referrals were soon coming from outside the hospital's sphere of service, straining the resources of the Foundation. It was thus decided in 1958 that, except for unusual and compelling reasons, only patients living within 10½ miles of the Foundation would be accepted.

Because it was located near the border of two counties, and because it was already providing exemplary service to a population of approximately 120,000 Bux-Mont residents in 1969, Penn Foundation was authorized by the State to function as the base service unit for *two* catchment areas—one in either county. Catchment Area 091 was by far the larger of the two, comprising eighteen townships and boroughs in upper Bucks County. Montgomery County Catchment Area 462 consisted of four townships: Salford, Upper Salford, Lower Salford, and Franconia. The Foundation's State-sanctioned responsibility for serving the residents of these particular municipalities went into effect in July 1969. At a Board meeting held just prior to this administrative watershed, Dr. Loux explained that Penn Foundation would soon "be under the Mental Health and Retardation Act so far as appropriations from the state and county are concerned. Allocations of funds will be made to the county, although the funds will still come from the state in the proportion of approximately 90% from the state and 10% from the county. There will be certain administrative responsibilities for which Penn Foundation will be responsible and will be reimbursed in full, such as child evaluation services, which will be entirely underwritten by the county program. It has been made clear to [County officials] that we are ready, able, and willing to proceed with our end of the responsibility, and we intend to hold to our ideals and maintain control of the clinical program."

Early in July 1969 Dr. Loux, Board President Russell Moyer, and Executive Secretary Marge Alexander traveled to Harrisburg to meet with Pennsylvania's Commissioner of Mental Health and the Administrators of the Mental Health Departments of Bucks and Montgomery Counties. At this start-up meeting, the goals, terms, and division of responsibilities under the new contract were discussed and (it was hoped) clarified for all parties. The Penn Foundation contingent noted with particular interest that "all State funding will now be coming through the Mental Health/ Mental Retardation Program: 60% from Bucks County and 40% from Montgomery County. A percentage of the fee for patients who are not able to pay the full fee will be paid, and funds also will be available for maintenance, heat, light, interest on mortgage insurance, etc." The arrangement purported to be something of a trade-off for Penn Foundation—assurance of steadier income would be gained at the expense of stricter government regulation and oversight. It was assumed that the former would ultimately outweigh the latter, paving the way for a major expansion in the Foundation's offering of services. Only time would tell if that assumption was overly optimistic.

Infusion of staff

With a new government contract certain to increase clinical activity, and a spacious new wing open for business, Penn Foundation needed a

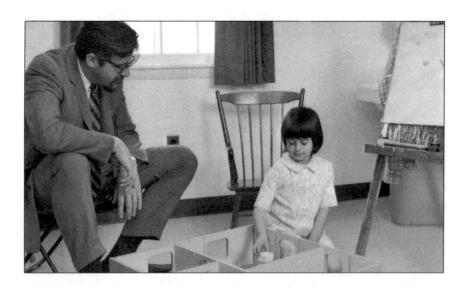

larger staff. The first hire after the September 7, 1969 Dedication was a registered nurse—Robin Morgan—engaged later that September to serve in the Day Treatment program. She was followed in July 1970 by no fewer than three appointees: pediatrician Perry Grossman, clinical psychologist Gerald Musselman, and psychiatric social worker Janet Medori. Mrs. Medori had been previously employed as a psychiatric social worker at Philadelphia General Hospital, while Dr. Musselman, a Montgomery County native, had most recently served as assistant professor of psychology at the University of North Carolina. The initial assignment of their colleague Dr. Grossman was to launch the "Comprehensive Diagnostic and Evaluative Service" envisioned as part of the "Child Development Center" in the new wing. Within weeks of his arrival, Penn Foundation was "providing a unique service—in particular consultation with parents of the mentally retarded and consultation with school personnel," Dr. Loux reported to the Board. Though mental retardation was Dr. Grossman's specialty, his Evaluative Service also addressed learning disorders, cerebral palsy, and language disorders.

As the "extremely busy" summer of 1970 drew to a close, Dr. Loux happily informed the Directors that the Foundation's recent hiring spree

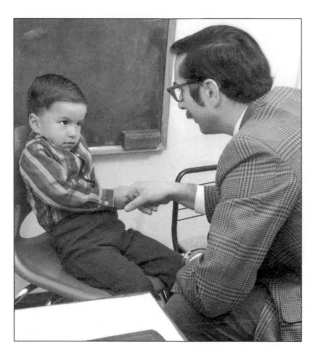

The two psychiatrists presiding over Penn Foundation's pediatric services in the early 1970s were Dr. John "Mike" Dunn (facing page), on staff since January 1960, and Dr. Perry Grossman (left), a relative newcomer following his July 1970 hiring. Dr. Dunn was instrumental in planning the "Comprehensive Diagnostic and Evaluative Service" offered in the new "Child Development Center" beginning in January 1970. Dr. Grossman was brought in to serve as the Center's Coordinator of Pediatric Services.

had "worked out unusually well. He commented on the splendid work being done by Janet Medori as a social worker in her contact with families. Jerry Musselman is also doing a good job, and Dr. Grossman has been exceptional in the field of pediatrics. In commenting on other members of the staff, Dr. Loux emphasized that the administration has been running exceptionally smoothly and that perhaps the only problem was that posed by an enlarged staff, namely, the inability to keep in close contact with each individual and their particular programs because of the constantly expanding program of the Foundation." Indeed, one of the challenges of the new era would be maintaining a sense of "family" among a larger, more diverse, and more changeable population of employees.

Another challenge would be responding to a sharp increase in drug abuse cases. Rarely encountered at Penn Foundation in the 1950s and 1960s, drug-related troubles washed into the clinic in an unexpected tide as the Woodstock Generation came of age in the Bux-Mont region. Of all the Foundation employees, Dr. Barbash felt the force of this influx most distinctly in its initial stages. His position as psychological consultant to schools and youth services placed him on the front lines of this emerging social crisis. The up-tick in his busyness was first noted by Dr. Loux in the spring of 1970, and the Foundation's Medical Director alerted his colleagues on the Board to this phenomenon. The gravity of the situation was further articulated when the Foundation hosted a workshop titled "Drugs and Adolescents: What's Going On?," led by two professors from the Temple University School of Medicine. For the time being, the escalation in drug-related cases at Penn Foundation could be absorbed by existing staff, but unless conditions took a turn for the better, it looked like it would be necessary to hire a Drug and Alcohol specialist in the not-too-distant future.

"A particularly fortunate financial situation"

As anticipated, the new State-regulated compacts with Bucks and Montgomery Counties gave Penn Foundation a fiscal shot in the arm. Both Counties came through with "substantial support" in 1970, their appropriations being the principal reason Board Treasurer Russell Moyer could report as of September that "the Foundation had been particularly fortunate in its financial situation during the current year and at the present time." The prospects for the immediate future looked good in that Bucks County's Mental Health/Mental Retardation Board had just approved an appropriation of $97,000 to Penn Foundation for the new fiscal year, which was in addition to $48,000 approved by County officials for the operation of the Foundation's Child Study Unit. Montgomery County agreed to contribute another $65,000 for services provided in Catchment Area 462. That was about six times what the County had appropriated for Penn Foundation before the State contract went into effect.

Financially invigorated, Penn Foundation continued its expansion of services and staff. In November 1970, the Board approved the establishment of a pre-school program devoted to early diagnosis, treatment, and preventive care for young children with severe developmental disorders linked to emotional or social problems. Dr. Grossman would direct the two-hour-per-day program, with newly-hired Ann Swayne serving as teacher and Winona Ondra as teacher's aide. Eager parents began enrolling their children in the program weeks before its January 1971 launch.

By that time the Penn Foundation family was one psychiatrist stronger. Dr. Carmela F. deRivas resigned as director of the 2,250-patient Norristown State Hospital in November 1970 to join the Foundation staff on a four-fifths-time basis. It was quite a coup for Dr. Loux to land someone of Dr. deRivas's stature. No less a personage than Pennsylvania Governor Raymond Shafer had recently lauded her "wise and compassionate leadership, her personal warmth, vitality and deep dedication and concern for others." According to one of Charles Hoeflich's press releases, Dr. deRivas was drawn to Penn Foundation because "its organization permits a maximum of patient contact," and because "new ideas for helping others are born here. 'Some of the plans being put together for the days ahead are so exciting, one wants to be a part of it all,' she says." In her new position, Dr. deRivas would spend one day per week at Norristown State Hospital, working with Penn Foundation patrons accommodated there.

A sustained growth spurt

The Foundation family continued its growth spurt in the summer of 1971. The hiring of psychiatric social worker Gary Beese in July and psychiatric caseworker Karen Kern in September generated less publicity than did Dr. deRivas's signing, but the long-term impact of these additions to the organization would be immeasurably greater. A 1968 graduate of Rutgers University, Gary found his way to the Foundation after stints at the Illinois Department of Public Aid, a half-way house, and the Eastern

State School and Hospital. He was something of a stand-out in this journey, ducking doorways and low ceilings because of his six-feet, four-inch height. Anticipating his arrival at Penn Foundation, a new colleague remarked that Gary "will almost literally see eye to eye" with Dr. Dunn, who had been the tallest employee to date. Karen Kern needed less of an introduction to the Foundation. She had grown up in Perkasie, best friends with Marge Alexander's daughter. After earning a Bachelor's degree in psychology at Southern Methodist University and working in Texas for a year, she was encouraged by Marge to apply for a job as case manager in the Foundation's emergent mental retardation program. There was nothing particularly auspicious about her appointment to this

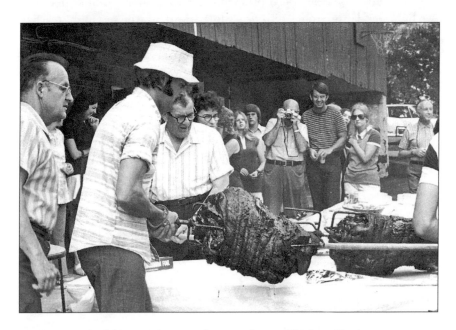

With upwards of thirty employees and an even larger collection of trustees, spouses, and children, the Penn Foundation family was so big by the early 1970s that new ways of fostering familiarity among its members were needed. In addition to launching a company newsletter—*IDKT!* (i.e. "I Didn't Know That!")—in August 1971, Foundation officers conducted the first Board-Staff Picnic at Norman and Esther Loux's farm on July 1, 1972. This event became an annual "Ox Roast" the following year, with Board member and MOPAC President Curt Moyer supplying the featured entrée. In this snapshot from a mid-1970s picnic, clinical psychologist Gerald Musselman wrestles some barbecued beef onto the carving table under the watchful gaze of Directors Harold Mininger (left), Roland Detweiler, Mahlon Souder (center), Charles Hoeflich (right), and a collection of hungry bystanders, including the Foundation's tallest employee, Acting Administrator Gary Beese.

position in September 1971, but it turned out to be the beginning of a remarkably long-lived and fruitful career at Penn Foundation.

Staff expansion was pressing on facilities less than two years after the Foundation had doubled its square footage. "Office space is at a premium," Directors acknowledged at their July 1971 meeting. For short-term relief, the Board directed "that the patio adjoining the business office be enclosed and used for an office for Mrs. Alexander." This would buy time while "realistic long-range plans for additional buildings" were developed in consultation with architect George Hay. Another effect of expansion—reduced familiarity among employees—was addressed in August 1971 through the publication of the first staff newsletter. This four-page, typewritten, and mimeographed "informational bulletin" was given the "temporary and admittedly hoaky name" of *IDKT!*, which (it was explained in an introductory note) stood for "I didn't know that!" In its pages employees could find updates on new and departing colleagues, accounts of staff participation in professional conferences, news of upcoming events, and humorous anecdotes involving members of the extended Foundation family. Published every other month for at least a year, *IDKT!*

Among the picnickers shooting the breeze in this post-meal snapshot were several trustees: Curt Moyer (on left), Elvin Souder, Roland Detweiler (second from right), and Harold Mininger (far right).

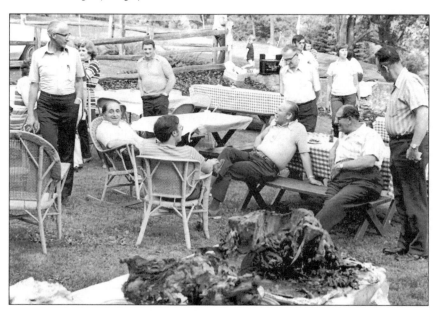

was soon lengthened to five pages, and then to six. Even so, its editors had to hold some items for inclusion in later issues.

The lead dispatch in the inaugural *IDKT!* reminded employees of a "planned 'happening' for the public, initiated by the Board and presented to the staff with infectious enthusiasm by Mr. Hoeflich" in early August 1971. Intended to "further community ties" and "inform [visitors] about the Foundation," this "happening" was tentatively scheduled for a Saturday in late September. Day Treatment staffers Art Isaak and Ruth Lefever were co-chairing the Organizing Committee, and they were fishing for volunteers among the pool of Directors, employees, and members of the Women's Auxiliary. Board minutes relate that Charles Hoeflich had run the idea of an autumn-welcoming "Lawn Party or Fiesta" past his fellow Directors at their July meeting, explaining that such an event would allow "our neighbors in the community to see the facilities available at Penn Foundation, hear about the various aspects of our program, and see displays of handicraft." The name "Fall Festival" was ultimately adopted for this affair, which went off on September 25. "It was a successful venture," the Directors agreed at their October 1971 meeting, "and should be repeated next year." Thus was born a tradition that would attract hundreds of Bux-Mont residents to the Penn Foundation campus one Saturday in September for many years to come.

With the Foundation's annual budget pushing half-a-million dollars, and upwards of thirty employees on the payroll, the Directors began discussing "the advisability of employing a Business Manager." They were ready by November 1971 to authorize the Executive and Personnel Committees to draw up a "job outline" and "work together in filling this position." Mid-way through December they retained the services of Sellersville native Albert Strehle Jr., formerly employed as program director for the Philadelphia-Montgomery County Tuberculosis and Health Association. Perhaps because the range of Strehle's new responsibilities had yet to be discerned (creating a management-level, non-medical position at Penn Foundation was, after all, a venture into unfamiliar territory), his employers stopped short of titling him "Business Manager." At least for the time being, he would serve as an "Administrative Consultant."

A "serious curtailment of funds"

Albert Strehle had barely organized his desk before Foundation officials received some distressing financial news. The eighty percent increase in state and county funding they had been told to expect for 1972 was not going to materialize. At best, appropriations would be only about nine percent higher than in 1971. There might well be no increase at all. This "serious curtailment of funds" (a grim Christmas present, indeed!) threw an elephantine wrench into the organization's projected budget, which Strehle and Marge Alexander were just then completing. Even a nine percent boost in appropriations—the "best case" scenario—would yield a $67,000 annual shortfall. The Foundation's fiscal team would now have to revisit every aspect of the budget, revising downward in light of the lowered expectations. Even if they managed to carve off a few hundred dollars here and there, there was still bound to be a deep deficit at year's end. The Directors quickly authorized an increase in "clinic fees" (several years had passed since the last adjustment), and began discussing more sweeping measures. Out of one of their discussions came a directive to the new Administrative Consultant "to work with the various charitable foundations, organizations, and other private sources of charitable contributions in an attempt to find new sources of financial support for the Foundation."

Three difficult months later, it was clear that Penn Foundation faced stiffer financial challenges than an Administrative Consultant could be expected to handle. Albert Strehle resigned, handing back many administrative and bookkeeping responsibilities to Marge Alexander, Dr. Loux, and their assistants. The organization could limp along administratively for a little while, but, as Dr. Loux insisted to the Board, the need for a full-time business specialist was growing ever more urgent. "Because of State funding, it is imperative that Penn Foundation be represented at the many meetings being called by the County Boards," he reminded the Directors at their March 1972 meeting. "This places an added burden on the schedules of many staff members."

This burden would weigh on the staff for another sixteen months, as the appropriations picture remained cloudy and the organization experienced an uncharacteristically high rate of employee turnover. Janet Medori, pre-school teacher Nancy Swartley, Dr. deRivas, Day Treatment nurse Janet Canouse, and veteran Day Care Coordinator Ruth Simpson all departed between April 1972 and June 1973. Their exits opened the door to the hiring of psychiatric social worker Esther Siderov, pre-school teacher Judith Hubbard, occupational and recreational therapist John Snyder, and Day Treatment Coordinator Sandra Trakat (John and Sandy would still be on staff three decades later, as Penn Foundation's fiftieth anniversary rolled around). Amid all of the comings and goings, the key position of Business Administrator remained unfilled. The wait was just about over, though. Psychiatric social worker Gary Beese had demonstrated a knack for administration in recent months as his duties diversified. Dr. Loux and the Directors concluded it would make more sense to promote this two-year staff veteran to a more business-oriented position within the organization than to import someone less familiar with Penn Foundation's culture. They presented the idea to Gary in May 1973, and he accepted the challenge of serving as the Foundation's first Administrator—in a preliminary "Acting" capacity—starting in July.

A propitious appointment

July 1973 turned out to be a red-letter month in the Foundation's history for yet another reason. Two former general practitioners who had been seeing patients part-time at Penn Foundation while completing psychiatric residencies at Temple University Hospital accepted full-time positions as staff psychiatrists at the Foundation beginning on July 1. The older of these doctors, Wheaton and Jefferson Medical College graduate Chester Schneider, would spend only nine months at the Sellersville institution before taking an appointment elsewhere. The tenure of his younger colleague—thirty-year-old Montgomery County native Vernon H. Kratz—would be *significantly* longer. When Dr. Loux first recommended Dr. Kratz to the Directors in November 1972, it was as an immediate replacement for Dr. DeRivas, not as the Medical Director's own potential successor. But this "outstanding person" who had "already had five years of medical [missionary] service in Africa" (as Dr. Loux noted in his introductory comments) would demonstrate remarkable staying power at Penn Foundation, and Dr. Kratz's distinguished career would, in fact, include a twenty-three-year stint as chief medical officer. Though neither he nor his employers could have foreseen such a future at the time of his hiring, there were already some striking parallels between Dr. Kratz's vocational development and Dr. Loux's. In a 2002 interview, Dr. Kratz recalled his journey to Penn Foundation as follows:

> I got the idea of going to medical school in my senior year at Lancaster Mennonite High School. I remember my biology teacher, Lois Good, pulling me aside and saying, "Did you ever think of going into medicine?" Of course, I never had.

I never even considered that a possibility. But Lois got me interested, and so I enrolled at Eastern Mennonite College in the fall of 1953 as a pre-med student. After one year at EMC I came home because my two brothers had been drafted—this was during the Korean War—and so I needed to be my dad's helper on the farm for two years. When I finished farming, I wanted to go back to school. I was going to go to Ursinus College, because our farm was in [the neighboring village of] Creamery. I wanted to stay home and commute. But then [Eastern Baptist College student and Mennonite minister John Ruth] got ahold of me and said, "Vernon, you ought to come to Eastern!" [in St. Davids, Montgomery County]. So I went to this "Eastern," and of course they took me in with open arms. They had never had a pre-med student there. They were very eager to build a science department.

When it came time to apply for medical school, Eastern had never had any student apply for medical school before, so I was the test case. I'll never forget when I went to Hahnemann Medical College for my interview, the professor of biochemistry was one of the interviewers. He said, "You know, my wife and I were just driving around St. Davids the other day, and I remarked to her that we had never had an applicant from Eastern Baptist College yet." Of course, this was 1959, and Eastern was still a fairly young college.

So I got into the program at Hahnemann. I actually worked at Grand View Hospital occasionally while I was a student at Hahnemann. This was in the days before they had emergency room physicians at Grand View. The emergency room was not nearly as big a deal as it is today. A group of us medical students would come out from Hahnemann, take our time on nights and weekends, and sort of serve as an in-house emergency team. When we needed it, we would call an on-call doctor. That was a good growing-up experience. The doctors were very happy to have us there.

I did my internship up at St. Luke's in Bethlehem. We still did internships in those days—one year of post-graduate work and then you were ready for family medicine. I was actually going to take a residency in internal medicine, but then I was drafted. I finished my internship on June 30, 1964, was married

five days later, and left on September 2 for Ethiopia on a
three-year term of [alternative] service with Eastern Mennonite Board of Missions. I served as a general physician in a
clinic there. At one point I was assigned to speak at an annual
missionary conference. My topic was "the emotional health
of missionaries." Talk about a challenge! I wrote to Norm Loux
asking for advice, and to Roy Harnish, one of my teachers at
LMH, who had gone on to Brook Lane [Psychiatric Center]
in Hagerstown. Corresponding with them kind of got my
juices going for psychiatry. When my term of service was
ending, and I was trying to figure out what in the world I was
going to do next, I decided to go into psychiatry. I wrote Norm
and I said, "I'm over here in Africa. What would you recommend as a training program?" He sent back a couple of suggestions. One was that I enter the program at Temple University
Hospital. I applied, and Temple accepted me without even
seeing me. We came back in June of '68, and I started my
residency in July.

Six months into it, the Board of Missions called and asked
if we would consider going back to Somalia for two years.
They really needed someone there. I told them we would go
if we could get out of our lease and get a leave of absence from
Temple with assurances that I could get back into the program
when we returned. That all worked out, so we went back to
Somalia for two years—1969 to 1971. I returned to Temple in
July of '71. I never thought I would end up here at Penn Foundation. One of my colleagues at Temple was very interested
in working for the Foundation, but I was kind of ambivalent
about whether to come back home to practice psychiatry. The
people at Philhaven [the twenty-year-old Mennonite-run private mental hospital northwest of Lancaster City] pursued me
pretty actively. But I had a really hard time thinking of practicing in a psychiatric hospital that was separate from an acute
care hospital. In East Africa we were closing down leprosy
hospitals and closing down TB hospitals and trying to pull
everything into community health care centers. It was strange
to come back to the States and find all these [autonomous]
psychiatric hospitals. So one of the things that really attracted
me to Penn Foundation was that it was part of a hospital

community. It operated independently, but it was very closely related to Grand View Hospital, and had access to all of the Hospital's services.

Of course, Norm [Dr. Loux] came after me pretty hard. And Dr. Peters, who I had worked with when I was a student at Hahnemann, said, "Vernon, you've been away long enough. You come back to your own right now. You've grown up." So I started full-time here as a staff psychiatrist in July 1973.

An administrative boon

With the hiring of Drs. Kratz and Schneider, Penn Foundation had a record six full-time psychiatrists on staff during the summer of 1973. The organization also had, in Acting Administrator Gary Beese, its first senior staff member devoted to administrative affairs. The benefits soon became apparent. Within months Gary had evaluated the institution's accounting practices and submitted to the Directors his recommendation for an overhaul. He had also prepared "a revised version of Personnel Policies" and presented this to the Board, which further authorized him to "initiate a study of both disability and pension plans." It was a new administrative day, indeed. Through Gary's promotion, the Foundation also acquired an able and enthusiastic spokesman. Inquiring reporters were now directed to him more often than to Dr. Loux or Charles Hoeflich. In a feature article titled "Know Your Community: Mental Health Foundation Growing With Community," published by a Bux-Mont newspaper in October 1973, all of the direct quotes were attributed to the Foundation's new Acting Administrator:

> "We like to view ourselves as a preventive place. We would like people to come to us before their problems get too intense. . . ."
>
> "We want to treat all ages. . . ."
>
> "'Success' [for Penn Foundation] is when the community sees us as a place for help. For the most part, the community [accepts] the Foundation very well. . . ."
>
> "We emphasize family involvement. Mainly, social workers work with the family. . . ."
>
> "[Our] emphasis is on community treatment of mental health and mental retardation. . . ."

The author of this October 1, 1973 article counted off the services and programs offered by the Foundation, paying particular attention to group therapy, the Day Treatment Program, in-patient services, the Child Development Evaluation Service, 24-hour emergency psychiatric service, and the Mental Retardation Program. There was no hint in the article of imminent program expansion, but there *could* have been. Several important improvements waited just around the corner. One of them, as reported in Doylestown's *Daily Intelligencer* a week later, was Penn Foundation's use of a special $21,000 allocation from the Bucks County Department of Mental Health/Mental Retardation to open a "therapeutic educational kindergarten" in the newly-renovated former farmhouse. News of this early-October opening was conveyed under the headline "Disturbed pre-schoolers get help":

> Sometimes a child who needs help asks for it straight out. Sometimes he shows it by his hurt feelings or confusion or by behavior that constantly gets him in trouble. But often, adults have to recognize the child's trouble and come to his aid.
>
> This is what Penn Foundation for Mental Health, Sellersville, does for children in Upper Bucks and Eastern Montgomery County in its Children's Psychiatric Service.
>
> Within a few days, the Foundation will offer a new service to pre-school children with emotional and social disturbances, behavior problems, neurological, visual-perceptual-motor impairment, and severe immaturity.
>
> A new therapeutic educational kindergarten has opened at the Foundation, certified by the state Department of Education and staffed by a certified teacher in special education, a certified assistant teacher, and volunteer aides.
>
> The kindergarten class of six to eight students will meet daily for two and a half hours, following the school calendars of the school districts in the Foundation's service area. Each new child and family will be evaluated by the Foundation's children's unit staff before admission into the class, and details on transportation and tuition fees will be arranged on an individual basis.
>
> David Clayton, clinical psychologist in charge of the kindergarten, explains the goals:

— therapeutic: promote general maturity, provide socialization to a small group setting with peers and adults.

— education: develop general readiness skills and provide specialized training in specific needs.

— diagnostic: observation on group and individual basis by trained professionals.

— parent counseling: parent groups will meet on a regular basis and there will be frequent parent-teacher communication and direct training of parents.

The therapeutic kindergarten is an additional service to children, carrying forward the Foundation's work with children which began in 1959. . . . A child study unit was established in 1969 to evaluate and treat a wide variety of developmental disorders in children, including mental retardation, learning disabilities, cerebral palsy, and neurological, psychiatric, and language disorders and multiple handicaps.

A summer recreation program, run as part of the child unit services, includes a wide variety of outdoor as well as indoor activities.

The outdoor activities in summer 1973 included swimming instruction and free swim, hay wagon rides, outdoor games, and field trips that took the youngsters to the Pennridge Airport in Perkasie, Trexler Animal Farm in Lehigh County, Mercer Historical Museum in Doylestown, and Washington Crossing State Park in Upper Makefield Township. The Foundation also runs a nursery school in which teachers work several days each week with one to three children.

The staff of the children's unit includes a child psychologist, child psychiatrist, pediatrician and social workers. Consultants also come into the Foundation for speech and hearing evaluations. There also are ear, nose, throat specialists, physical therapists, orthopedic surgeons, public nurses and such special consultants as geneticists, endocrinologists and neurosurgeons who are not available in the immediate community.

"Anyone who cares about children can refer them to us," says Clayton. "They may be parents, family doctors, children's agencies, probation officers, or ministers. "They ask us, 'What's wrong? Help us fix it!"

The prospect of a "group home for retarded children"

The Foundation's Mental Retardation program also appeared primed for a major expansion in November 1973. As was the case with the kindergarten's addition, the anticipated boost in Mental Retardation services derived not from a surplus in Foundation revenue, but from a special, earmarked allocation. Dr. Loux had raised the prospect of Penn Foundation operating a "group home for retarded children" at the September 1972 Board meeting. After pointing out that "funds are available from state and federal sources, to be distributed through county Mental Health/ Mental Retardation programs, which would provide 100% funding for small group homes," he observed that "apparently, the money is there for the asking, and some private profit organizations seem to be getting into the field of this activity." Beyond encouraging "Penn Foundation to support this program," Dr. Loux suggested the Directors "even give consideration to sponsoring a home of this kind, on the assumption that it could be done with very little financial outlay on the part of the Foundation."

This prospect became a lot less theoretical the following November when Penn Foundation received a $30,000 gift from Montgomery County realtor Lawrence Yerk, "to be used in establishing a Group Home for retarded persons within the requirements of the State of Pennsylvania" (as noted in Board meeting minutes). "Mr. Yerk has a special interest in contributing to such a project because of a son who is rather severely retarded and, therefore, he is interested in contributing toward the establishment of a group home which would be able to take care of severe cases requiring continuing nursing care and proximity to a hospital." The ensuing months were filled with deliberations in-house and with Grand View Hospital officials, because, as Dr. Loux noted, "the provision of medical care [would be] a most important aspect of such a facility, and [such a] service could only be provided with the complete cooperation of Grand View Hospital." The number of consulting parties was eventually expanded to include parents of mentally retarded children living in the Bux-Mont region.

By the fall of 1973, the initiative had reached a point where Foundation officials were drafting "a charter and by-laws for an organization devoted to the care of the mentally retarded," and Directors Harold Mininger and Paul Souder were "looking into the availability of land for such a project adjoining Penn Foundation." These and other related developments were reported in a flurry of local newspaper articles, such as one published on November 14 under the headline "Retarded Children 'Group Home' May Be Built in Sellersville." "The Sellersville area may get one of the first 'group homes' for retarded children in the state," its author began. "One proposal under consideration is for establishing a life support center for at least 20 children on land adjacent to the Penn Foundation for Mental Health headquarters, Sellersville. 'The site is not yet assured,' said Dr. Norman Loux, the foundation's medical director. 'But this area is going to get at least one group rehabilitation home and possibly several. There is no question of that,' he added. Because of the foundation's progressive approach in the field of mental health, it has been generally expected to become a leader in the new venture."

When it became apparent that constructing a "life support group home" for severely retarded children on Sellersville Heights would cost several hundred thousand dollars, it also became clear that Penn Foundation's contribution to the venture would have to be limited to consultation, administration, and staffing. Despite the Yerk bequest, the Foundation wasn't close to being able to fund a major construction project. The point was rendered moot, anyway, as the parties involved in the initiative concluded that it made more sense to establish an independent not-for-profit organization to build and administer the group home. The new corporation, named Community Foundation for Human Development (CFHD), would work closely with Grand View Hospital trustees and Penn Foundation personnel in getting the project off the ground. Penn Foundation's Directors resolved at their February 19, 1974 meeting to "support the Board of Grand View Hospital and the Board of the [CFHD] in their efforts to develop a building site on the grounds of Grand View Hospital for a Type 1 facility to serve the severely mentally retarded individuals of this community." Foundation officials would ultimately pass on the unspent $30,000 Yerk endowment to the CFHD, and these funds would be added to several other sizable bequests to open the Ridge Crest group home on the Grand View Hospital campus in 1977. Two years later, the Mental Retardation Case Management Program Penn Foundation had been administering for Bucks County would be reassigned to the CFHD. The extremely complicated but ultimately successful unfolding of the group home project stands out in retrospect as a particularly poignant example of Foundation and Hospital officers working together to deliver an important community service. "The potential was there for the Hospital to hold us at sword's point after the balance of power swung over to them mid-way through the project," Dr. Loux remarked recently. "But they remained magnanimous throughout the process. That kind of cooperative spirit has been vital to us over the years. I can hardly emphasize that enough."

Give and take

As a base service unit under contract to Bucks and Montgomery Counties, Penn Foundation had to live with the reality that Counties gave, but they also took away. They almost always assumed the lead in the tango of funding agency and service provider, and the Foundation was left to respond as creatively and energetically as it could. In good times, this collaboration resulted in the offering of new services or the expansion of existing programs at Penn Foundation. A special grant from the Bucks County Department of Mental Health/Mental Retardation in November 1974, for instance, funded the Foundation's establishment of a Crisis Intervention Program, equipped with a hot-line and crisis-trained personnel. A year later, the same Department provided one year's worth of funding for a Community Outreach Program. Headquartered in the old Nurses Home on the Grand View Hospital campus, and staffed by a social worker, a nurse, and secretary, the program "sends psychiatric social workers out on home visits to individuals who are unable or unwilling to come to the center for treatment," a local newspaper reporter explained in a November 1975 article.

Bucks County also contributed $7,500 in July 1976 toward another round of "major repairs" to the Foundation's farmhouse, so that facility could accommodate an expanded Kindergarten Program. That would be the brighter face of a two-sided coin, however. The flip-side came to light two years later when the County abruptly withdrew funding for both the Kindergarten *and* the Pre-school Programs, throwing five Foundation employees—two teachers, two teacher aides and a part-time speech consultant—out of work. "Naturally upset" Program Director Mike Dunn was quoted in a June 14, 1978 newspaper article as saying "a federal law passed about a year ago mandates that public educational systems assume the responsibility of education for handicapped children down to the age of 3." Dr. Dunn assumed that, in light of this new legislation, Bucks County had decided to withdraw funding from Penn Foundation and "funnel state funds into the Bucks County Intermediate Unit, which will then establish pre-school education programs. For the immediate future [however], 3- and 4-year-olds [in central and northern Bucks County] do not

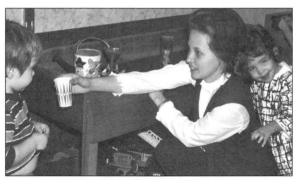

Notes jotted alongside these snapshots in the 1971–74 Penn Foundation Kindergarten scrapbook indicate that the photo below was taken during a December 1972 Christmas party, and the undated photo on the left showed a teacher and two students engaged in "water play."

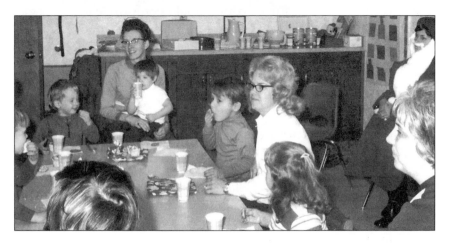

have special schools available. At this point, our program is closed, and that's it."

Reduced appropriations represented one set of teeth in a vise squeezing Penn Foundation's finances ever tighter in the mid-1970s. The other set was represented by an old nemesis: uncollected fees. Because the percentage of clients paying partially, late, or not-at-all remained fairly consistent year after year, the Foundation's success in serving more patients had the frustrating effect of swelling the income deficit. The paradox of treating record numbers of patients (such as in 1973, when 650 new clients pushed the total patient load to more than 1,700) was that a record income deficit was bound to result. This dilemma was examined repeatedly by the trustees in consultation with Dr. Loux and Acting Administrator Gary Beese, not only because the Foundation officials themselves were concerned, but because administrators in the County departments were registering alarm. At the April 16, 1974 Board meeting, for instance,

Gary Beese "commented that County authorities were [again] bringing pressure about fee collection. It was agreed that [responsibility for] collection must remain with [Penn Foundation] and that an appropriate method to follow up on past due accounts must be found. Grand View Hospital has set up a corporation made up of staff members to serve as a collection agency, and this method has been most successful. The chairman appointed Paul Souder to work with Dr. Loux and Mr. Beese on this matter. It was suggested that financial matters be discussed with the patient at an early date."

While uncollected fees would weigh heavily on Penn Foundation for years to come (Treasurer Russell Moyer would notify his fellow Directors in October 1975 that "$93,000 was at least 120 days overdue"), the overall accounting picture brightened considerably under Gary Beese's ministrations. Gary worked with the Foundation's accounting firm to devise a manual system of bookkeeping which would "provide much necessary information on program costs" and "lend itself to computerization at a later date" (as reported in April 16, 1974 Board meeting minutes). The Directors approved the new system and authorized Gary to hire a full-time bookkeeper to implement it as soon as possible. In June 1974 Gary traveled to Elkhart, Indiana to observe "the administrative set-up, methods of establishing costs, and fee schedules" employed at Oaklawn Psychiatric Center, the outpatient and day treatment facility established eleven years earlier by the Mennonite Central Committee. Penn Foundation's Acting Administrator reported upon his return that he had been "much impressed" by what he saw at Oaklawn, especially the method of "establishing the fee schedule, which reflected actual cost of service. He suggested that a cost study be made at Penn Foundation so that a more equitable fee for services could be established." Gary's employers affirmed his initiative and performance by removing the "Acting" qualifier from his "Administrator" title as of July 19, 1974.

Celebrating two decades of pioneering service

There were affirmations aplenty for the entire organization in 1975, as Penn Foundation marked its twentieth anniversary. Weeks before the scheduled November anniversary event, the public expressed its support by attending the Fifth Annual Fall Festival in record numbers. The crowd of 2,000 milling about the Foundation's campus on Saturday, September 20 was nearly twice as large as the previous year's turnout. Attendance was also strong at the two-part, free-admission film series presented by the Foundation "in the interest of the drug and alcohol project" the following November 5 and 19. As announced in local papers, the featured attractions of this series were *The Secret Love of Sandra Blain* ("a portrayal of the developmental symptom of Alcohol Addiction; discusses ways women in similar distress may obtain help") and *A Time for Decision* (a "documentary focusing on a family in search of help"). Audience members were invited to stay after the screenings to participate in "discussion groups led by Drug & Alcohol Specialists" (including Richard Kardon, the Foundation's first D&A expert, approaching the end of his second year on staff).

The day after the first of these cinematic presentations, Penn Foundation mounted a Twentieth Anniversary Luncheon and Seminar in the multi-purpose Grundy Auditorium. The two-part observance—held on Thursday afternoon, November 6, 1975—demonstrated that while the Foundation was now just one star among a constellation of community mental health centers operating across the country, it still held a special place in the hearts of certain psychiatric VIP's. Lending their considerable weight to the commemoration of the Foundation's first two decades were no fewer than four former presidents of the American Psychiatric Association: Drs. Kenneth Appel, Leo Bartemeier, Daniel Blain, and Francis Braceland. Rounding out the cast of visiting dignitaries were Dr. Abram M. Hostetter, President of the Pennsylvania Psychiatric Society; Dr. David B. Bernhardt, Executive Director of the Mental Health Association of Southeastern Pennsylvania; and Dr. Edward Auer of St. Louis University. Any one of these heavyweights might have been the guest of honor on another occasion, but the spotlight was trained during the Anniversary Luncheon on Sellersville's adopted son and Grand View Hospital's Chief of Medicine, Michael Peters. Dr. Bernhardt rose after the meal to present Dr. Peters with a citation from the Mental Health Association of Southeastern Pennsylvania, recognizing the sixty-seven-year-old internist's indispensable contributions to the launching of Penn Foundation. Dr. Hostetter followed with a similar award from the Pennsylvania Psychiatric Society, which included recognition of Dr. Loux's vital role in bringing Dr. Peters' dream to fruition. The Luncheon concluded with the announcement that Penn Foundation's annual lecture series—about to kick off its thirteenth year, still funded by the Lemmon Pharmacal Company—would thereafter be known as the Michael A. Peters Seminar Series.

The inaugural lecture of the 1975-76 series was delivered later that afternoon by Dr. Braceland in the second event of the Twentieth

Anniversary observance. The Editor of the *American Journal of Psychiatry* turned his audience's attention to the future in a lecture titled "Psychiatry, the Next Decade." As it was summarized in a newspaper article published the following day, Dr. Braceland's address called for the psychiatric profession to make a "rapid return to medicine, in an age when a great many therapists are providing a wide variety of services" without a strong medical orientation. "Suggesting that divorce and other problems in society, including poverty, do not cause mental illness, he urged emphasis on the relationship between the mind and the body" (this exhortation was music to the ears of Drs. Peters and Loux).

At the same time, psychiatrists and medical doctors alike needed to recognize that society was experiencing an "upheaval" that "may force further change in the [mental health and medical] professions. Things are happening to the whole structure of society—things that none of us have faced [before]," Dr. Braceland observed. "Unprecedented problems of the nation have left the confidence of the people rudely shaken. People who feel that order has collapsed . . . may be secretly homesick for a world of tranquility and security not available anywhere in the world." Spoken near the end of a year that had begun with the conviction of four White House staffers in the Watergate conspiracy, and that had later included the evacuation of American forces from South Vietnam, a subsequent North Vietnamese take-over in that country, and two attempted assassinations of President Gerald Ford, Dr. Braceland's commentary needed few illustrations. It was also admittedly light on answers. The future of the mental health care industry—let alone the nation—was as unforeseeable as it had ever been.

8

TRANSITIONS AT THE TOP

The first year of Penn Foundation's third decade (which happened to coincide with the nation's Bicentennial) began portentously with Dr. Loux calling a special meeting of the Executive Committee. The Foundation's hard-working Medical Director was approaching his fifty-eighth birthday, so no one attending the January 16, 1976 meeting was surprised to learn he had been contemplating his eventual retirement and its ramifications for the organization. These ponderings had led him to develop a five-year plan which he now asked the Executive Committee to consider. Secretary Ruby Horwood summarized the six major components of Dr. Loux's proposal as follows:

(1) His retirement from the position of Medical Director five years hence [when he would be 61½ years old].
(2) The establishment of a position of an Assistant Medical Director in 1976.
(3) Recommendation that Dr. Lyons be considered for that position.
(4) Within the next five years the establishment of an adequate retirement plan for all eligible employees.
(5) The development of a half-way house and other alternative living arrangements for the emotionally ill in our community.
(6) The establishment of an Executive Committee of a managerial level comprised of the Executive members of the Board of Directors, the Medical Director, Assistant Medical Director and the Administrator to meet monthly for major policy decisions.

In its customary manner, the Executive Committee subjected these points to "lengthy discussion" before agreeing to present them to the full Board at the Annual Dinner Meeting of Directors and employees at the Indian Valley Country Club four days hence. Dr. Loux's vision was widely affirmed on that occasion as each of the six principal points of his plan were approved or acted upon. The earliest outcome was the appointment of Dr. Lyons—in his fourteenth year as staff psychiatrist, and recently named Fellow of the American Psychiatric Association—as the Foundation's first Assistant Medical Director. Hard on the heels of this promotion came the first meeting of the new Executive Managerial Committee in February. It was a sign of the times that monthly meetings of personnel responsible "for major policy decisions" were now deemed necessary. The challenges of riding herd on a rapidly expanding organization would be further underscored the following year when the full Board began meeting every month rather than every three months.

Near the top of the "Challenges" list for Foundation officials in 1976 was accommodating an ever-growing staff and spectrum of services, even as monthly shortfalls gnawed at the organization's framework. Somehow, somewhere, room had to be acquired for physical expansion. The answer appeared to lie in private donations from major supporters, which were typically earmarked for conspicuous "special projects" so both the donors and the public could see and celebrate the philanthropic results. Indeed, the Grundy Foundation had offered money for use in constructing "additional offices and a conference room" at Penn Foundation as far back as 1972. But the Grundy grant would have covered only a quarter of the projected construction costs, leaving the remainder to be generated through other channels. Even with that caveat, building committees met with architect George Hay several times between 1972 and 1976 to discuss "the feasibility of adding a new wing to the present building." Each committee ultimately concluded that—at least in financial terms—the time was not yet right for a major undertaking.

Another series of meetings held with Mr. Hay early in 1976 resulted in an updated set of building plans and a renewed sense of anticipation. But by August, "expansion" was back "on hold," as the Board decided to "delay action" in light of "the present financial situation." The holding pattern persisted through the remainder of the year, which saw the "financial situation" degenerate to the point where the Board's Nominating Committee set aside the notion of cycling new officers into the Executive Committee. At the December 21, 1976 Board meeting, Paul Souder simply reported that "the Nominating Committee had met and recommended that, due to the fiscal crisis and concurrent clinical pressures, the present officers should continue for another year."

The financial picture remained murky in 1977, but the *other* crisis—caused by cramped conditions—escalated to the point where Foundation officials could no longer delay the inevitable. They would have to bite the bullet and proceed with expansion. Out came the building plans, in came new cost projections, and by June the trustees had the information they needed to make a decision. After Building Committee member Curt Moyer "presented the plans of the new wing and reported on progress with the architect" at the June 21 Board meeting, President Harold Mininger "asked for a consensus of opinion to proceed with the project. . . . Based on the demand for service and the lack of space for programs, a motion was made, seconded and approved, that the [building] project should be continued to meet that need." Some last-minute touches were applied to the building plan, the project was put out to bid, and in November a construction contract worth $155,709 was awarded to builder Robert M. Koffel.

The new wing of staff offices, meeting rooms, and group therapy facilities, dedicated at the Fall Festival on September 23, 1978, project southward (to the right) from the 1962 core structure in this aerial photo gracing the cover of the *Penn Foundation for Mental Health Annual Report 1980.*

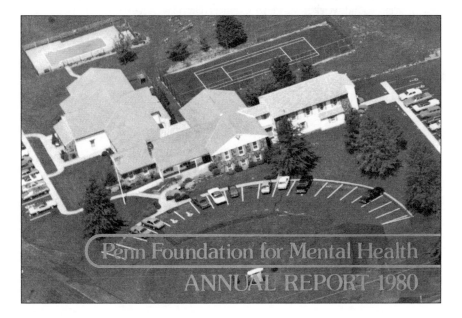

"First satellite program"

As the building project finally got off the ground in the fall of 1977, Penn Foundation pressed forward with a kind of expansion that would not require additional facilities: providing on-site psychiatric services to area hospitals. Contracting with medical institutions would have the added benefit of ensuring full and timely payments for services rendered. The Foundation's long-standing partnership with Grand View Hospital had been particularly amiable and productive. Why couldn't strong and mutually beneficial working relationships be established farther afield? The most obvious candidate for collaboration was Quakertown Hospital, not only because it lay a mere eight miles to the north, but because a precedent for partnering had been set there four years earlier when Dr. Kratz began "providing consultant services to patients on a one day a week basis for the number of hours required" (as noted in July 1973 Board meeting minutes). While Dr. Loux had affirmed this arrangement "as a positive step in establishing better working relationships with Quakertown Hospital," patients treated in this manner were billed by Penn Foundation directly, so the potential for non-payment or late payment was still there.

Now, in the summer of 1977, Foundation officers were eager to implement a more extensive and financially secure practice. They arranged with their Quakertown Hospital counterparts to have a Penn Foundation psychiatric social worker serve in Quakertown twenty-five hours per week, under terms outlined as follows in an August 26, 1977 newspaper article:

> The cost that Penn Foundation will bill Quakertown Hospital is $1,600 a month. The social worker providing the direct service will be given supervision, team support and consultation from the Penn Foundation staff. The worker will conduct interviews and therapy programs at Quakertown Hospital, Penn Foundation, and possibly in the patient's home or social agency. Gary C. Beese, administrator of Penn Foundation, said yesterday it is his group's "first satellite program." He explained that Penn Foundation has had a working relationship with Grand View Hospital in Sellersville for years where 13 beds are normally set aside for psychiatric patients and where Penn Foundation psychiatrists are on the hospital's medical staff. Beese said, "The general hospitals in Bucks County are in the process of developing psychiatric units." He

sees the agreement as the beginning of a psychiatric unit at Quakertown. James S. Crawford, Quakertown Hospital administrator, commented, "Quakertown Hospital has a great many patients for physical causes who have emotional and psychiatric problems."

The psychiatric social worker appointed by Penn Foundation to initiate the satellite program in Quakertown was thirty-four-year-old John M. Goshow, a 1961 graduate of Christopher Dock Mennonite (High) School who had gone on to earn a B.A. degree in sociology at Eastern Mennonite College and a M.S.W. degree at Virginia Commonwealth University. For six years leading up to his Penn Foundation employment, John had served as a psychiatric counselor and social services coordinator at the Wayne-Holmes Mental Health Clinic in Wooster, Ohio. After the arrival of their second child, he and his wife Janet (also a 1961 CDMS graduate) were ready to return to the Bux-Mont region to be closer to relatives. John recalls that his first job offer from Penn Foundation had involved conducting a grant-funded "study of the geriatric needs in the community." But as he was getting ready to leave Ohio, he got a call from Gary Beese telling him the grant had fallen through, taking the job prospect with it. All was not lost, however. Within days Foundation officials had decided that John could be even more productively employed as their satellite launcher in Quakertown.

By mid-October 1977, John had re-located to Perkasie and commenced his duties at Quakertown Hospital. Along the way he had also received a crash course in Penn Foundation's history, philosophy, and program, with which he was happy to identify himself. That message came through loud and clear in his comments to a reporter, quoted in a November article in Quakertown's *Free Press*:

> Goshow, who says he is enthusiastic about his appointment to the [Quakertown] hospital staff, explained that this program is unique for the hospital. "In the past, any doctor who felt his patient needed mental health care had to have him sent to Grandview Hospital or to the Penn Foundation Clinic in Sellersville. This often meant that patients and family doctors were forced to go out of their way for consultation and services." Now, Goshow said, many problems can be dealt with right in Quakertown.

"The Penn Foundation is considered a forerunner in the concept of 'home environment' and its importance in treating mental health problems," he continued. "We feel it is extremely valuable to keep patients in an everyday, home-type atmosphere as much as possible. We want to help people cope with life and feel that the best way to do that is through the combination of expert professional care as well as contact with family, friends and normal life happenings."

One of his main objectives is to involve the family of the patient and to keep the patient's actual hospital stay to a minimum. Dr. Norman Loux, medical director for the Penn Foundation, explained one of the programs now being instituted at Quakertown Hospital. "The program is called 'partial hospitalization,' and what this means is that the patient in this hospital would go to Penn Foundation Clinic during the day for roughly eight hours, returning to the hospital at night. When the patient is released from the hospital, this program would continue on a day basis."

Goshow, for his part, is concerned with the hospital patient who suffers from depression, tremendous anxiety, has family problems or worries that make him unhappy and can prolong recovery from the physical illness for which he was hospitalized. "I have heard it said that as high as 75 percent of all physical illnesses are the direct or indirect result of a mental illness. That figure may be high," he said, "but the point is valid." He continued, explaining that the mind can be over-worked and over-taxed, just as the body can. A serious physical problem can cause a patient to have a mental problem such as depression and worries about the ability of family and friends to cope.

Goshow said a reverse situation also is true. "A serious mental problem can cause serious physical problems—ulcers, high blood pressure, nervous breakdowns and many more. "I'm here to work with the hospital and for the patient. This is a comprehensive program to treat the sick of this community—whether mentally, physically, or both."

Hospital physicians and Penn Foundation doctors will contact Goshow and ask him to determine if psychiatric care is necessary for a patient. "Whatever the problem, the important thing is that I am here to be contacted. There is no treatment if there is no one skilled to perform it, so I'm at Quakertown Hospital 25 hours a week to provide that treatment and make the cure possible."

Goshow believes that having a psychiatric social worker on the staff is a direct benefit to the entire community, and not only the physically or mentally ill portion of it. He is now in the process of planning educational seminars to be offered to the whole community. The programs will deal with real-life situations that just about everyone is faced with at some time in his life, Goshow said.

He said that one of the difficult problems he wants to tackle is changing the attitude surrounding mental health care. "Mental illness doesn't mean that everyone who suffers from it is a psychotic," he said.

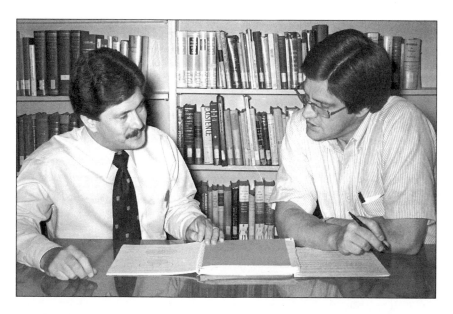

Two of Penn Foundation's early emissaries to Quakertown were comparing notes when this picture was taken in the mid-1980s. Psychiatric social worker John M. Goshow (on right) moved back to Pennsylvania in October 1977 to serve as the Foundation's agent at Quakertown Community Hospital. Quakertown native Wayne R. Schantzenbach was hired as a family and marriage counseling specialist in August 1979. A year after joining Penn Foundation, Wayne was appointed Team Leader of the organization's first satellite clinic, housed in Quakertown's First United Church of Christ.

John Goshow's groundbreaking efforts were so warmly received that only five months into the satellite venture "representatives of Quakertown Hospital, schools, and churches" called a meeting with "Penn Foundation staff and board at the hospital to discuss establishing increased psychiatric services in the Quakertown area," according to a March 27, 1978 newspaper article. The "discussion centered on Penn Foundation establishing in-patient and emergency psychiatric services at Quakertown Hospital by Sept. 1 under a contractual arrangement," the article continued. "Dr. Norman Loux, director of Penn Foundation, said, 'I am aware that the time has come when Quakertown Hospital needs more than it has in terms of (psychiatric) service. This is a matter of working out the details—you will find no resistance on our part for that.'" Whoever worked out the details would have to come to grips with "shrinking state and federal dollars coming into the Foundation," and the fact that there were "few staff members available to apply for government funding for new programs." Hospital Administrator James Crawford suggested at the meeting that a "community development agency" be created in the Quakertown area "to obtain funding for Quakertown Hospital, Grundy House, Quakertown School District and Penn Foundation." Dr. Loux and his colleagues certainly had no resistance to *that* proposal, either. In the end, the parties agreed that Foundation and Hospital officers should "meet frequently to hammer out the contract for services."

And so they would. It might have only taken a few weeks to fashion an agreement, but a major development at Penn Foundation delayed the negotiations. Administrator Gary Beese unexpectedly submitted a letter of resignation on April 22, 1978, four days after returning with Dr. Lyons and Harold Mininger from a series of meetings with Mennonite Mental Health Services personnel in Canada. Gary had brought back with him two strong recommendations: first, that Penn Foundation "finalize [its] affiliation with the Mennonite Mental Health Services" as soon as possible; and second, that the Board seriously consider adopting "an alternative management structure [like that] used by the majority of the agencies currently enrolled in the Mennonite Mental Health Services." That structure involved "an Executive Director reporting directly to the Board, with support from an Administrator focusing on financial and business matters and a Medical Director who focused on the clinical issues."

The Directors had barely begun considering this new model when Gary's letter of resignation arrived. He and his wife were finally acting on a long-felt impulse to re-locate to California and adopt a simpler life-style.

His last day on the job would be May 19, giving Foundation officials four short weeks to find a replacement. Everyone agreed that the drafting of the contract with Quakertown Hospital "should not be completed at this time but should be delayed until the new administrator has a chance to review it and have input into the process." This interruption added urgency to the search for the Foundation's second Administrator.

New administrative energy and vision

Fortunately, this search turned out to be mercifully short and rewarding. Dr. Loux quickly drew a bead on another native son whose education and training in mental health administration had taken him far afield. Henry D. Landes had stood to inherit a place in his family's central Montgomery County plumbing and heating business, but his intellectual fires were sufficiently fanned at Christopher Dock Mennonite (High) School (where he was President of the Class of 1964) that he set off to study history and ultimately social work at Goshen College in Indiana. A social work field placement at Oaklawn Psychiatric Center in nearby Elkhart proved critical in steering Henry's vocational trajectory. After serving two post-college years of Voluntary Service as Director of Mennonite Central Committee's Appalachian Unit in Kentucky, Henry found himself "attracted both to management jobs and to community mental health services," as he related in a 2002 interview. He continued:

> I applied to graduate schools in social work administration
> and program planning, thinking the role of Oaklawn founder
> and Administrator Robert Hartzler would be an interesting
> one. Running a community mental health center would be a
> way for me to combine my interests in management and
> entrepreneurial development. I received a National Institute
> of Mental Health fellowship at the University of North Carolina at Chapel Hill to train me to work in community mental
> health administration. My first graduate field work placement
> was with the Wake County Community Mental Health Center
> in Raleigh. My second field placement was with the Office of
> Personnel for the State of North Carolina where I joined the
> staff as a management trainer and consultant after completing
> my Master's. After two years, I went on to seminary at [Associated Mennonite Biblical Seminaries in] Elkhart, and worked

at Oaklawn part-time doing management training and consultation with [former Brook Lane chaplain-therapist] Chet Raber and Oakwood Associates.

Like Penn Foundation, Oaklawn was a pioneer in the community mental health movement, with strong roots in the Mennonite community. I directed Oaklawn's Consultation Department, doing a lot of consultation with community organizations, the police department, the sheriff's department, schools systems, and businesses—which was out at the very edge of the community mental health field in those days. We were doing all sorts of interesting things—continually moving, developing, elaborating. I thought I'd have a long and happy career at Oaklawn.

Then I got a call from Dr. Loux who I had learned to know fairly well while we served together on the Goshen College Board. We used to visit together in the O'Hare airport after Board meetings—I was flying back to Kentucky and he to Pennsylvania. [Henry had other connections with Dr. Loux, including one cemented in 1968 when Henry married the daughter of Penn Foundation charter trustee Marcus Clemens.] When Norm called, I was flat on my back, recuperating from back surgery. I couldn't even get off the couch. He said, "I'd like you to consider coming to Penn Foundation."

I had deep respect for Dr. Loux and the national reputation of Penn Foundation, which included a highly regarded affiliation with Grand View Hospital. Unlike many other community mental health centers, Penn Foundation was able to attract and retain quality psychiatrists and other professionals.

Well, as soon as I got back on my feet, I interviewed at Penn Foundation. It felt like a good fit to me, even though I was only thirty-two years old. When I think about it now, I was really in over my head. I mean, I wasn't even the *Assistant* Administrator at Oaklawn, but I was eager and interested. I figured I could learn. And they hired me.

Two days before he was scheduled to step into the Administrator's shoes, Henry was introduced to his new colleagues at the Annual Staff and Board Ox Roast at Dr. Loux's farm. This July 22, 1978 affair was also an opportunity for employees to meet the first two additions to Penn

Foundation's Board of Directors in six years. Perkasie realtor Harold O. Gross Jr. had been appointed to the Board three months earlier when charter member and twenty-three-year veteran Mahlon Souder retired (and was named the Foundation's first "Director Emeritus"). Dr. Raymond P. Landes, Chairman of Grand View Hospital's Department of Medicine, had been elected to the Board a month later. Like Mahlon Souder before him, Dr. Landes was also a Hospital trustee, so he now served as an important human bridge connecting the executive echelons of the Lawn Avenue institutions.

Additions to Penn Foundation's administrative team did not have the luxury of easing into their positions in the summer of 1978. The business at hand was extremely pressing. Henry Landes' inherited to-do list included finalizing a contract with Quakertown Hospital; preparing for the Fall Festival, which would feature a dedication of the new wing; vetting a new set of "personnel policies involving retention, review of work, and handling of grievances"; developing "a viable middle management structure at Penn Foundation"; and, above all, finding a way to balance the books.

Appointed in July 1978 to fill the Administrator role vacated by Gary Beese, Henry D. Landes (left) inherited a daunting to-do list. In tackling it, he worked closely with Board President and Foundation co-founder Harold Mininger (right). "There were some important contributors on the Board at that time," Henry would later observe, "but Harold really was the glue that held everybody together. He and I would have lunch together once a week—because he was my supervisor—and I learned so much from him. Harold is one of my heroes."

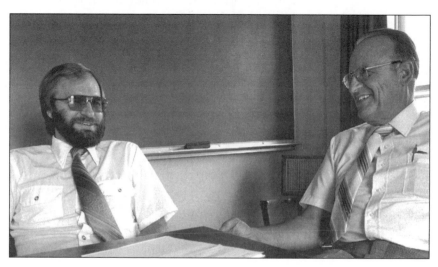

"Coming to work was a little like stepping into a cold shower," Henry would say of his first months on the job. "At first, there wasn't even an office for me. We had to clear out a secretarial area to create a temporary office. That sort of made me wonder where I fit. There was one part-time assistant for the Administrator. It seemed like I was always discovering something else. Like, we were losing $25,000 a month while a big addition was being built! The funding for the Kindergarten and the Pre-school Programs had just been withdrawn by the County. I was thinking, "Wow! How did all this happen? I didn't know what I was getting in to.""

A promising track

As he settled into his new position, Henry also discovered plenty of evidence that Penn Foundation was on a promising track. A contract with Quakertown Hospital was signed in mid-August, ensuring the Foundation of $5,000 in monthly income from that collaborative effort. The first psychiatric patient was admitted to the Hospital under Dr. Kratz's care on September 1. By that time, the farmhouse had been renovated yet again, this time for occupancy by the Case Management Program under a new fee-for-service contract with Bucks County (as this development had been explained to the Directors a couple of months earlier, "a person will be trained by Penn Foundation to function as a County employee and to assist clients or patients of the Foundation to make application for MH/MR funding"). Then, on September 23, the Fall Festival was expanded to include a dedication ceremony for Penn Foundation's new wing. The facilities crunch was eased, at last. Equally relieving to the new Administrator was the arrival, four days after the Dedication, of Betty Caroff, whom Henry had been authorized to hire as a "fiscal officer" (i.e. business manager). "Betty brought financial strength and discipline to her job," Henry remarked recently. "She really knew how to work with the system." A busy and hopeful autumn was capped off by the adoption of a new fee schedule ("to cover increasing costs"), the signing of a psychiatric services contract with Grand View Hospital (similar to the Quakertown Hospital agreement), the report of Treasurer Russell Moyer that "November figures revealed a profitable operation in the amount of $9,000 for the month." and the subsequent recommendation by the Directors of "a 7% salary increase [for all employees] effective January 1, 1979."

Penn Foundation's future took on an even brighter cast that winter through a pair of major administrative developments. First, Dr. Lyons resigned as Assistant Medical Director at the close of 1978 in order to practice privately. This opened the door to the appointment of a new Assistant Medical Director who—even more importantly—stood to inherit the position of Medical Director when Dr. Loux retired in a couple of years. It didn't take long to identify the man for the job. Vernon Kratz had demonstrated remarkable leadership skills, creativity, and tirelessness since his arrival in 1973. His talents had become even more conspicuous to Dr. Loux and the Directors following his promotion to Director of Day Treatment in March 1977 (when Dr. Richards left to join the Emergency Service of Grand View Hospital). Now, in the winter of 1978–79, Dr. Kratz stood "head and shoulders" above the other employees as a candidate for the Foundation's top medical position, as trustee Harold Mininger recently recalled. "Vernon could have gotten a substantial pay increase if he would have gone to another institution. But his 'heart work' was here, so he stayed and did it. We believed he would stay, and the Foundation would be in good hands. Our only concern was that he'd work *too* hard and wear himself out. Just watch sometime how he walks from the Foundation over to Grand View. He *moves!* That tells you what type of guy he is."

Dr. Kratz was appointed Assistant Medical Director on February 1, 1979, with Dr. Loux's projected retirement less than two years away. The vacated position of Day Treatment Director was filled the following July by John Goshow, who had spent the previous two years serving as the Foundation's point-man at Quakertown Hospital. In yet another auspicious appointment, former psychiatric caseworker Karen Kern was named "Coordinator of Emergency Services" and given responsibility for the Foundation's new round-the-clock emergency coverage program, staffed by non-medical therapists with support from psychiatrists. Karen's employers were so convinced she was a "keeper" that they had picked up her tuition for two years while she earned a M.S.W. degree at the University of Pennsylvania. Now, less than a year after her return to full-time employment, Karen was eager to reward their confidence by assuming greater responsibilities.

With some key posts newly filled, Penn Foundation pulsed with fresh energy in the months leading up to its Twenty-Fifth Anniversary celebration. The new administrative team worked hard through the remainder of 1979 and the first half of 1980 to pull the Foundation's finances back into the black by adjusting the fee schedule, adopting "both capital and expense budgeting systems in order to project and control future cash needs," retaining a collection agency, and—where it could not be avoided—cutting personnel (when "the subject of staff reduction" was raised at the March 22, 1979 Board meeting, the Directors were in "unanimous agreement that the Medical Director and the Administrators be given a free hand to take the steps necessary to achieve the desired result"). The cost-cutting measures had the desired effect. By October 1979, Russell Moyer was able to report that "our net is now on the plus side for the month and year-to-date." In his year-end statement, the Treasurer confirmed "a turn-around in our [financial] situation, with an excess of receipts over expenditures."

Other signs that Penn Foundation was shifting into a higher administrative gear included the distribution of a comprehensive Personnel Handbook to each of the thirty-five employees in November 1979, the concurrent development of a "personnel classification system" by which "each job at the Foundation was classified into a pay grade category," and the publication in February 1980 of the first issue of *Horizons*, a four-page, offset-printed institutional newsletter heralding the arrival of Penn Foundation's Twenty-Fifth Anniversary year. In addition to a profile of Dr. Loux's

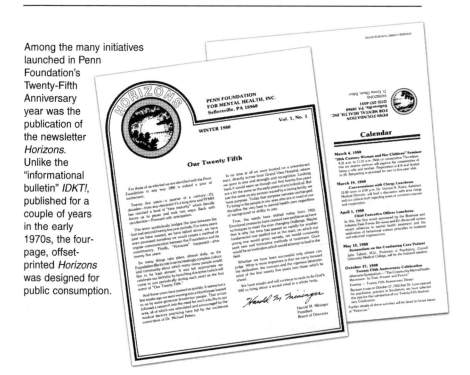

Among the many initiatives launched in Penn Foundation's Twenty-Fifth Anniversary year was the publication of the newsletter *Horizons*. Unlike the "informational bulletin" *IDKT!*, published for a couple of years in the early 1970s, the four-page, offset-printed *Horizons* was designed for public consumption.

career (which had recently been crowned by his appointment by Governor Thornburgh to the Pennsylvania Advisory Committee for Mental Health and Mental Retardation), the inaugural edition of *Horizons* announced the formation of five task forces charged with "investigating present and future needs, and making program proposals" in the areas of Business and Industry, Children and Youth, Churches and Pastors, Continuing Care, and Older Adults. Henry Landes played a prominent role in creating these task forces. "The fundamental vision of Penn Foundation was being maintained," he explained recently. "But fundamental visions sometimes need to be refreshed, and I think Norman brought me in partly to refresh the Foundation's vision—with *his* very active involvement, of course. Forming the task forces as part of our Twenty-Fifth Anniversary was a way of saying, 'We're going to rekindle the innovation around here.'" Comprising trustees, professional staff, and community representatives, the five committees would meet regularly in the spring and summer of 1980 as they organized public events (luncheons, lectures, workshops, etc.) and worked to draft longer-term program recommendations prior to the "capstone" event of the Twenty-Fifth Anniversary, scheduled for October 27.

Two employees who had been with Penn Foundation for most of its first quarter-century would be absent as the second quarter-century dawned. Dr. Barbash, who had begun serving as a clinical psychologist on a part-time basis in 1961, and had moved into a full-time position seven years later, retired on disability in February 1980. His departure was followed in June by the retirement of executive secretary Marge Alexander, a lynchpin in the organization's framework for twenty-three years. Her long tenure concluded with the Board's welcome announcement that "a Penn Foundation for Mental Health, Inc. Pension Plan has been adopted."

Some old friends made their way to Sellersville that fall, as the Foundation orchestrated a "Twenty-Fifth Anniversary Symposium" followed by a "Twenty-Fifth Anniversary Celebration" on Monday, October 27 at the Indian Valley Country Club. Among the visiting dignitaries were Dr. Francis Braceland, Dr. Edward Auer, and Dr. Daniel Blain, all of whom had participated in earlier anniversary celebrations (Dr. Blain had barely missed the first annual Penn Foundation dinner meeting way back in 1957). Two other distinguished guests making return visits to Sellersville were Dr. Howard Rome, Senior Mayo Clinic Psychiatrist and former President of the World Psychiatric Association, and Dr. Shervert H. Frazier, Professor of Psychiatry at Harvard Medical School (both men had lectured in the Foundation's Seminar Series in 1976). They and their eminent colleagues were featured speakers in the afternoon Symposium, titled "Community Mental Health: The Promise, the Accomplishments, and the Vision." During the dinner program, they sat back with 340 other celebrants and enjoyed the home-grown flavors of less-formal proceedings. The dominant tones of reflection and congratulation modulated at the end of the day into expressions of hope. Even in honoring Dr. Loux "for his foresight and years of service," the Directors and staff placed their emphasis on the future as they announced the establishment of the "Norman Loux Fund for Research and Development." Designed to "provide perpetual benefits to be used in underwriting new programs according to Dr. Loux's vision," the Fund had already been seeded by an anonymous donor to the tune of $10,000.

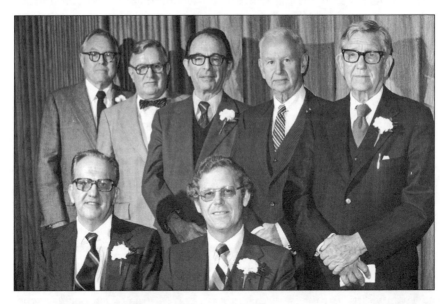

Dr. Loux (seated on left) and the man groomed to take over as Medical Director (Dr. Kratz, seated in center) welcomed some distinguished guests to Penn Foundation's Twenty-Fifth Anniversary Symposium and Celebration, held at the Indian Valley Country Club on October 27, 1980. In the caption for this photo, published in the Foundation's new *Horizons* newsletter, the visiting dignitaries and old friends posing with Drs. Loux and Kratz were identified as (from left) Shervert H. Frazier, M.D., Psychiatrist in Chief, McLean Hospital, Belmont, Massachusetts; Edward T. Auer, M.D., Clinical Professor of Psychiatry, University of Pennsylvania; Howard P. Rome, M.D., Professor of Psychiatry Emeritus, Graduate School of Medicine, University of Minnesota, Mayo Foundation; Francis J. Braceland, M.D., Editor, *The American Journal of Psychiatry*, 1965–1978; and Daniel Blain, M.D., First Medical Director, American Psychiatric Association.

9

INTO OVERDRIVE

Identified on the last page of Penn Foundation's Twenty-Fifth Anniversary program in October 1980 were forty-one persons currently constituting the Foundation's staff. If the names of former employees had been added to this list, the tally of Foundation family members between 1955 and 1980 would have just topped one hundred. Fast forward a second quarter-century, and one finds as an appendix to this Fiftieth Anniversary retrospective a list of more than 1,600 past and present employees, including approximately three hundred persons presently on staff! Equally impressive evidence that something extraordinary unfolded at Penn Foundation during its second quarter-century is provided in accountings of annual revenues and expenses. These numbers soared by *a factor of twelve* between 1980 and 2004—revenues from $1 million to $12 million, and expenses from just under $1 million to $11.6 million. It is also intriguing that in eight of those years—including four straight years from 1988 through 1991—not only did expenses exceed revenue, but the average annual shortfall was in the neighborhood of a quarter-million dollars! What lay behind these eye-catching statistics?

The doubling of the Bux-Mont population in the latter decades of the twentieth century, and the Foundation's mandate to function as a base service unit for the area's burgeoning townships and boroughs, only partly accounts for the sharp increase in activity at 807 Lawn Avenue between 1980 and 2005. Much more consequential were the initiatives launched as part of the Twenty-Fifth Anniversary celebrations, spearheaded by task forces addressing the needs of Business and Industry, Children and Youth, Churches and Pastors, Continuing Care, and Older Adults. A sixth and equally consequential task force, focusing on Chemical Dependency, would be formed a couple of years later. Out of the dreaming and recommendations of these committees would spring robust programs— some of them immediately successful, others requiring one or more (sometimes painful) adjustments.

The chief medical officer presiding over all but three years of Penn Foundation's expansive second quarter-century was the indefatigable Dr. Vernon Kratz. His predecessor and mentor, Dr. Loux, stepped down as Medical Director on January 1, 1981. "I have given up my clinical administrative duties," the Foundation's sixty-two-year-old progenitor declared in a Winter 1981 *Horizons* article, as well as "the Chiefship of the Department of Psychiatry at Grand View Hospital." Dr. Loux would remain intimately involved in Penn Foundation, however, seeing patients in his new role as Senior Psychiatrist, and "leading in the development of a psychogeriatric service" (the latter responsibility devolving from his service as Chairman of the Older Adults Task Force). Dr. Kratz assumed the mantle of Medical Director at Penn Foundation as well as that of Chief Psychiatrist at Grand View, where he too would take his turn (in the mid-1980s) serving as President of the Hospital's Medical-Dental Staff.

A Quakertown "mini-clinic and drop-in center"

Dr. Kratz was a key player in the first expansion episode of Penn Foundation's second quarter-century, inaugurated just weeks after the Twenty-Fifth Anniversary Symposium. Having met periodically over the course of a year with Quakertown area residents and community leaders "very clear about their wanting to see an outpatient program developed in Quakertown by Penn Foundation" (as an adjunct to the inpatient program at Quakertown Hospital), Dr. Kratz and his colleagues on the "Ad Hoc Committee for Psychiatric Services for the Quakertown Area" organized the opening in November 1980 of the Foundation's first field office. Several rooms attached to Quakertown's First United Church of Christ became a Penn Foundation "mini-clinic and drop-in center" (as one journalist dubbed it) every Wednesday and Thursday, under the direction of recently-hired social worker Wayne R. Schantzenbach. The field office quickly became "like a second home to between 15 and 20 Upper Bucks residents who have chronic mental illnesses," the aforementioned journalist reported seven months after opening day. "[They] come to the drop-in center to have their medication checked, see a psychiatrist, or just to chat over coffee with staff members or other people who have similar problems. In the past, such people might have faced long periods of hospitalization. . . . Besides the drop-in center, an outpatient adult and child psychiatry clinic and a counseling and support program for drug and alcohol abuse are offered at the Quakertown location. Since those services began, 110 people have made use of them—many of them on a continuing basis."

A year into this venture, Penn Foundation's Quakertown clinic was in such demand that the service schedule was expanded from two days per week to five. In a local newspaper article announcing this development, the reporter noted that the number of patients seen weekly when the field office was open only two days per week had grown from forty-five in November 1980 to seventy-nine in November 1981. A month after office hours were stretched across the entire work week, the weekly patient count stood at 138. Foundation staff responsible for accommodating this population explosion were identified as follows:

> Team leader Wayne Schantzenbach is aided by other Penn Foundation staffers who share time between the Sellersville and Quakertown offices. Included is Dr. Vernon H. Kratz, medical director and psychiatrist for marital and family problems, drug and alcohol addiction, and parent-child relationships. Schantzenbach, who spends 40 hours a week at the Quakertown office, sees most of those with marital problems. Social worker Priscilla Crawford handles the drug and alcohol abuse program, including a group therapy session that has some 10 participants. Dr. John M. Dunn, a child psychiatrist, deals with child-parent relations. Sandra Trakat, a registered nurse, runs a one-hour-a-week program for chronic care patients with the help of Dr. Kratz and volunteers. This is for chronic patients not included in the active case load who drop in each week.

Day treatment activity back at the main office also spiked around this time, as Partial Hospital Program Director John Goshow increased the number of days each week Penn Foundation therapists worked with psychiatric patients from Grand View. As John explained in a recent interview:

> The Partial Hospital Program is a therapeutic day program for both patients living at home and hospitalized patients who

need more than outpatient treatment—more than, say, one hour of therapy once or twice a week. Some patients may be in the hospital, partly for their own protection, because they're really so sick that they can't be safely treated as outpatients. They spend their nights and weekends in the hospital, then come over to Penn Foundation certain days from nine in the morning till three in the afternoon for psychiatric evaluations, for their medications, for group therapy, occupational therapy, that kind of thing. I really think this is the best way to do it. It's *normalizing* for patients. They get out of their beds. They dress up. And over here we have more facilities for therapy than are available at the hospital.

When I became Director of the Partial Hospital Program in 1979, I was bringing between ten and twenty patients across the street on Tuesdays, Wednesdays, and Thursdays. Sometimes we walked, but that could be a little dangerous, so other times I drove a van. There were about five staff members to work with the patients. They did this three days a week, and spent the other two days planning and consulting. That was just the way things were set up, and everyone was comfortable with it. The staff paid more attention to individual patients that way. It meant that every Monday morning, for instance, all the doctors, all the social workers, all the clinicians could gather in the library to report and talk about patients that were in our care. It was really a good way of caring.

Well, as part of our financial recovery strategy, [Administrator] Henry Landes asked me to expand the Partial Program from three to five days per week. He was going to lots of meetings with other mental health organization administrators and hearing how their Partial Programs were doing well financially. Since we only had a three-day-a-week program, he figured there was potential there. So I turned it into a five-day program pretty quickly. It really irritated some of the staff. Their world changed dramatically. They were used to a more relaxed work environment. Those days were over. With those five staff members, or maybe one or two more, we bumped it up to five days per week, and soon increased the daily census to about forty-five patients. No one ever told me how much the Partial Program began contributing to our bottom line, but I have a feeling it was a pretty significant amount.

Two years down the road, Penn Foundation's Partial Hospital Program would be expanded again to accommodate "chronic mentally ill patients who need long-term care ranging from six months to two years," as Director Goshow explained in a July 1983 *Horizons* article. "We strive to help the patient understand and live realistically with his or her illness. We teach social skills to the patients, thus enabling them to widen their support system. And we support the patient's growth toward independence." When this article was published, twenty-eight patients had already enrolled in the new Continuing Care Partial Hospital Program.

"Financial recovery" and program expansion

Another economic boost was provided in the early 1980s through the development of an Employee Assistance Program (EAP). The most substantial product of the Business and Industry Task Force's work, this Program was initiated with part-time staffing in the fall of 1981. As future Program Director Bill Killgore related in a 2002 interview: "John Goshow, Karen Kern, and Henry Landes were instrumental in pushing the idea for Penn Foundation to develop an EAP. The Program is designed to extend counseling services directly to employees of companies with whom we contract, so it provides a more immediate reaction and response to individuals who are having difficulty. Plus, it makes entry into the system much easier, because we don't deal with insurance [paperwork]. There's really not a lot of red tape. It's purely an employer-paid benefit. That means it's relatively easy to get the people the assistance they need." The types of assistance provided through the EAP were described in a December 1981 newspaper account identifying Penn Foundation's first EAP client: Horace W. Longacre, Inc., a Mennonite family-owned poultry processing firm headquartered in Franconia Township:

> Kenneth A. Longacre, president of Horace W. Longacre, Inc., recently announced a new benefit for all Longacre employees and their immediate family members—an Employee Assistance Program. This is a program whereby Longacre employees and their immediate family members can receive short-term counseling, diagnostic and referral services

from a trained, professional employee counselor for personal problems such as alcoholism, drug abuse, and emotional stress. These counseling services will be paid by the Longacre Company. In announcing the program to employees, Longacre stated the Longacre Family is always concerned for the welfare of their employees, [and] recognizes [that] personal problems often prevent employees from successfully carrying out their jobs. The company also recognizes that many of these problems can be treated by existing medical and therapeutic methods. This Employee Assistance Program has been adopted to assure that through appropriate professional intervention, the employee will again be enabled to contribute to company goals.

In the coming months, other major employers in the area with strong Mennonite connections signed up for Penn Foundation's EAP program. Among them were Moyer Packing Company, Union National Bank, Bergey's Inc. (automotive sales and service), and Hatfield Packing Company (pork products). Significantly, the Presidents of both Moyer Packing Company and Union National Bank (Curt Moyer and Charles Hoeflich, respectively) were also Penn Foundation Directors. Hatfield Packing's Executive Vice-President John W. Clemens was appointed to the Foundation Board in June 1981. The EAP had grown so large by the close of 1982 that former intern Lesley McGarvey, having recently earned a Masters degree in counseling at Villanova University, was appointed full-time EAP Director. Under her supervision, and with a major impetus from Director of Marketing Carol Washko, the Program continued its steady ascent. A profile of the Foundation's EAP penned in 1995 would reveal that "57 satisfied client corporations" and "17,000 employees" were then being served. The Program's Director as of August 2002, Bill Killgore, noted that "we have contracts with about sixty-six different companies. Most of them have at least a headquarters in this region. About eighty-five to ninety percent of the employees are in Bucks, Montgomery, and Lehigh Counties. We also serve a relatively large population in northern New Jersey. Some are in New York, and out on Long Island. We work with one company that has a plant in Mexico, another in Missouri, and another in California. It's hard to say how many states we're in, because one of our larger companies has a sales force throughout the entire Midwest. We don't know where some employees are located until they call in. If they're in an area where we don't have a clinician, we go and find one. I've got three full-time staff members and four or five part-timers, and we all travel quite a bit."

While the Business and Industry Task Force was laying the groundwork for an Employee Assistance Program in the early 1980s, the Continuing Care Task Force was "reviewing the needs of psychiatric patients who require long-term support and medical supervision of psychotropic drugs" (as reported in the Winter 1980 *Horizons*). "Many of these patients have been hospitalized in a state institution or community hospital. A wide variety of community supports, including residential, vocational, and socialization, [are being] considered." The Task Force concentrated initially on meeting the most immediate need of clients with chronic mental health disabilities: dependable shelter. The committee applied for and received a grant in September 1980 that would fund the Foundation's leasing of apartments in the Sellersville area as accommodation for adults with long-term mental illness. The next step in establishing a "Community Residential Rehabilitation Program" (CRR) was the appointment of a Residential Coordinator (former caseworker Gloria Cocron, in December 1980) and

Each of the six task forces formed at the dawn of Penn Foundation's second quarter-century to identify and address unmet community needs spun off a new program. The principal product of the Business and Industry Task Force was an Employee Assistance Program (EAP), rolled out with part-time staffing in the fall of 1981. By the time this picture of EAP Counselor Peter Bullock meeting with human resources personnel was taken in 1988, the Program had become a full-time effort for several employees, and a dependable generator of revenue.

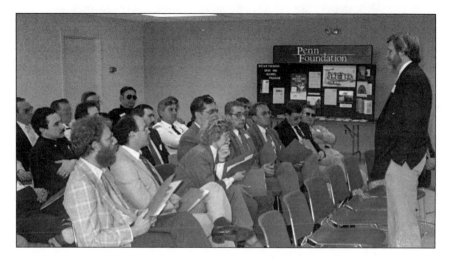

the forming of a "Continuing Care Team" comprising Cocron, Medical Director Vernon Kratz, Continuing Care Team Leader Karen Kern, Socialization Coordinator Sandee Trakat, and Case Manager Patricia Vandegrift. Under this Team's care, the first "minimum supervision" consumer moved into a Foundation-leased apartment in March 1981.

When Gloria Cocron left to take a position in the Lenape Valley Foundation's Maximum CRR program the following August, an experienced psychiatric counselor, case manager, and supervisor named Christine Shannon was hired to take her place. It was the beginning of another decades-long and immeasurably fruitful career at Penn Foundation. Reflecting recently on the this career—in the early stages of which she was promoted to CRR Program Director, and helped expand the Program to include "Moderate" and "Maximum" components as well as additional housing units in both Bucks and Montgomery Counties—Chris remarked:

> I only had one person on my staff when I started, and seven residents. Now we have twenty-one residents when all of our beds are full. We also serve around fifty active alumni. We lease two-bedroom apartments, and we have three people in each apartment. All of our consumers are residents of either Bucks or Montgomery County, and they all have some major form of mental illness, such as schizophrenia, schizo-affective disorder, bipolar disorder, major depression, border-line personality disorder, or dissociative identity disorder.
>
> When the Residential Program was getting started, we leased apartments in Sellersville, Perkasie, Telford, and Souderton. At first, we only had to work with draft licensing regulations from the State. But then they became formal regulations, and our program had to become licensed, and the apartments we leased had to be L&I approved. Only one of our landlords was willing to bring his apartment up to code. We had to move out of the other places. That's when we got into the Southgate apartment complex in Perkasie. One of Penn Foundation's Board members was Harold Gross of Fretz, Gross, and Spanninger Real Estate in Perkasie, the company that managed the Southgate Apartments. Some of the apartments had already been built, but others were still under construction. Through Harold's connection we were able to

move into a few new apartments. We gradually moved more of our program to Southgate, and we've been there ever since.

Chris and her staff added "Moderate Community Residential Rehabilitation" services to Penn Foundation's menu when the first Southgate units were occupied in November 1983. Two years later, the Foundation leased several more Southgate apartments and began offering "Maximum" CRR services. Caseworker Donna Duffy, on staff for less than a year, was promoted to Coordinator of the new department, which provided residents with a much higher degree of supervision, and thus required its own divisional Coordinator. Like the women who recommended her promotion (Chris Shannon and Continuing Care Team Leader Karen Kern), Donna would flourish in her elevated role, demonstrating executive skills that would earn her a promotion, five years down the road, to Director of Mental Health Case Management Services, and then to Rehabilitation Services Director in 1997. A glimpse into the work and mission of the CRR Program during Donna's term as Coordinator of Maximum services was published in a Foundation flyer in May 1990, under the title "Gretchen Finds a Supportive Place to Live." Key excerpts of the profile read as follows:

> In a dimly lit hotel room, Gretchen stares blankly at the bare walls. Instant soup is slowly heating on a hot plate. It's another night in an endless series of nights spent alone. At least tonight won't be so cold. There's a mattress and a donated blanket. She listens to her endless thoughts. It's the end of the week . . . $75.00 room rent paid today . . . $10.00 left for food this month . . . ration the milk . . . need meds . . . laid off job . . . no car . . . last pair of jeans ripped yesterday . . . the voices are coming back.
>
> In today's fast-paced world with its high-tech conveniences and quick fixes, the simple necessities of life are often taken for granted. For millions of persons with chronic mental health disabilities, however, meeting practical needs such as shelter can be an overwhelming and often an insurmountable task. These persons are not only faced with financial constraints and limited housing options but, in many cases, their disabilities have also precluded their development of the living skills necessary to successfully pursue and maintain a stable residence.

In response to this dilemma, the Penn Foundation founded a Community Residential Rehabilitation (CRR) Program in 1981. The purpose of the CRR Program is not only to provide housing but to create an atmosphere which facilitates skill growth and maximizes residents' potential to transition successfully to independent community living through instruction and support. Consumers in this program gain a sense of competence and confidence in their ability to lead meaningful lives as valued, contributing members of society. Further, since the program is based in local apartment complexes and offers three progressive levels of supervision, it provides a unique opportunity for persons to practice and integrate newly developed skills in a realistic setting while still living in a supportive community.

To live in the CRR Program is a participatory experience where the relationship between staff and residents is not one of teachers to students but rather persons to persons. This egalitarian atmosphere allows staff and residents to see beyond each other's limitations, promotes feelings of mutual respect and acceptance, and allows for individual growth. Along with these feelings, however, comes a shared sense of expectancy. Residents not only expect honesty and trustworthiness from staff and each other, but all persons are expected to be active members of the CRR community in whatever capacity they are able. Programmatic functioning is not meant to be a professional, administrative process but rather the personal responsibility and ownership of each member.

Another long-term expectancy of the CRR Program is increased participation in the larger community. Mental health disabilities, like many problems, often pull persons into themselves. Involvement in the community is not only a way to become more "other-centered" but it also assists residents in gaining a sense of giving back to the community. . . .

While the CRR Program is not appropriate for all persons with mental health disabilities, it is one viable alternative. For many, it is the first step in a life-long process of coping with their disabilities. It's a place to learn, a place to share, a place to come home.

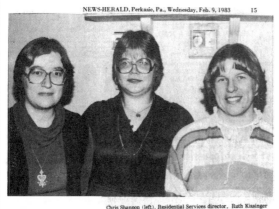

NEWS-HERALD, Perkasie, Pa., Wednesday, Feb. 9, 1983   15

Residential Instructors

Chris Shannon (left), Residential Services director, Ruth Kissinger (center) and Patricia Gordon (right), residential instructors, provide supervision to Penn Foundation for Mental Health's newly established Moderate Supervision Residential Program. Housing for six individuals and their supervisor have recently been obtained for the program which assists persons in learning to live independently within the community.

Penn Foundation Photo

Penn Foundation Announces New Program

It could be said that the history of Penn Foundation has been published in Perkasie's *News-Herald*— one article or press release at a time, over the course of fifty years. In the February 9, 1983 issue, the Foundation's "recently opened Moderate Supervision Residential Program" was given a quarter-page of coverage, including a photo of Residential Services Director Chris Shannon (on left) with Residential Instructors Ruth Kissinger and Patricia Gordon.

More Task Force fallout

The work of the Churches and Pastors Task Force culminated in the establishment of a Pastoral Services Institute in October 1981. This program launch coincided with the hiring of Lamont A. Woelk—a Mennonite pastor with twenty-seven years' experience as a pastoral counselor, including a recent stint at Brook Lane Psychiatric Center—to serve as Pastoral Services Institute Director. The mission of the Institute was "to train pastors of the Pennridge, Quakertown, Souderton-Telford, and Upper Perkiomen area in providing pastoral care, a term used to describe the spiritual support pastors give when individuals or families have emotional and spiritual problems," according to a newspaper article published several months after Lamont's arrival. The article continued:

> Those problems include ministering to a family after a relative dies, making hospital visits, marital counseling, visiting shut-ins and occasionally intervening in a crisis situation such as a suicide attempt. [Director] Woelk called pastors the "front line of defense" in the community. He said the pastors are the people to whom fifty percent of the population go to first for help. Pastors who are highly-trained in pastoral care can sometimes eliminate the need for a person to visit a

psychiatrist or psychologist, such as those at the Penn Foundation, or can refer people to the proper mental health care personnel, Woelk said last week. . . . "When a person gets sick, he goes to a general practitioner first, not a specialist," he said. "When a person has a problem, the first person he goes to see usually is a pastor."

Using practical workshop training rather than academic training often provided at theological seminaries, the Institute intends to bring in experts in the health care field, including medical doctors and psychiatrists, to train pastors. And the Institute will bring together pastors to share their knowledge about pastoral care. Pastors will witness each other administering pastoral care in clinical settings and evaluate each other, Woelk said. Pastors usually administer pastoral care without other pastors present, so they have doubts whether they are performing properly; thus bringing pastors together for workshops would be helpful. . . . "Most of the pastors have the right hunches about providing pastoral care, but they're simply guessing sometimes. They often have the most difficult experiences ministering to children," Woelk said. "A pastor knows what to say to an adult, but what do you say to a child?"

Woelk, who worked with the mentally-ill at Topeka State Hospital in Kansas, said pastors sometimes have difficulty ministering to the mentally ill. "Pastors who were very capable preachers in other settings were scared to death in the wards," he said. Pastors' main strengths in pastoral care often are called upon during a family's bereavement, Woelk said. "That's the kind of thing that hits a pastor squarely," he said. "It hits them early in their career." Although pastoral training programs date back to 1925, Penn Foundation's Institute is unique because it has broad-based community involvement, Woelk said. The Institute is operated by the Penn Foundation, but a community committee advises the Foundation. A representative from five area ministeriums and Grand View and Quakertown Hospitals sit on the committee.

Before the Pastoral Services Institute was a year old, Director Woelk earned certification as an Acting Supervisor by the Association for Clinical Pastoral Education, authorizing him to add Clinical Pastoral Education

(CPE) to the Institute's program. CPE was described in Penn Foundation's *1983–84 Annual Report* as "training for pastors and seminary students, designed both to give an understanding of and support pastoral care. 'Pastoral care involves giving people a religious perspective for looking at and dealing with problems,' says Rev. Woelk. 'During CPE, clergy learn to be better givers of pastoral care by ministering in the hospitals, where there is a constant need.' During the past year, Grand View and Quakertown Hospitals have welcomed Rev. Woelk and the CPE students as team members who can make a special contribution to health care. 'Both hospitals and pastors strive to bring soundness and health to other people. Through CPE, patients begin to consider their emotional and spiritual as well as physical needs. We try to integrate all the elements that make up a healthy person into the healing process.' Directing CPE also means being a teacher, and Rev. Woelk guides his students with the same care and understanding he encourages them to learn. [His] high regard for people is a reflection of Penn Foundation's dedication to sharing treatment of 'whole people' throughout the community."

Bump in the road

In his message "From the Medical Director" in the *1983–84 Annual Report*, Dr. Kratz reaffirmed his commitment to a building program more ambitious than any yet attempted in the Foundation's forty-year history. Plans developed by Dr. Kratz, Administrator Henry Landes, new Board President Charles Hoeflich, and other members of the Long-Range Planning Committee called for nothing less than construction of a $6.5 million, fifty-bed, 35,000-square-foot psychiatric hospital on a twenty-three-acre tract just south of the Foundation's Lawn Avenue complex. The inpatient facility would be "a product of a cooperative alliance between Penn Foundation, Grand View, North Penn, Quakertown, and Doylestown Hospitals," Dr. Kratz explained, "and it will be called Penn Foundation Hospital Associates. Expanding our services to include a state-of-the-art psychiatric care facility will complete the continuum of care we now offer. The new hospital will enable us to address a much broader range of mental health concerns than in the past. A hospital designed to provide the best physical environment for patient care also means an experienced staff entirely devoted to caring for patients with psychiatric illness. Now, with the cooperation of these four area hospitals, we are extending our same high quality of service to an entire region."

More than two years of negotiating and planning had already been lavished on the hospital project by the close of 1983. Excitement had been building with each major stride: the filing of a letter of intent with the Health Systems Agency of Southeastern Pennsylvania in April 1983; the presentation of construction plans to West Rockhill Township the following June; the securing of Township approval in August; the submission of an application for a Certificate of Need from the Pennsylvania Department of Health, first by Penn Foundation alone, then in partnership with the four area hospitals. In the latter application, the signatories cited the "need to provide comprehensive psychiatric treatment services in the area," and stressed that "the five sponsors [would] have a shared responsibility for all community mental health center services now provided by the Foundation and the new hospital" (as reported in a February 1984 newspaper article). Designed to "include a chemical dependency unit along with a general psychiatric unit," the proposed facility would "not eliminate the need for approved psychiatric beds, which exist at Doylestown and Quakertown hospitals."

When this article was published, Foundation officials predicted construction of the psychiatric hospital could begin "as early as August." "We were quite optimistic," Dr. Kratz confirmed two decades later, adding:

> We went to all kinds of hearings—in Philadelphia, in Harrisburg—covering all the bases. We had legislative people involved. We had bylaws written. We had the Board composition worked out. Each hospital and the Foundation was going to have a certain number of representatives on the Board. We really took this project right up to the threshold of breaking ground.
>
> And then—I'll never forget it—we had a final hearing with the Secretary of Health [in May 1985]. We made this elaborate presentation using all kinds of drawings. I mean, this thing took a lot of energy! When we finished, he said (and I can still almost hear him say these words), "You know, this is really a wonderful idea. But I can't approve funding for it. There are already enough beds available at Grand View, and North Penn, and Doylestown. Take this idea and your cooperative spirit, and put them to use in one of those hospitals, in an *existing* structure."

That was it. The project was done. There was no way to appeal.

Talk about disappointment! We went into a sort of institutional depression when we had to withdraw our application. As I look back on it now, though, I think it was a godsend that we didn't proceed. The method of medical care reimbursement had just been changed. Instead of getting paid retrospectively for services, hospitals were getting paid *prospectively*. So if a patient came in with pneumonia, for instance, the hospital would get paid $5,000 regardless of how long the patient stayed in the hospital. Under those conditions, hospitals started discharging patients earlier. All of a sudden Grand View's occupancy, which had been around 105 percent, dropped to 85 percent. The same thing happened at the other hospitals. That's why the Secretary of Health turned down our application to add fifty beds to the mix. And it's probably a good thing he did. If we had built our hospital under those circumstances, it could have been a financial disaster, especially with competition for patients really starting to intensify.

BreakThrough

Out of the ashes of the psychiatric hospital plan rose a building project of smaller dimensions, but still carrying significant financial risk. Indeed, the phoenix-like emergence of a new expansion strategy in the mid-1980s would come to appear, for several unnerving years, like a proverbial jump from the frying pan into the fire. The focus of the revised scheme was Penn Foundation's Drug and Alcohol Program, an array of control and rehabilitation services rolled out in the summer of 1985 after three years of planning by the Chemical Dependency Task Force. Under newly-appointed program director Elizabeth F. Reach and clinical director Dr. Mark H. Bernstein (the Foundation's Assistant Medical Director since January 1984), the D&A Program partnered with Grand View Hospital to make a six-bed unit in the Hospital available for patients in need of detoxification and rehabilitation therapy. The six-day program of treatment—given the modernistic moniker "BreakThrough" in February 1986—included daily therapy across the street at Penn Foundation. Had the Foundation's drive to build a psychiatric hospital on the east side of Lawn Avenue not been halted, BreakThrough clients (and all other patients needing inpatient psychiatric services) would have been given beds in that new facility.

The fifty-bed hospital dream had been dashed, but the prospect of more fully integrating psychiatric services—and tapping into a reliable revenue stream—continued to energize Foundation officers. That potential, they concluded, might still be at least partly realized through the construction of a smaller inpatient facility, built specifically for the BreakThrough program. To test the waters for such a project, Penn Foundation launched an aggressive promotional campaign in the summer of 1986, orchestrated by Henry Landes and Community Relations Director David Birkey. A series of newspaper advertisements, public service radio announcements, and visits with corporate executives in markets from Philadelphia to Allentown attracted the desired attention. Monthly D&A admissions at Grand View Hospital jumped from the low thirties to the mid forties. Convinced that BreakThrough's profile was sufficiently elevated, Penn Foundation officials hired a new program director, Frank R. King, in April 1987, and announced plans to build a twenty-three-bed D&A residential rehabilitation center in the field behind their headquarters. They broke ground for the $1 million, 10,750-square-foot facility the following September.

Raising construction funds and building the BreakThrough Center turned out to be relatively easy tasks compared with the challenge of establishing within the new structure a program that would at least pay for itself, let alone generate much-needed revenue. It was something of an ill omen when Henry Landes—the Foundation's first Vice President following an executive reorganization in January 1988—resigned a couple of weeks after the June 12, 1988 BreakThrough Center Dedication. On a much-needed post-Dedication vacation, Henry had decided the time had come for him to launch his own consulting business. It would fall to Dr. Kratz—now serving as the Foundation's President and CEO—and newly-appointed Vice President and Administrator John Goshow to preside over the deployment of the BreakThrough Center. They were in for a rocky ride. Several years and several changes in program leadership would be required to get the Center on course for profitability, as recalled by current Drug and Alcohol Services Director J. Todd Barlow in a 2002 interview:

> I started working at Penn Foundation as an intern in April
> 1987, and I became an outpatient drug and alcohol counselor
> the following January. The outpatient program was located in

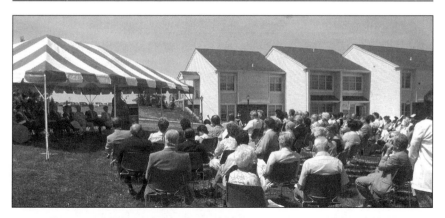

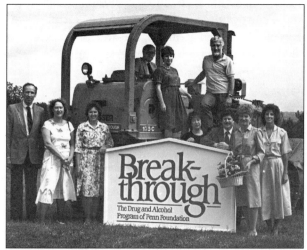

Ten hectic-but-hopeful months transpired between the September 10, 1987 groundbreaking ceremony for the BreakThrough Center (left) and dedication exercises held on the lawn in front of the new facility on June 12, 1988 (above). Among the many groupings of staff, building project personnel, and well-wishers posing around the ceremonial bulldozer at the groundbreaking was this collection of employees comprising (from left, on lawn): Gerald O'Brien, Karen Schmoyer, Sandy Landis, Pat Trauger, Mickey Bernstein, Peg Emerick, Donna Duffy-Bell; (on bulldozer) Bob Ferrell, Pat Vandegrift, and Art Isaak.

the long building at the southern end of the campus [one of the two former Pennridge Medical Arts buildings purchased by Penn Foundation in the fall of 1983]. Frank King was the D&A Director at that time. He had developed our outpatient program where clients would be able to go to work during the day, then come in for therapy three or four nights a week. They would stay in the program for three or four weeks and then phase down into an aftercare program. There were no inpatient accommodations yet. We were in the process of building the inpatient facility. There was lot of hope and energy, because the inpatient program was going to feed the intensive outpatient program. The new building was envisioned purely as an inpatient building, and we were going to run the outpatient services down where we were.

This was the heyday of the D&A treatment world. There had been a boom during the Seventies and Eighties in the development of twenty-eight-day inpatient D&A programs. The insurance companies basically paid for everything, so it could be very lucrative. If someone looked like they needed the program, his insurance company would cover the full twenty-eight days of treatment. Well, all of a sudden things started to get out of control financially, and insurance companies began developing more of a "managed care" mindset. They began to limit how long a person could stay in treatment, rather than automatically pay for twenty-eight days. That switch occurred just as we were building the Break-Through Center.

We never saw it coming. In the first months that the Center was open, we had censuses of three, or five, or maybe ten patients—in a twenty-three-bed facility! You can imagine that within six months we were starting to get a little scared. And then, within a year the Center had lost a significant amount of money. Penn Foundation wasn't that large, and when they took this jump into inpatient services, they were thinking the program would be able to pay for itself very quickly. That clearly wasn't happening. I still have employees who remember having only two or three clients in there during the Christmas season. Here was this big building, and only two clients! Those were some scary times.

Frank King left after about a year. Things didn't get much better under the new Director, and he only stayed a year. It was during that time [1989] that we moved the outpatient program up to the inpatient facility. We did it out of a desperation, but in hindsight it was a brilliant move. It set the stage for our turnaround.

I had been moving into an outpatient coordinator position, and Kathy Wisser was more or less running the inpatient program on a day-to-day basis. When the second Director left,

Kathy and I became interim overseers of our departments. There was not a big hurry to hire a Director, because the census was so light. Well, that's when Kathy and I really began to talk and work together as a team. We realized we had to give up hope on the fully-insured population. All the other rehabs catering to insured patients were seeing their censuses drop.

We had just signed fee-for-service contracts with a couple of counties to provide inpatient care to uninsured D&A clients. They were trying to move people out of the incredibly expensive hospital detox units into non-hospital facilities, which were much more economical. At the time, we didn't really see these new contracts as a priority, because they didn't generate as much revenue as the insurance system. But we got to thinking: maybe we should concentrate on serving uninsured and disadvantaged populations. We've certainly learned how to run an economical program. So we went out and visited county referrals, and told them how we were approaching inpatient treatment. They liked it. They began referring people to us, and we handled them well. As we made more and more contracts with more and more counties, our census began to increase. After about four or five years we were averaging eighteen patients per day, up from twelve.

As competition increased, we needed an even more refined niche. Kathy and I were debating what this should be, and I said, "Look, Penn Foundation has been about mental health for thirty-five years. Why not use our strength and specialize in dual-diagnosis, which involves both mental health and drug and alcohol treatment?" The dual-diagnosed patient is someone with a primary addiction as well as a serious emotional problem—maybe depression, or a thought disorder, or even a personality disorder. Kathy and I continued our debate, but eventually we began to cater more and more to dual-diagnosed clients. The counties noticed that we were getting pretty good at it. They also liked that we were right next to a hospital, so if a patient needed medical attention, he could be sent to the hospital right away. The fact that we'd been handling psychiatric care here at Penn Foundation for many years meant we could tap into a great wealth of experience. That really helped us move into the dual-diagnosis niche. We contracted with more and more counties. We now have contracts with about thirteen different counties, and we drive as far as two hours away to pick up clients.

After four straight years in the red, Penn Foundation's finances crept back into black in 1992, as the D&A program approached its own economic "breakthrough." That terminology was no longer current, however. Back in November 1989, when the inpatient program—and perhaps the fate of Penn Foundation itself—appeared to be hanging in the balance, the "BreakThrough" label had been scrapped in favor of the more business-like "Recovery Center." That turned out to be the first of many steps in the right direction for the infant program, which would "break through" to its own balanced budget for the first time in 1994.

10

RESILIENCE

The financial crisis of the late 1980s and early 90s did not prohibit Penn Foundation from cultivating new ground. The organization was committed to meeting the behavioral health needs of its catchment areas, and that meant adapting or expanding services as new needs were identified or existing needs intensified. Economic viability was a key concern as the Foundation felt its way into an uncertain future, but decisions regarding program adjustments or expansion would continue to be made within the larger mission-oriented framework of "community service."

So even while the Recovery Center's shaky launch was weighing on the budget, several major initiatives were pushed forward, two of them involving facilities located some distance from the Penn Foundation campus. The "Penn Gardens" building project on the southern outskirts of Sellersville even carried a hefty million-dollar-plus price tag. The lion's share of the tab was picked up, however, by a federal agency, and the way was further paved by a sympathetic landowner. Who were Penn Foundation's partners in the Penn Gardens venture? The Department of Housing and Urban Development (HUD) and the Rockhill Mennonite (retirement) Community—strange bedfellows, in the eyes of some observers. The creative collaboration of these three service-oriented parties resulted in the construction of two one-story apartment buildings on a 2.84-acre parcel off Route 309, each building containing ten one-bedroom units. The accommodations were designed, in the words of a *News-Herald* reporter, "to provide long-term housing for those with mental disorders capable of living on their own, but unable to afford housing in the area." HUD covered a million dollars in construction costs, while Rockhill Mennonite Community agreed to lease the site to Penn Foundation for $1 per year.

That still left the project about $100,000 short of full financing. The challenge of closing that gap fell mostly to Vice President and Administrator John Goshow. "We ended up getting a loan from the Pennsylvania Housing Finance Authority," he would later recall, "and some from [a couple of private benefactors]. I applied for a grant from the Grundy Foundation, and they pitched in. We also got some assistance from a Bucks County Development Block grant. It took a number of sources to finally get that project done."

Upon its opening in the spring of 1992, Penn Gardens became "home" for almost all the alumni of Penn Foundation's Minimum Supervision Community Residential Rehabilitation Program, which ceased operations with the opening of Penn Gardens. Funds previously used for housing these residents in scattered apartments were now available for developing an alumni program.

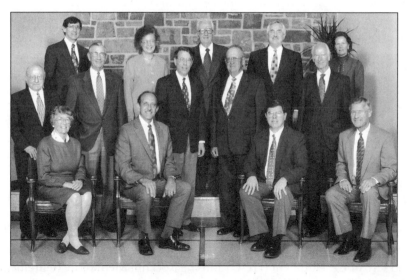

Expanded from fifteen to eighteen members in the fall of 1988, the Penn Foundation Board of Directors comprised fourteen regular members and four Directors Emeritus when this portrait was taken for inclusion in 1995's Fortieth Anniversary flyer. Three of the regular members in this photograph had been with the Foundation since its inception (their names are marked with an asterisk). The Directors are (seated, from left) Secretary Dorothy M. Williams of Quakertown, Chairman Thomas K. Leidy of Souderton, Vice Chairman David G. Landis of Telford, Treasurer Merrill S. Moyer of Souderton; (standing) Elvin R. Souder* of Souderton, Dr. Ronald Souder of Sellersville, John W. Clemens of Hatfield, Carol Washko of Hatfield, Member-at-Large Dr. J. Phillip Moyer of Green Lane, Dr. Norman L. Loux* of Souderton, Member-at-Large Harold M. Mininger* of Telford, Mark G. Garis of Souderton, Curtis F. Moyer of Harleysville, and Elizabeth B. Meredith of Quakertown. Directors Emeritus in the fall of 1995 were Charles H. Hoeflich, L. Ruby Horwood, Russell M. Moyer, and Paul F. Souder.

Simultaneous with the opening of Penn Gardens was the re-activation of Penn Foundation's Mental Retardation Case Management program, dormant since Bucks County had transferred MR Case Management responsibilities from the Foundation to the new Community Foundation for Human Development back in 1979. Now, in March 1992, the County was ready to return responsibility for this service to the organization that had played a leading role in its early development. Reflecting on the significance of this reunion in a note to the author a dozen years after the fact, Director of Rehabilitation Services Donna Duffy-Bell would observe:

> Because Community Foundation for Human Development (now known as LifePath) was a provider of direct services to persons with developmental disabilities, and to avoid the perception of a conflict of interest, MR Case Management services were returned to Penn Foundation when Early Intervention services were first offered in Bucks County through the Office of Mental Retardation. Early Intervention services are state-mandated services for children from birth to three years of age who exhibit at least a twenty-five percent developmental delay in physical or cognitive functioning. When it rejoined Penn Foundation in March 1992, the MR/EI department, with a staff of five, was housed in an office on West Market Street in Perkasie. The department was re-located in 2000 to join Mental Health Case Management at 712 Lawn Avenue, just south of the Grand View Hospital campus. Today, Penn Foundation enjoys a reputation as a premier provider in Bucks County of MR/EI Case Management services (now known as "supports coordination services"). A sixteen-person staff delivers these services to over five hundred consumers each year.

In a broader, philosophical context, the return of MR Case Management services to Penn Foundation in 1992 was a reflection of parallel paradigm shifts in mental health and mental retardation service delivery. Following the deinstitutionalization movement of the 1970s and 80s, the focus of both mental health and mental retardation service providers shifted away from *disabilities* and *segregation* toward *functioning* and *community integration*. Just as people with mental health disorders were being discharged from state hospitals, people with developmental disabilities were being discharged from intensive care facilities for the mentally retarded. Through Medical Assistance waiver funding, services and supports were made available to these people in their homes and natural community environments, rather than solely through agency site-based programs. The delivery of Mental Retardation Case Management services and the implementation of Early Intervention services in the early 1990s reflected a recognition that people with developmental disabilities have a right to live "everyday lives." Rooted in the concept of self-determination, an "everyday life" is a life filled with choices and opportunities to have and do ordinary things that people without disabilities take for granted. The vision for people with developmental disabilities was no longer that they merely *live* in the community but that they meaningfully and actively *participate* in it.

It was a similar vision that had led over a decade earlier to the development of Community Residential Rehabilitation programs for people with mental disorders. After that came the realization that CRR programs and traditional treatments

---

The Mental Health Case Management staff nearly doubled during its first sixteen months back under Penn Foundation's umbrella (March 1992 through August 1993). Posing on the porch of the multi-purpose farmhouse in the latter month are (front row, from left) Rhonda Krolikowski, Stephanie Degaitis, Kelly McGuire, Cindy Moyer, (rear) Donna Duffy-Bell, Vince Grimm, Melanie Masin-Moyer, and Gayl Brunk. Not pictured is Germaine Hornig.

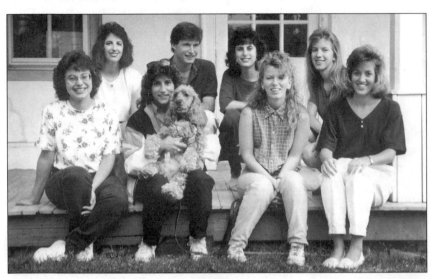

could not be the only community-based rehabilitation options for people with serious and persistent mental illnesses. Some of these people could not access the programs because of long waiting lists. Others didn't *want* access to such programs, and still others had needs that couldn't be met by such programs. There was also widespread recognition of something that Penn Foundation long held as a philosophical tenet: the importance of the home environment in treating mental health problems. CRR and traditional treatment programs could not be the be-all and end-all of people's recovery options. There was thus a state-wide and a national shift toward providing rehabilitative services to people in their homes and natural environments (such as schools). There was recognition that community support, resource acquisition and coordination, and continuity of supportive staff relationships with people with mental illness and their families was imperative if people were truly going to be empowered to live successfully in the community and have an enhanced quality of life.

Penn Foundation had its finger on the pulse of this shift, which was also highly congruent with our philosophical roots. We participated fully in the development and implementation of Mental Health Targeted Case Management (TCM)—that is, Intensive Case Management (ICM), introduced in 1988, and Resource Coordination in 1993. This was one of the pivotal periods in the Foundation's history, as it was in the State and nation's behavioral healthcare history. It laid the groundwork here at Penn Foundation for the development of services to people in their homes and natural environments, including Wraparound [discussed below], Mobile Engagement Services, Rehab At Home, and Family-Based Services. Major contributors to the proliferation of ICM services at Penn Foundation were Germaine Hornig (the first full-time ICM staff member) and Stephanie Degaitis, who joined the staff in 1990 and remains a TCM supervisor today. Our Mental Health Case Management staff has grown from five persons in 1992 to twenty-three in 2005.

A few months after Penn Foundation resumed administration of MR/El Case Management for Bucks County in the spring of 1992 came another stirring announcement. Plans for a "psychosocial clubhouse"—germinating at the Foundation ever since an Administrative Committee brainstorming session back in 1979—were about to blossom thanks to a $190,000, two-year development grant awarded to the Foundation by the Philadelphia-based Pew Charitable Trusts. When the first installment of this funding was made available early in 1993, Foundation officials hired Lucille Mauro, a native Philadelphian who had spent nearly a decade working in "clubhouse" settings in the City, to serve as the Foundation's first Clubhouse Director. As Lu recalled in a 2002 interview:

> From 1988 through 1993 I had worked at the Open Door Clubhouse operated by Co-MAHR in the Kensington section of Philadelphia. This was the first Fountain House-style clubhouse in the City. The original Fountain House was established in 1948 in New York City by former patients of Rockland State Hospital. It was truly visionary, and it really grew over the years. There are about seven hundred members of that program today. They tried to proliferate this model throughout the U.S., but like a lot of innovative ideas, it had some economic and systemic structures that made it hard to push forward in many settings. That's what happened here in Pennsylvania. A few groups tried to start clubhouses, and squeeze in ideas from the New York model, but they never really took off because the public funding was more limited here. Most of the money in Pennsylvania was going to mental health initiatives with a strong medical orientation, not to programs aimed at social or vocational rehabilitation.
>
> Then, in the 1980s, new medications were becoming available that could stabilize people for longer periods of time, and allow them to function at a higher level. At the same time they were closing down state mental hospitals. I was working at the Open Door Clubhouse when Byberry [a.k.a. Philadelphia State Hospital] started closing its doors [in the late 1980s]. Here was this major metropolitan hospital releasing severely institutionalized individuals into the community. It was a *very* challenging time. There were some structured housing programs and some residential rehabilitation programs, but clubhouse programs were particularly appealing to these individuals because a lot of them didn't necessarily fit well into

traditional Partial Hospital programs where they would be expected to go and talk in groups or participate in group therapy, that kind of thing. So a lot of these people started coming to our Open Door Clubhouse in the late 1980s and early 90s. It was just a whirlwind of activity.

Part of being a Director of a Fountain House-style clubhouse is being trained at the original Fountain House. You go there for three weeks and you get immersed in the program, which has a very specific philosophy and a way of working with people. It was really transformative for me to be up there in Manhattan with those folks who were so incredibly passionate about what they were doing. They were really zealous, and I liked that a lot. I like having a specific philosophy and mission. That way you always know where you're going. I've seen some programs that aren't sure where they're going, and they get kind of lost from not having a focus.

Penn Foundation really picks up on things that are cutting-edge. Long before I came along, they had gone up to Fountain House to see the program. Board members went up, and family members of some of the potential consumers of the program went up. They all decided they wanted this type of program at Penn Foundation, and they had started raising money for it. That's a big reason why I applied for the Director position. I wanted to be part of a program that involves certification and training, and has a lot of integrity.

When I was hired in May 1993, they said, "You have $190,000 over the next two years. You have to find a building, hire the staff, purchase everything." So it was really neat. At the time, the Continuing Care Team was really moving the project along. Just like the Fountain House folks, they could see that clients were recovering, remaining stable, and now they needed something more to help them regain their ability to function and have a regular life. So I joined the Continuing Care Team. I asked them to recommend some consumers who would be interested in helping me create the program. Right from the beginning I tried to establish the idea that consumers and staff would work on this together (we actually call clubhouse consumers "members" because it's like they're members of a club—a totally destigmatizing way of thinking about it). They recommended five consumers and we started meeting twice a week—looking for buildings, devising plans, going to seminars, and educating everybody on campus about the Fountain House model. It was pretty challenging, but there's always a lot of support around here.

Then something sort of providential happened. We were looking at a house down along Lawn Avenue, and we went to a zoning hearing where the neighbors were very concerned about us putting in a parking lot down there. And one of the women there said, "Why don't you ask Grand View Hospital if you can use their farmhouse up there on the old Stump farm?" [Grand View had recently acquired this property, comprising a two-story farmhouse and accompanying barn on a large tract of land bounded by Lawn Avenue and the Route 309 Expressway, for storage and potential expansion purposes.] So John [Goshow] called up [Hospital President] Stewart Fine, and Stewart said "Sure you can use it. We'll lease it to you for a dollar a year. Do whatever you need to with it." The house was pretty dirty, because it hadn't been used lately, and it was full of medical equipment. But you could immediately see it had potential. It was so homey. It had a kitchen and a beautiful community room. Clean it up, and it would be just perfect.

The Pew Charitable Trust has a rule about their money, that it cannot be used for capital or anything like that. You cannot purchase or renovate buildings. Because we were using this property for free, they permitted us to use some of the money to upgrade the house. We had to widen doors for wheelchair accessibility. We had to put in a ramp to make at least the first floor accessible. There were other kinds of licensing and inspection kinds of improvements. We also had to get permission from West Rockhill Township to do this. They were very open to what we had planned. We also worked with the Bucks and Montgomery County offices of Mental Health and Mental Retardation, which provided additional funding for operations.

We had a contest to name the Clubhouse, and one of our members came up with the winner: "Wellspring." We opened in April 1994, and within four months we had about forty-five members. Now [in August 2002] we have about seventy-five. It's just been awesome to see people with severe and persistent mental illnesses being completely integrated into the community. We have employment programs and all sorts of things to help them get back into their normal roles— going back to school or getting a job or returning to being a parent. In some ways Wellspring is like a lot of other clubs, like a veterans' club with a lunch program and a newswire. Our club happens to be for people who share the experience of having a mental illness. Our members come into a completely non-judgmental environment where they don't have to recount their history and all their problems and all their failures and all their delusions. They're asked to come and tell us what they can do. We focus on their talents and strengths and abilities. We ask, "Can you cook? Can you clean? Can you garden? Can you enter data into a computer? What can we teach you? What interests do you have?" And then the Clubhouse is organized into departments that focus on specific skills. We have kitchen and agriculture maintenance, clerical, education and employment. The people gravitate to the

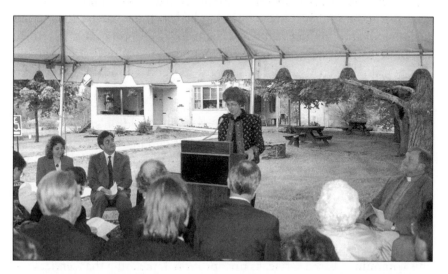

Continuing Care Team Leader Karen Kern takes a turn at the podium during the dedication of the Wellspring Clubhouse in April 1994. Awaiting their chance to address the audience gathered in front of the renovated farmhouse are (seated on left) Vice President and Administrator John Goshow and Clubhouse Director Lucille Mauro.

departments in the Clubhouse that interest them. They do real work that contributes to the running of the Clubhouse, not pretend work. They really enter data. They really cook lunch. They don't just talk in a group about nutrition—they *cook a nutritious lunch*, which is completely different. We ask them to expand their comfort zone from "talking" to "doing." And we hope that action begets more action, generates more energy until pretty soon they're focusing on what's right and good about themselves.

Director of Rehabilitation Services Donna Duffy-Bell points out that "the introduction of Clozaril in the early 1990s enabled people with long-term mental illness not only to live successfully and more independently in the community but to begin to develop interests in the vocational, educational, social, and advocacy aspects of their lives. They began to have a real voice, which allowed them to direct the evolution of programs. That was the basis for the development of Wellspring Clubhouse. As one former Penn Gardens resident put it, Clozaril had caused an awakening in him, a feeling that he was 'all dressed up with no place to go.' Cutting-edge medication, integration into the community, and consumer empowerment through services like the Clubhouse had given him the ability to start seeing beyond his illness, and kindled in him a desire for a more meaningful and productive life." Recognizing Wellspring's role in returning hope to persons with long-term mental illness, the Pew Charitable Trusts has renewed its Clubhouse grant to Penn Foundation every two years for ten years running.

The Foundation's other major program launch of the early 1990s was also enthusiastically received. Rolled out by the Children's Unit in 1993, Wraparound Services "represented the latest trend in children's behavioral healthcare services," according to a brief description published in Penn Foundation's Fortieth Anniversary flyer (1995). The explanation continued: "Working closely with school districts which identify 'at risk' youngsters, Wraparound adopts a highly individualized approach which addresses each of the life domain needs of children from birth to age 21. Utilizing an empowerment approach which focuses on a child's strengths, this community-based service is unconditional, meaning that services are never denied because of severity or circumstance. The child benefits from the services of a community team which includes, at a minimum, the child's parents, school personnel, community support agencies and Penn

Foundation professionals. Services include, but are not limited to, intensive one-to-one interventions in community settings, behavioral consultations, 'mobile' psychotherapy, creative arts therapies, and school-based interventions."

Wraparound Services were initially offered only to residents of Bucks and Montgomery Counties, and its charter staff worked out of an office in one of the former Pennridge Medical Arts buildings. As Wraparound proved its worth, however, school superintendents in adjoining Philadelphia, Berks, and Lehigh Counties took note and asked Penn Foundation to expand its coverage into their districts. Foundation officials complied, establishing a Wraparound office in a school building in Red Hill Borough for the Upper Perkiomen School District in the winter of 1994-95. Then, as John Goshow related in a 2002 interview, Penn Foundation was "invited to go out to the Reading area and help them start their own Wraparound program. They didn't have anything like that in Berks County. So one of our employees went out there and trained their people. Since we had a presence there and already had a couple of clients in the area, we decided to open a satellite office [in Sinking Spring, outside Reading]. After a while we had a number of clinicians working there."

The seduction of satellites

Over the course of several years in the mid-1990s, Penn Foundation added half-a-dozen outpatient clinics to its stable of satellite facilities. This piecemeal expansion was part of a broader strategy to keep the organization afloat—and perhaps even sail it briskly onward—in seas churned up by the "managed care" tempest. Private health care insurers faced with skyrocketing costs were abandoning the traditional fee-for-service practice—by which health care providers billed patients or their insurance companies for each service provided—in favor of alternative coverages known collectively as "managed care." Where conventional insurance plans simply underwrote whatever treatments doctors prescribed for their patients, the new forms of coverage were designed to encourage "wellness" or "health maintenance," recognizing that it is much less expensive to prevent an illness than it is to treat it. Under managed care contracts, insurers paid primary care providers a specific amount every month for each client enrolled in a coverage plan. It was then up to the providers to deliver or coordinate the delivery of all health care services required by plan participants.

Private insurers—many of them constituted as "Health Maintenance Organizations" or HMOs—led the charge in the managed care revolution, but state governments eventually also turned to managed care to help with the Medicaid program, and the federal government ultimately introduced a managed form of Medicare. Amid the restructurings, new health care contracts worth many millions of dollars were put up for grabs, and medical organizations were forced to react. Much could be gained from playing ball with insurance companies and government agencies. Indeed, smaller providers like Penn Foundation had to wonder if they could even *survive* without doing so. Director of Rehabilitation Services Donna Duffy-Bell remembers the industry-wide mindset of "wanting to be ready for managed care, and thinking that if you weren't a big provider—if you weren't able to get all of these managed care contracts—you were either going to get sucked up by a bigger organization, or you'd go bankrupt. So we were trying to be pro-active at Penn Foundation. We wanted to be aggressive in the managed care market."

That eagerness dovetailed nicely, it turned out, with the desire of the region's largest insurers to give Penn Foundation as much behavioral healthcare work as it wanted. Medical Director Vernon Kratz remembers officials of US Healthcare, Keystone East, and Allegheny Health System (to name some of the major players) approaching the Foundation and saying "Hey, you people do good work! You really ought to get involved with us. Why don't you take over this contract [for mental health services under our managed care plan]?" This succession of overtures "looked to us like a tremendous opportunity," Dr. Kratz would later recall. "We thought, 'Hey, we've really earned our standing in the marketplace. This is something we can do!' So we were seduced into opening up satellite operations around the region—first in Newtown [southern Bucks County], then in Doylestown, then in Langhorne [southern Bucks County], then in Reading. After a while we had outpatient offices in Lansdale, North Wales (both in central Montgomery County), and up in the Bethlehem area. And the Board supported us. I still remember [Board President] Tom Leidy saying repeatedly, 'We'll support the expansion and going into new communities, *provided* we keep the center of the organization strong. We don't want to get out there and then just wither.'"

The potential for withering was altogether real, as evidenced several years into this "satellite era" when, in 1999, the Foundation's expenses exceeded its revenue by nearly half-a-million dollars. That shortfall was dwarfed the following year by a loss surpassing one million dollars. "The expansion stretched us in a way we weren't ready to be stretched," Dr. Kratz has since conceded. "It all just happened too fast for us to get the many administrative details channeled through our system, and to give absolutely everything a full financial analysis. The satellites began to drain off our energy, drain off our time, drain off our resources." Looking back on this period, John Goshow has observed that "the satellites never really fit with our mission, which is to serve our community. When you set up an office in a new community, you need to find people in that community who will take a vested interest in it. We weren't always successful at that. Plus, we have a very hands-off style of administration. If you don't have a strong leader running something, it doesn't run well. In some cases, we just weren't able to find the right personnel to make the satellites function smoothly."

"But we kept thinking, 'We've *got* to make it work!'," John recalls. "We probably should have pulled the plug on the satellites long before we did, but we had all those clients to consider. Shutting down an office isn't like shutting down a hotdog stand. You've got a thousand clients counting on you. Where are they going to go when you leave? You have to make sure they have ongoing care, and that took some time. Eventually we gave notice to our managed care companies. They really wanted us to continue, but we said 'We're sorry, we just can't.' So we closed up the offices one by one, and we've been out of the 'satellite' business ever since. We got back to doing what we do best." Dr. Kratz has added: "Once we took care of all the transfers, got rid of the properties, got out of the leases, we could see there was life on the horizon. Our recovery really went better than we might have imagined. There was a sense of renewal, of renewed commitment and ownership in our mission. It was like we were starting over. There was a different tone as we stopped worrying so much about simple survival and started thinking about our long-term future again. After a while, we were saying, 'Hey, it sounds like we're planning to be around for a *long* time!'"

"Back to what we do best"

Part of "getting back to what we do best" was a two-phase building project on the Lawn Avenue campus, with Phase One commenced in the midst of the "satellite era," and Phase Two concluded in 2002 (the Foundation's third consecutive year in the black). Penn Foundation was urged into this particular venture by the Bucks County Office of

Community Development, whose program director brought a team of County officials to Sellersville in 1993 to propose establishing a dual-diagnosis residential facility that the Foundation would administer. As the program director explained through a local newspaper reporter, "Counselors at the Red Cross homeless shelter in Bristol told me that they could place people with mental illness and people with addictions, but not people with both problems in a substantial way." His search for a means of accommodating the County's dual-diagnosis population led him to Penn Foundation's Recovery Center, which had demonstrated in recent years an unusual enthusiasm and effectiveness in this area. If Penn Foundation would build and manage a dual-diagnosis residential facility (as he and his colleagues suggested), the County would provide or help pull together construction funds, and then also underwrite operational costs.

Foundation officials agreed to this partnership, and drew up preliminary plans by the spring of 1994 that called for "an eight-unit dual diagnosis [ranch-style] facility to be built on 2 acres owned by the Foundation between the Holiday House swimming pool complex and the West Rockhill Elementary School [to the rear of the Recovery Center]," as reported in an April 27 newspaper account of a West Rockhill Township Board of Supervisors meeting. The article went on to relate that one of the Supervisors "was concerned about the closeness of the home to the school and swimming pool," and that the "chairman of the supervisors" had added that he could "visualize public hearings on this [matter]."

The coming months would prove the Supervisors' apprehension well founded. Foundation officials, concentrating on design issues and acquiring the necessary permits and construction funding that would lead to groundbreaking, discovered in the fall of 1995 that word of the dual-diagnosis house's proposed construction—which had not yet been approved by the Township, and had therefore not been widely broadcast—was spreading among the Foundation's next-door neighbors and among parents of West Rockhill Elementary School students. Spreading with it was a tone of alarm. One "worried, anxious, angry" parent was quoted in a December 5, 1995 newspaper article as inquiring "What if one of the addicts decides to have a binge or go off the wagon? It just seems like you're asking for some kind of trouble." In this same article, the school's Principal was reported to have pointed out that "within the past five years there have been two patients from Penn Foundation who have walked over here into the school building. Nothing happened except that it scared a few people,

[but] you can't guarantee that residents of the group home are not going to just wander off [and pose a more serious risk to the students]." She indicated that "the school district will try to stop construction of the home by opposing the matter at a West Rockhill Township Zoning Hearing Board meeting."

Penn Foundation's Public Relations Coordinator since August 1992, former *Souderton Independent* publisher W. Brooke Moyer, was contacted for a response, and he was quoted in the December 5 article as assuring the public "there will be no violent offenders and no sex offenders at the home. The residents will pose no threat to students. They will be in the latter stages of treatment, preparing to enter the community. Many will have jobs. These are not high-risk individuals, at all. The whole [program] has been carefully thought out." In some ways, "the opposition to the group home illustrates the *need* for [such a facility]. These people are stigmatized," Moyer said, "and so they often can't find a place to stay."

After a series of meetings with West Rockhill Township officials and concerned citizens, Penn Foundation earned approval for the project by shifting the construction site to the center of its campus (several hundred yards distant from the elementary school, with access provided from Lawn Avenue), and also agreeing to institute round-the-clock supervision of residents. Township Supervisors endorsed the project in July 1996, then ten more months elapsed while the last of the construction funding was secured from the Bucks County Office of Community Development, from

A tent awaits a crowd of well-wishers on Dedication Day for the Men's Dual Diagnosis House, November 12, 1997.

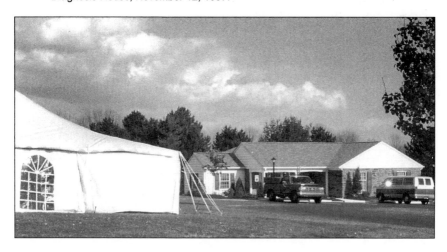

HUD, and from the Grundy Foundation. Between May and November 1997, contractors erected the "family-setting facility [with] four resident bedrooms [with two beds each], staff quarters, five full baths, a powder room, laundry area, kitchen, living room and office," according to a newspaper article reporting on the facility's November 12, 1997 dedication. Speaking at the dedication ceremony, Penn Foundation's Director of Housing Development since 1992, Wendy Simmons, stressed that the dual-diagnosis residence "is a Bucks County program, with operational expenses provided through the Bucks County Office of Mental Health/Mental Retardation. The men will be referred by case managers from Bucks County base service units and also homeless shelters." Vernon Kratz added that "hopefully the [clients'] experience of being part of a family will be an important part of their recovery."

These hopes were amply rewarded, and the success of the men's dual-diagnosis house was such that Penn Foundation and its partner agencies decided to construct a matching facil-ity nearby for women. The doors of this building were opened in January 2002, as the Foundation was enjoying its post-satellite re-invigoration. By that time, the new emphasis on using "people-first language" in behavioral healthcare circles had inspired Foundation officials to discard the term "dual-diagnosis house" in favor of the longer but more appropriate "supportive housing for people who are homeless and have co-occurring mental health and substance abuse disorders." The program itself was renamed "Village of Hope."

Also emblematic of the "renewed commitment and ownership in our mission" energizing the post-satellite era was the resurgence of the Pastoral Services Program, which had foundered following the death of Director Nancy Lapp in 1998, barely two years into her Foundation tenure. The fiscal crisis of the latter 1990s had delayed the hiring of a new Director for the non-revenue-generating program, but the appointment of Easton Hospital chaplain Carl Yusavitz to the Directorship in October 2000 turned out to be worth the wait. Fully certified as a Clinical Pastoral Education supervisor, Carl reaccredited the Foundation's CPE Program and breathed life back into the Pastoral Services Institute. He also expanded pastoral services to include direct care to Foundation clients at the Recovery Center, in the Partial Hospitalization Program, at the Wellspring Clubhouse, in the Community Residential Program, and at the behavioral healthcare unit at Grand View Hospital. As he explained in a September 2002 interview:

Pastoral care attends to the *whole* person, including his or her spiritual side. With some of the people who come to Penn Foundation for help, it might be that they have a kind of "soul sickness," something which disturbs them about their relationship with God, no matter how they name God. They need help, they need guidance, they need some clarification. The pastoral counselor will attend to that, listen to the person, let them try to affirm what can be affirmed, and contradict what needs to be contradicted. In that way we keep an eye on the spiritual side of a person's health.

We wanted to look at how we could structure into all the major programs here an opportunity for people to attend to that part of who they are. So I began to do spirituality seminars or "spirituality groups." They were very successful, particularly in the Partial Program. People really wanted to talk about their spirituality, about their faith. I also went over to the Recovery Center and asked if I could be helpful as an ordained person. They said, "Well, we bring ordained folks in when we need them, like the priest to hear confessions, and we've never really had an ordained person on staff. But some recovery centers do, so let's see how it goes. Let's see what you can come up with." I had worked in recovery programs before, so I knew that the second step of the Twelve-Step Program is clearly about a higher power who can restore us to sanity. In that way, there was already attention being paid to the recovering client's spiritual side. I came up with a curriculum of six spirituality groups or seminars so that when people rotate through the Recovery Center they will hear the material at least once. We later cut back the number to five. The first session is on negative and positive aspects of spirituality. The second one is on the movement from fear to trust. Another one is from self-pity to gratitude. In general, we work with moving spiritually from negative thinking and negative behaving to positive thinking and positive behaving. Those seminars have become mandatory in the Recovery Center.

A Catholic sister who had done some work in recovery came to me and wanted to volunteer at Penn Foundation. So I got her involved in pastoral care at the Recovery Center. She really liked it, and they liked her; we were able to find some limited money to give her a stipend for that. She's actually doing the work in the Recovery Center now, while I continue to work in the other Programs. That takes up about a third of my time. Another third goes to clinical pastoral education with seminary students, and the final third goes to working with five ministeriums and another clergy group in community education, peer review, and continuing education.

In July 2003, Carl was instrumental in launching Dayspring, a "Christian-based counseling program for people of all ages and religious backgrounds" (as described in the Foundation's Summer 2003 *newsletter*). The program's three charter counselors—Wallace Wolff, Lois Halsel, and Tedd Bradford—stood ready to "use passages from the Bible, prayer, and other religious methods, along with their clinical skills, to treat people who have issues in their personal lives that interfere with Jesus' desire that we 'live life and live it to the fullest.'" In the course of its first well-received year, Dayspring's staff was increased by two counselors, "grief" and "caregivers" support groups were added, and the Program earned a license from Pennsylvania to accept insurance payments.

The half-century mark

It is fitting that the years leading up to Penn Foundation's Fiftieth Anniversary have been highlighted by a renewed emphasis on pastoral care and, by extension, attention to spiritual health across the Foundation's spectrum of services. It was, after all, through a divine impulse to "love your neighbor as yourself" that the organization was conceived, and Foundation officials past and present have recognized the fingerprints of God on corporate twists and turns taken en route to the half-century mark. The Foundation's religious underpinnings are unabashedly proclaimed in a progressive mission statement drawn up for the twenty-first century. The multi-part declaration is given its own page on the organization's brimming Internet website:

Central Purpose

Penn Foundation believes in the resilience of the human spirit and provides a safe place where people of all ages can grow, develop, or recover to their fullest mental, emotional, and spiritual health.

Our Philosophy

. . . Born of community need, Penn Foundation brings together the finest aspects of the mental health profession with the caring values and qualities of the Mennonite tradition. The deeply held personal beliefs of its founder and Board help Penn Foundation remain accountable and worthy to serve its neighbors while setting a standard of excellence for psychiatric care. Four basic tenets continue to shape Penn Foundation's vision and direction; (1) individuals and their families are served with dignity, compassion, and integrity; (2) treatment is provided to achieve a whole mind in a whole body: ideally one cannot be treated without the other; (3) mental and emotional illness is treated within the supportive milieu of the community, as in any other medical specialty; (4) addiction is addressed as a disease within the context of the 12-step program philosophy emphasizing the importance of family involvement in recovery.

Core Values

Penn Foundation provides compassionate holistic services that are grounded in Christian values and open to all.
Penn Foundation respects the dignity and rights of all individuals who come for help, regardless of their socioeconomic status.
Penn Foundation employees are competent and hard-working individuals who are committed to the community's well being.

Courageous Goal

Penn Foundation strives to become a national leader and regional model for evidence-based, community-centered comprehensive behavioral healthcare treatment and services.

Descriptive Future

Penn Foundation will be recognized as an innovative national leader in the field of comprehensive behavioral healthcare and case management services—a community of hope and energy where everyone is welcome. This community will include providers, educators, advocates, and researchers who are committed to the holistic care of anyone who seeks long-term stability in their lives. As conscientious of human potential and solid financial resources, Penn Foundation will offer compassionate and creative care to everyone we serve.

Will Penn Foundation be "recognized as an innovative national leader in the field of comprehensive behavioral healthcare and case management services" as its second half-century unfolds? The organization certainly appears positioned to meet the challenges of the immediate future, and it continues to demonstrate a corporate "resilience of spirit," a willingness and ability to adapt to changing circumstances. The Foundation will, however, be sailing into its future without the steadying executive leadership of Dr. Kratz, who retired as Medical Director in January 2003. A whimsical sign reading "Caution Psychiatrist Crossing" was planted by a friend beside Lawn Avenue in recognition of the estimated 22,5000 times Dr. Kratz had crossed the road dividing Penn Foundation from Grand View Hospital in the course of serving both institutions. "He made that trip at least three times a day for the past thirty years," President and CEO John Goshow observed in the Summer 2003 *newsletter*. "His patients always come first, and his caring and commitment are the hallmark of his work." Dr. James G. Showalter, a Child and Adolescent Psychiatrist on the Penn Foundation staff since January 2000, was given the challenge of filling the outgoing Medical Director's well-worn shoes.

With the retirement of Dr. Kratz, there remain only two senior executives—John Goshow and Director of Mental Health Clinical Services Karen Kern—whose tenures reach back to the era when Norman Loux and a dozen charter Directors were still in charge. Physical connections to Penn Foundation's formative years are fading fast in this Fiftieth Anniversary year. The organization's humble birth in a borrowed Souderton townhouse a decade after World War II is a distant memory for those involved, and it is hardly fathomable to latter-day employees accustomed to a three-hundred-person staff, annual revenues approximating $12 million, and an operating budget with forty closely-monitored "cost centers." That should change with the publishing of this chronicle of Penn Foundation's first half-century. It is here for all to read how this pioneering community mental health organization became "a model for the country and the world."

A Penn Foundation Album

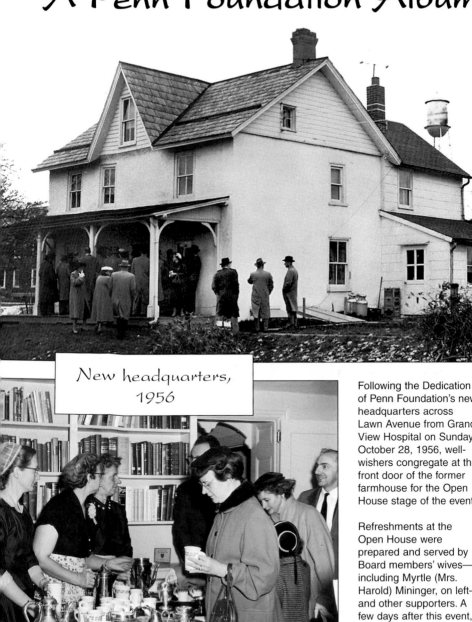

New headquarters,
1956

Following the Dedication of Penn Foundation's new headquarters across Lawn Avenue from Grand View Hospital on Sunday, October 28, 1956, well-wishers congregate at the front door of the former farmhouse for the Open House stage of the event.

Refreshments at the Open House were prepared and served by Board members' wives—including Myrtle (Mrs. Harold) Mininger, on left—and other supporters. A few days after this event, some of these women began forming a Ladies Auxiliary, which would be officially organized midway through 1957.

Penn Foundation had to find a new home in the summer of 1956 because its first headquarters—a vacated residence at 15 West Chestnut Street in Souderton—was only on loan until it was time to build a new municipal parking lot. The demolition phase of that construction project is underway in this southward-looking photograph, taken in September 1956. Penn Foundation's former accommodations—the three-story brick building just above and left of center—is one of several structures still awaiting the wrecking ball.

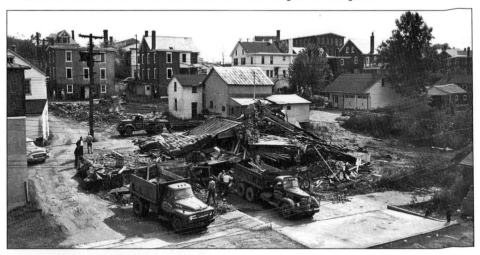

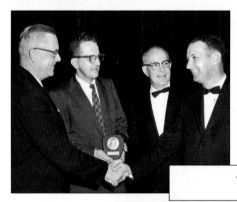

Board President Marcus Clemens (on right) shakes the hand of Dr. Lauren Smith, Physician in Charge of Administration of Pennsylvania Hospital, who was one of the guest speakers at Penn Foundation's first annual dinner meeting, held on Saturday evening, September 21, 1957 in the Lower Salford Elementary School auditorium. Looking on are Dr. Loux (holding the Benjamin Rush Award for 1957) and State Commissioner for Mental Health Dr. Robert Matthews.

First Annual Dinner, 1957

Board members and their wives flank the visiting dignitaries at the head table in this photograph taken during the first annual dinner meeting, which marked the organization's second anniversary.

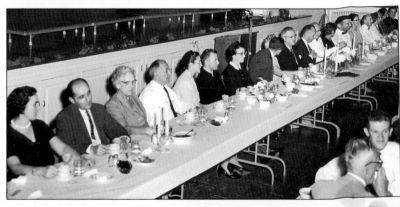

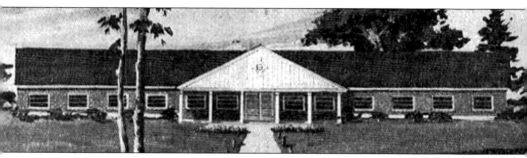

From the "What Might Have Been" archives: This artist's rendering of the proposed day care center was unveiled at Penn Foundation's second annual dinner meeting on November 8, 1958. When the Directors decided eighteen months later to decline federal funding because it would have required the inclusion of inpatient facilities, this building plan was scrapped and a less expensive, more compact two-story alternative was adopted.

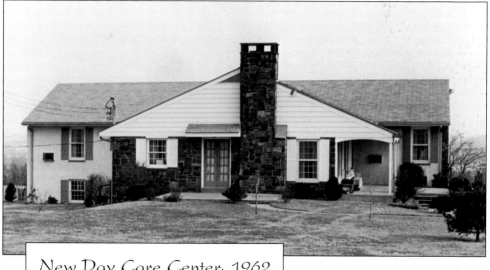

New Day Care Center, 1962

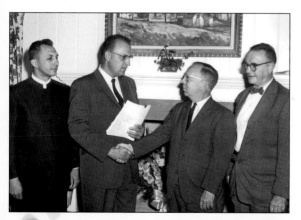

This was the view of the new Day Care Center from the north shortly after the facility's June 17, 1962 Dedication.

Board President Harold Mininger (second from left) thanks Congressman Willard Curtin and Dr. Kenneth Appel for their participation in the Dedication of the new Day Care Center. Mennonite Bishop and educator Richard C. Detweiler (on left), who had just delivered a memorable keynote address, rounds out the quartet of dignitaries assembled in the Center's spacious reception area.

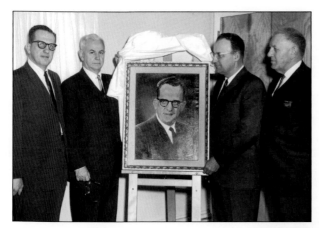

In a surprise luncheon ceremony conducted during a March 16, 1965 visit by Dr. Francis J. Braceland, editor of *The American Journal of Psychiatry* and Psychiatrist-in-Chief at the Institute of Living in Hartford, Connecticut, Dr. Braceland (second from left) unveils a portrait of Dr. Loux (far left) painted by Dr. Kermit S. Black (far right), one of Dr. Loux's colleagues on the Grand View Hospital staff. Helping with the presentation is Penn Foundation Board President Harold Mininger.

Art Isaak, Director of Occupational and Recreational Activities, demonstrates the operation of a hand loom on the ground floor of the Day Care Center for the benefit of Edna Francis (center), a Jamaican psychiatric social worker visiting Penn Foundation through a fellowship provided by the Pan American Health Organizations. Day Care Coordinator Ruth Lefever watches the November 28, 1967 demonstration.

Among the groups posing with a ceremonial shovel during groundbreaking exercises for the first major addition on August 8, 1968 was this collection of officials, comprising (from left) Grand View Hospital President Arthur Alderfer; Penn Foundation Board President Charles Hoeflich; Pastor Ellwood Reitz of Sellersville's St. Michael's Lutheran Church; Building Committee members and trustees Harold Mininger, Raymond Rosenberger, and Roland Detweiler; Grand View Hospital's Chief of Medicine Dr.Michael Peters, and Medical Director Norman Loux.

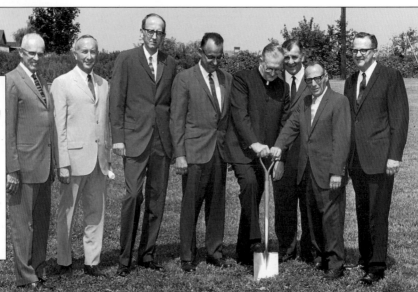

Breaking Ground for First Major Addition, 1968

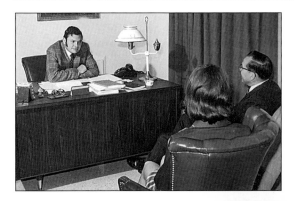

All of the pictures on this page were taken for promotional purposes around 1970. Here Director of Social Services and marriage counseling specialist Larry Landes works with a couple of "clients," one of whom is portrayed by his colleague, psychiatric social worker and children's specialist Bill Swartzendruber.

Penn Foundation "At Work," circa 1970

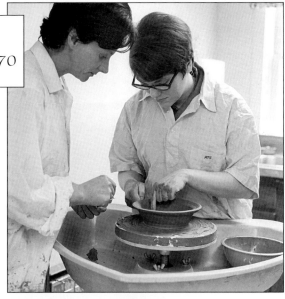

Day Care Coordinator Ruth Simpson (left) and Registered Nurse Robin Morgan demonstrate how a potter's wheel is used in recreational therapy.

Part-time Demonstration Project Officer and Board member Ruby Horwood points out the Foundation's catchment area for a visiting group of mental health workers.

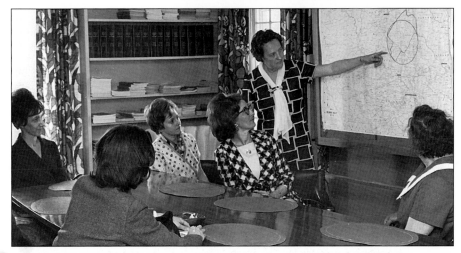

A Monday morning staff meeting in the library around 1970 brings together (from right) Dr. Wilbert Lyons, Dr. John Richards, Bill Swartzendruber, unidentified, Art Isaak, Dr. Loux, Ruth Simpson, and Larry Landes.

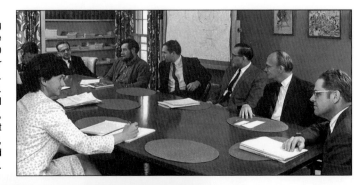

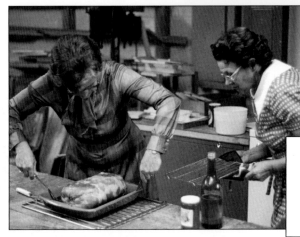

In the workshop, preparing for the Twentieth Anniversary Luncheon on Thursday, November 6, 1975, are Dr. Loux's wife Esther (on left) and Peg Detweiler, wife of trustee Roland Detweiler.

Twentieth Anniversary Luncheon, 1975

Dr. Edward Auer offers remarks at the Twentieth Anniversary Luncheon, which concluded with the announcement that the Foundation's annual lecture series would thereafter be known as the Michael A. Peters Seminar Series. Dr. Peters and his wife Maybelle are seated on the right at the head table, along with (from right) Dr. Loux, Dr. Leo Bartemeier, Dr. Francis Braceland, Dr. Daniel Blain (seated across from Dr. Auer, his back to audience), and Dr. Kenneth Appel.

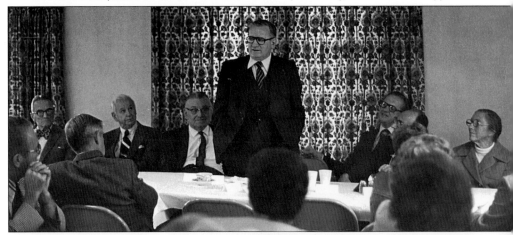

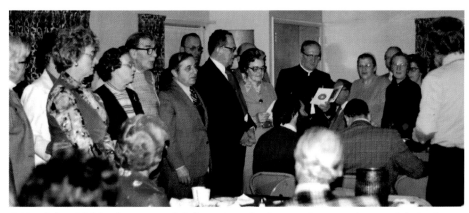

Art Isaak (on right) leads a group of staff members, trustees, and spouses in a carol during the annual Staff-Board Christmas Dinner at the Foundation on December 23, 1975.

Staff members enjoy a light moment during a training session in the Grundy Auditorium during the mid-1970s.

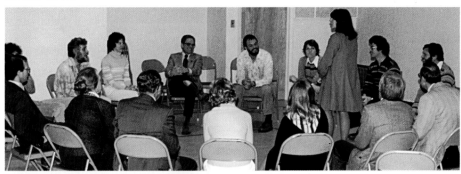

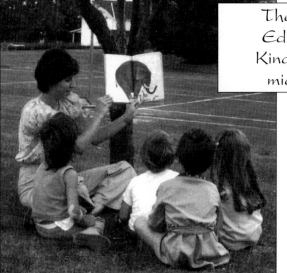

Therapeutic Educational Kindergarten, mid-1970s

An unidentified teacher reads to a quartet of kindergartners on the lawn beside the tennis court in the mid-1970s. Opened in the renovated farmhouse in October 1973, the Foundation's "therapeutic educational kindergarten" had to close its doors in June 1978 when new legislation impelled the Bucks County Intermediate Unit to withdraw federal funding in order to establish its own pre-school services.

Participants in this circa-1985 Board-Staff meeting include (from left) trustee Curt Moyer, Administrator Henry Landes, trustee Elizabeth ("Betsy") Meredith, social worker Wayne Schantzenbach, and Deputy Administrator Wayne Mugrauer.

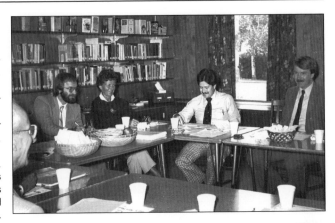

Medical Director Dr. Vernon Kratz addresses a crowd in the tennis court during a Fall Festival of the mid-1980s.

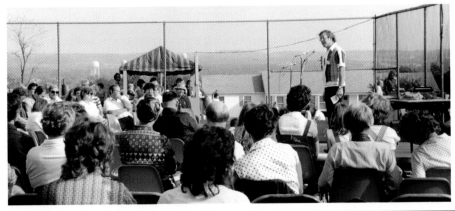

Penn Foundation Campus, 1980

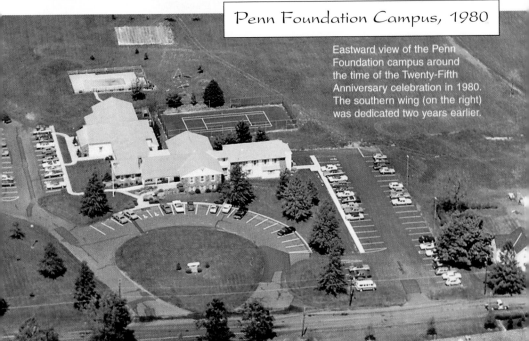

Eastward view of the Penn Foundation campus around the time of the Twenty-Fifth Anniversary celebration in 1980. The southern wing (on the right) was dedicated two years earlier.

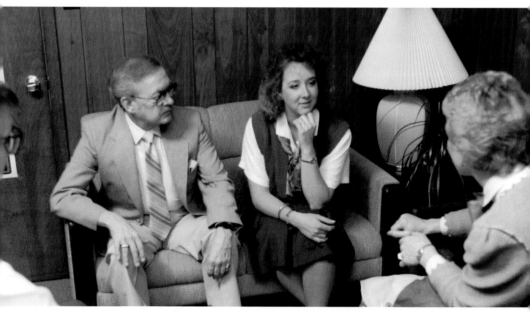

This "counseling session" scene was staged by Foundation staff members for pictorial use in the 1986 campaign to promote the BreakThrough addictions program. One of the campaign's creators, Community Relations Director Dave Birkey, sits in on the far left. Addictions Counselors Bob Ferrell (on sofa) and Grace Timins (far right) help fill out the cast, with an unidentified fourth participant.

Lecturer and best-selling author M. Scott Peck signs books, flyers, and other autograph-worthy documents proffered by fans at the second annual Penn Foundation Autumn Conference, held at the Indian Valley Country Club on September 10, 1987.

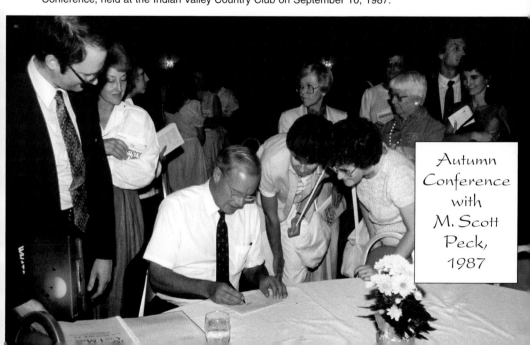

Autumn Conference with M. Scott Peck, 1987

Administrator Henry Landes (center, rear) chairs a roundtable of staff members, trustees, and building project personnel hammering out final details of the June 12, 1988 Dedication of the BreakThrough center. Henry is conversing at this moment with architect Phil Lederach.

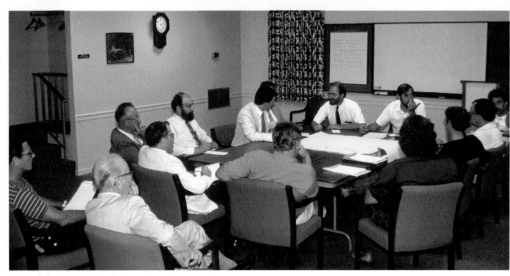

A client reflects on his struggle with addiction in a bedroom of the new BreakThrough center. Eighteen months after its opening, the facility —which was itself struggling with low patient censuses—was renamed "The Recovery Center."

The BreakThrough Center, 1988

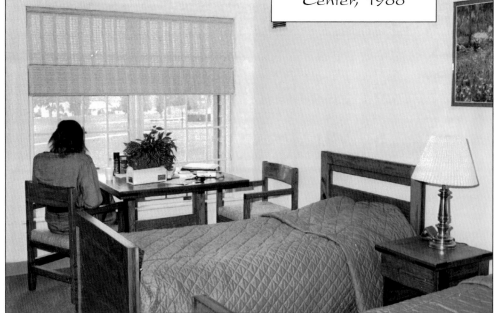

Penn Foundation Auxiliary members display some of the items they will offer for sale at the second annual Christmas Barn, to be conducted in Norman and Esther Loux's barn on November 5, 1988. The women are (seated, from left) Judy Leidy, Elaine Souder, Emily Clemens; (standing) Dorothy Williams, Elizabeth Kratz, Mim Derstine, and Molly Derstine (Auxiliary Chair).

2nd Annual Christmas Barn, 1988

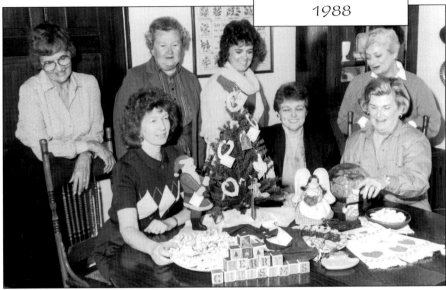

Wearing the hats of President, CEO, and Medical Director, Vernon Kratz (far left) presides over a meeting of support and maintenance staff in the mid-1990s. Other participants in the meeting include (from left) Vice President and COO John Goshow, unidentified, unidentified, Ken Gross, Earl Landis, Peggy Emerick, and, partially visible in the foreground, Pat Trauger and Bonnie Caroff. The most veteran employees were Pat (on staff since 1959), Peggy (1966), and Earl (1970).

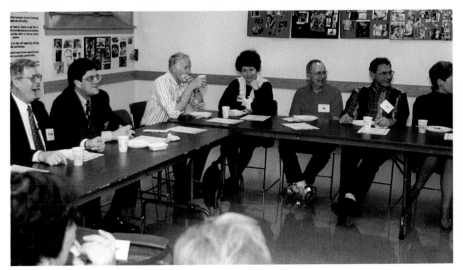

Partial Hospital clinician Bill Killgore appears to be facilitating a group therapy session in this staged photo from the mid-1990s. The "clients" are also members of the Partial Hospital staff.

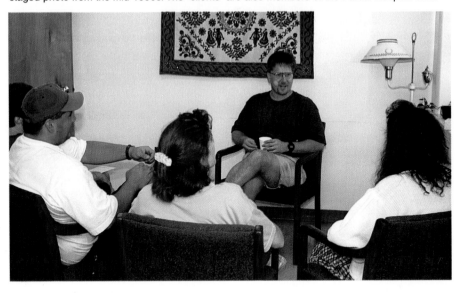

1994
Staff Dinner

There's fun for all at "Rancho Grundy" during the entertainment portion of the February 1994 Staff Dinner in the Grundy Auditorium.

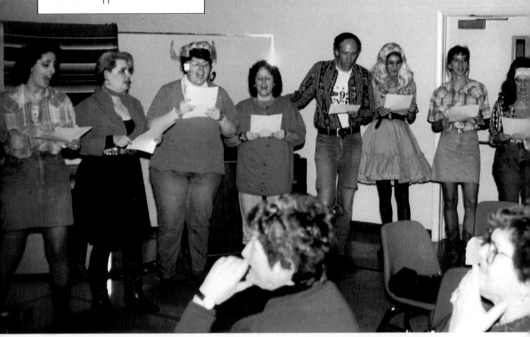

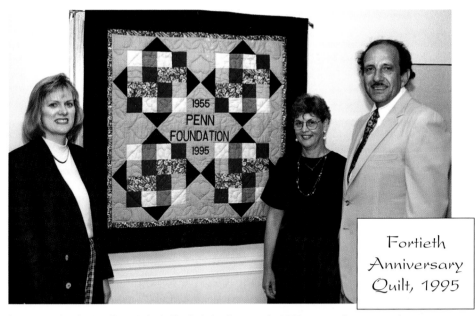

Fortieth Anniversary Quilt, 1995

In preparation for the Foundation's Fortieth Anniversary in 1995, an employee committee was charged with developing a new logo for the organization. The committee sorted through suggestions offered by staff members, and settled on this quilt design, which was said to represent "the bringing together of an array of specialized services which, when carefully pieced and interwoven, become the unique and caring environment that is Penn Foundation." This logo was incorporated into a Fortieth Anniversary Quilt, displayed here by (from left) LeeAnne Kingsbauer, President of the Penn Foundation Auxiliary; Sandee Trakat, Chair of the Quilt Project; and Thomas K. Leidy, Chairman of the Board of Directors.

The new quilt logo was also incorporated into a smart new metallic sign that replaced a weathered wooden predecessor on the Foundation's front lawn.

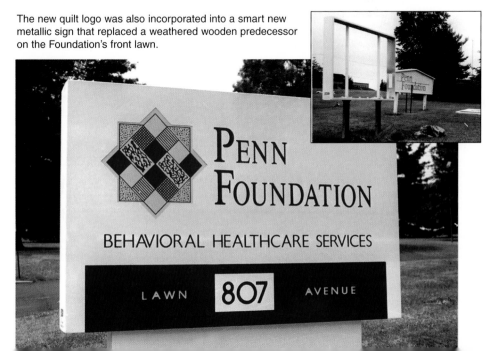

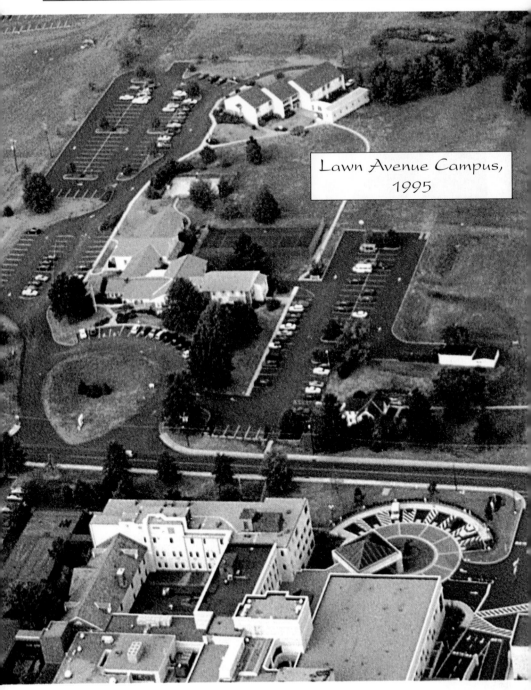

Lawn Avenue Campus, 1995

Penn Foundation's Lawn Avenue campus in 1995, the organization's fortieth year of operation.

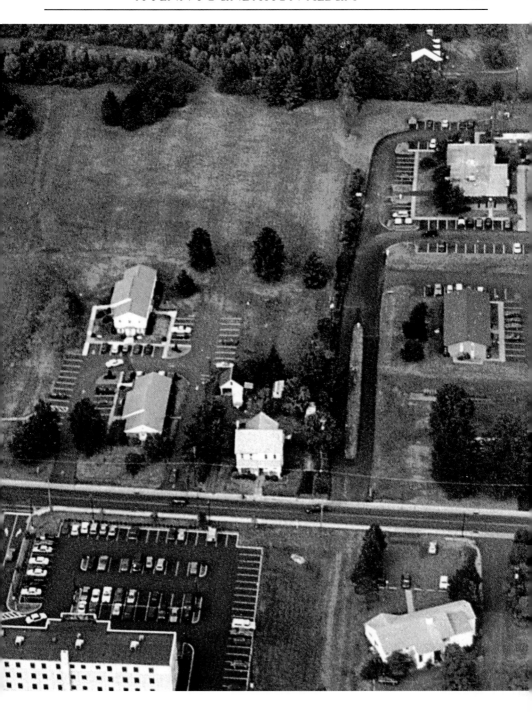

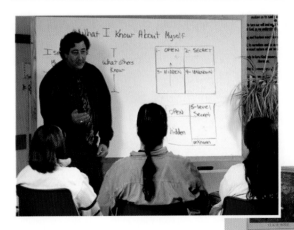

The Recovery Center
circa 1999

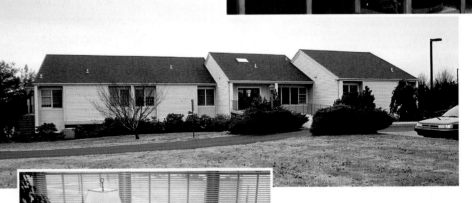

These photos were taken in and around the Recovery Center for potential use in a 1999 brochure. Addressing fellow employees sitting in as "clients" are (top left) Associate Director Bill Blumenthal, (above right) Director of Drug and Alcohol Services Todd Barlow, and (left) Admissions Representative Jo-Ellen Darling.

Afterword

ONE CLIENT'S TESTIMONY

This chronicle of Penn Foundation's conception and first fifty years began with an imagined but factually supported description of "the entrance of the first patient into the organization's first facility for the first session of treatment offered by the organization's first paid employees" in October 1955. Treatment was then, and it continues to be, the Foundation' raison d'etre. While that fundamental fact has underlain every step taken during the past half-century, individual accounts of treatment—or, better yet, healing—have been largely omitted from this narrative. This is so primarily because personal stories remain hidden behind a curtain of confidentiality. It is also so because Penn Foundation was conceived, shaped, and operated not by clients but by the members of its staff and Board of Directors.

It is worth remembering, however, that the Foundation's story is much more complex, and its work has been far more consequential, than any recounting of administrative evolution, service expansion, facilities development, and staff contributions can convey. Thousands of Bux-Mont residents distracted or overwhelmed by the storms of life have found refuge and healing at 807 Lawn Avenue, or at one of the Foundation's satellite facilities. Not only they, but their families and friends have benefited in untold—perhaps even unperceived—ways from the compassion and psychiatric expertise that have propelled this remarkable institution through its challenging days. We conclude, then, with the testimony of one client among thousands, offered anonymously to the author on an afternoon in August 2002.

I've been coming to Penn Foundation for over twenty years. Karen Kern and Dr. Kratz consider me one of their success stories, I guess. I have a long-term inherited illness—manic-depression or bipolar disorder—and

I'm on a fair amount of medication. I do pretty well on it. I've been able to do some really nice things in my life, even earn a national award for teaching. I've received a lot of help from Penn Foundation. I'm pretty quiet about coming here, though. My family knows I see a counselor. My husband's family knows I see a counselor. And my best friends know I see a counselor. But that's it. Nobody at work knows.

There was a history of biological and social problems in my family. There was mental illness on my father's side of the family, and then my parents were divorced when I was five. So I had some baggage, and sometimes I had trouble figuring out how to handle things on my own, how to make the right social decisions. I had two years of therapy with a psychologist before I moved to Pennsylvania. That therapy was good, but it was very intense. The doctor was really trying to work with my biggest problems. It was exhausting, and it put a lot of stress on my marriage. I moved to this area from the Midwest in the late Seventies, and I found myself really needing emotional support. I talked to my family doctor, and he recommended I come over here to Penn Foundation. So I started coming in here for counseling every two weeks.

My therapy here has been calmer, more low-key. I told Karen I didn't want to go through heavy therapy again. I just wanted to get counseling and make moderate gains. And I've done that. Now I come every six weeks or so. Or I can call in, if I want to. I still talk about my social and emotional problems, family adjustments, and that kind of thing, but I've worked through a lot of issues in twenty-plus years. So it's been very helpful. Of course, I also take advantage of opportunities in my own community, and I've got supportive friends.

I'm involved in creating my own therapy program. Every month or so, I sign a form where Karen has written down the objectives for my therapy, and I read that and then sign it. The objectives change. Right now I'm working on getting more exercise—walking mostly—and looking to other people, trying to talk to other people, rather than being isolated. I tend to not want to dump my problems on other people. But there should be a balance. Sometimes it's good to go to people and look for emotional support. So that's another one of my current objectives—to make stronger connections with my family. Karen asks different questions. She's got, of course, this tremendous knowledge of my family history and how I've had to deal with different things. A lot of times in our counseling sessions she has the objectivity to see where I've grown and where I still need to grow.

Now, one of the most important things for me to do is to come and get check-ups for my medication. They're finding that a lot of problems that people have can be helped if you have the right chemicals to balance things out. I remember when they suggested I go on medication. It was after I had a really strong reaction to surgery for a pituitary tumor. I was upset because I didn't like to think I had something that was so bad that I needed medication. But I've gotten over that, and now I've tried to educate myself a little bit about my illness. My husband's also tried to educate himself. The general feeling is that I'm doing a very good job, and I'm being respectful of the fact that I need the medication. I'd rather do it *without* the chemicals, but I've got enough evidence to know that it's been helpful. There are side effects to taking any kind of medication, somewhere down the line. In my case, the side effects are that I get a very dry mouth, and it has caused some dental problems and stuff like that. But I think that's much better than having severe depressions.

Even with the medication and counseling, there have been times when I was pretty suicidal, and nobody knew it was coming because I kept everything inside. I didn't want to frighten Karen, and I didn't want to frighten my husband. I didn't tell them till I was out of it. Then they were worried, and they talked it over with each other. But there's only so much other people can do. You have to want to stay alive yourself.

My husband and I can talk about a lot of things, but if I'm feeling extremely depressed, it frightens him, so I don't tell him. Lately he has told me that he *wants* to know, so he can help me. So I'm trying to be more honest with him, but sometimes you just need professional help. It's good to have somebody to talk to who's trained and up-to-date with the latest advances in psychiatry. I'm sure Karen gets in-servicing, since that's the thing nowadays. Plus there's the strong medical connection with Dr. Kratz. He's going to conferences and staying up-to-date in his field.

At Penn Foundation there's a very healthy respect for both counseling and medication. I can see that in the relationship between Karen and Dr. Kratz. At one time Dr. Kratz felt I was doing okay, but Karen sensed that I had gone a little downhill. So she made a pretty good argument with him that we needed to get together and talk it over. She and Dr. Kratz and my husband and I sat down and had a good conversation. It was very helpful.

Being a schoolteacher and very involved in the field of education, I do a lot of training in diversity education and how to help children with social and emotional needs. My experience at Penn Foundation has definitely made me a lot more sensitive and more knowledgeable in dealing with my students and fellow teachers. It's ironic that, with all I've gone through, I'm known for giving a lot of social and emotional support. That makes me feel very good.

Penn Foundation has really been an anchor for me. There's not a whole lot made about the [organization's] religious connection, but I know there is one. It comes across in the sincere way the staff handles clients. They've got a fairly conservative approach to giving support, but it's a very sensible approach that involves working with whatever you have to help you better interact with the people that you love and live with. It's obviously an approach that has worked well for me.

Appendix 1

ADDRESS BY PASTOR
RICHARD C. DETWEILER

Delivered at the Dedication of Penn Foundation's New Facility at 807 Lawn Avenue, Sunday, June 17, 1962

(as presented with an introduction in the
July 5, 1962 edition of Perkasie's *News-Herald*)

Three weeks ago, the Penn Foundation for Mental Health at Sellersville dedicated its beautiful new day care center with impressive exercises attended by many. Rev. Richard Detweiler, Perkasie, was one of the speakers at the occasion. The foundation's supporters said that seldom, if ever, has the aim of the Penn Foundation been described as well. For this reason, the text of the pastor's address is reprinted.

By Rev. Richard Detweiler, Pastor, Perkasie Mennonite Church, Bishop, Franconia Conference Mennonite Church

The measure of any community service is community acceptance. Penn Foundation for Mental Health is unique in that it has become a prophet with honor in its own country. This is a tribute both to the Foundation and to the community. The result has been an expansion of facilities and services that we are to dedicate here this afternoon.

The dollars and cents given this project have been weighed and not found wanting. However, there is a greater cost to pay if the work of Penn Foundation is to fulfill its purpose. It is toward the payment of this cost that I wish to challenge our dedication, and especially the use of these facilities and the ministry of those who serve thru them.

You would expect me to use a Biblical setting for this address and being a dyed in the wool preacher I would not miss the opportunity.

Upon occasion our Lord Jesus Christ sought to explain His ministry among men. In the Gospel of Luke, Chapter 15, His words in story form have marked out for us three concerns that should characterize the dedication of these facilities. Together these concerns also compose the cost we must pay if this building is to become a community symbol of health and wholeness. May I read for us the first:

"What man of you, having a hundred sheep, if he lose one of them, doth not leave the ninety and nine in the wilderness, and go after that which is lost, until he find it?"

We dedicate this center, its facilities, its staff and its services, first, to the task of finding the one. If health and wholeness are to be maintained among us we must pay the cost of breaking through our mechanical living to find the one. The 20th century has created masses and lost the individual. We are today people without a face. Even our family faces have become an anonymous blur as we pass each other on the run, dipping in and out of our endless activity. It is only the house, the car, the pool, and the boat of the man next door that matter, not the man next door who is our neighbor. The result of all this facelessness, this impersonalness of our living is that we find we ourselves no longer matter. And when a man no longer matters to himself he has lost his purpose for living.

The staff of Penn Foundation must provide community leadership to help us do two things [in order] to regain ourselves as meaningful individuals. First, they can help us to count our ninety-nine. The remarkable thing about the shepherd in our Lord's story is not only that he knew one was lost, but that he knew the number of ninety-nine that were in the fold. In fact, because he had counted the ninety-nine by one's, he discovered the one that was lost. And if he was a typical Eastern shepherd he knew that one by name. Through parent-teacher meetings, church group discussions, testing services, leader's workshops, and clinical counseling, Penn Foundation has already given significant service in helping us to understand how we count as individuals and the role each of us has to play for our health and the happiness of others.

It has begun to dawn upon us anew that a wife and mother must be counted as more than a household slave, that a husband and father is more than a bean counter, that sons and daughters are individuals, responsible beings to be respected and yet not bowed down to, that an employer is not merely an order book and that a neighbor is more than a landscape object next door. In fact, Dr. Loux and his associates have done as much to enable the ninety-nine of us to understand ourselves and our inter-personal relations as they have to restore the lost ones. This preventative of community education is an avowed goal of this staff and has already become worth many pounds of cure.

The second thing the staff here must do is to help us find and restore the lost one, the one who has lost touch with reality and is emotionally at sea. We need help as family members, ministers, teachers, counselors, employers, and friends to identify and understand the lostness of individuals who become unwell. We need someone to point us the way to help lost ones home. Penn Foundation services are as a safety director standing at the crucial crossroads of our mental health problems. The accident rate should go down as with this dedicated help, we count the ninety-nine and find each lost one.

May I read the second concern as spoken by our Lord in His second story:

"What woman having ten pieces of silver, if she lose one piece, doth not light a candle and sweep the house, and seek diligently till she find it?"

It is not enough to find the one. To achieve sound health, he must be restored to something to live by some measure of life in which he can trust. The woman who lost one piece of silver illustrates the person whose life is no longer complete and satisfied because of lost values. Our age has created not only faceless man, but also neutral man—without conviction of right to live by. One of the most penetrating criticisms of American life has come from a Chinese visitor who said it seems to him that Americans no longer have anything they are willing to die for. I know I am on delicate ground here, for I am speaking of values beyond the freedom of democracy, values beyond the slogans that litter the futile battlefields of the world. If we are to revitalize our generation, we must pay not only the cost of regaining our individuality—we must pay also the costs of finding the eternal precepts of the truth that sets us free. We must confess in humble faith that there are unchanging standards of mortality and eternal principles of life that are basic to health and happiness and that are woven into the very warp and woof of man's existence. We believe that truth has been absolutely revealed and that it can be known. We believe, as the Christian scriptures declare, that man has not been left in darkness, but that upon him has shone the light of life. In other words, we call upon the professional services of Penn Foundation to be basically in harmony with the postulates of divine revelation and the assumptions of the Christian faith. We look to the staff of this center, not only to neutralize inner conflicts and expose hidden fears and remove false guilt, but to assure persons that even in the 20th century of modern man there are trustworthy absolutes to live by.

Now this does not mean that we are suggesting naive and superficial answers to the deep-seated problems of the mentally and emotionally ill. Neither are we recommending that those who minister here should tear apart the personal fabric of every man's creed and exploit the sacred right of a man to his religion. But we do expect that this center will function on the promise that there are universal laws by which man has been ordained to live and that those laws have their being in the wisdom and love of a personal God who can be known.

We dedicate this center, therefore, under the lordship of Him who said, "I am the Way, the Truth, and the Life." If we are to restore health to human society, we must pay the cost of reaffirming our faith in the revealed Word of the living God. This is the piece that is lost.

Now may I yet read for us the conclusion of Jesus' third story in this same chapter of Luke's Gospel, for therein lies our third concern.

"This, my son, was dead, and is alive again; he was lost and is found." Men have searched for the one word that can change the face of the world. I believe I know what it is. It is forgiveness. We must find the one and restore to man his face; we must find the truth and restore to man his conviction; but more than all else, we must find and share forgiveness and restore to man the healing of his broken relationships.

You have noticed that the first story pictured ninety-nine and one; the second, nine and one; but the last story concludes with one and one. In the final analysis, life boils down to two things—you and God, and you and me, face to face, in our one-to-one relationships.

My friends, if there is one thing human experience has taught us, it is that when those one-to-one relationships are broken, husband-wife, father-son, friend-and-neighbor, life is no longer whole. There life stands or falls; there face to face, life becomes pleasure or pain, success or failure, hope or despair. God knew this too. Therefore He offered once and for all the ground of forgiveness to all men to pave the way for their healing. We dedicate this center to helping persons with broken relationships to be forgiven and to forgive, for therein lies the healing of human society. This is the highest calling on earth to the art of healing. It is the divine approach to the restoring of the brokenness of man. We can dedicate ourselves and the work of Penn Foundation to nothing less and nothing greater than the healing of forgiveness.

I know there is a symbol for the physician's art. I confess my igno-rance as to whether there has yet been adopted a symbol for the task of ministering to mental health. There is perhaps a symbol that encompasses it all. It is the cross.

I congratulate you—members of the staff and board of directors of Penn Foundation for Mental Health—upon your service to us, the families of this community. May the grace of God enable you to carry forward this ministry of healing among us. To this end, we dedicate in sincere gratitude these facilities.

Appendix 2

PENN FOUNDATION DIRECTORS

(charter Board members in bold)

Anders, Marvin A.
  7/1/2003 - present
Clemens, John W.
  6/23/1981 - 12/31/1997
Clemens, Marcus A.
  1/1/1955 - 12/31/1961
Derstine, Vernon H.
  5/28/1968 - 3/24/1990
Detweiler, Roland M.
  1/1/1955 - 5/1/1994
Garis, Mark G.
  1/1/1995 - 12/31/2000
Gross, Harold O.
  3/21/1978 - 12/31/1994
Hillegass, Russell M.
  1/1/1955 - 11/14/1972
Hoeflich, Charles H.
  1/1/1955 - 1/1/1989
Holbert, John W.
  12/21/1982 - 1/1/1986
Horwood, L. Ruby
  1/1/1965 - 1/1/1987
Kratz, Vernon H., M.D.
  7/1/2000 - present
Landes, Ray P.
  5/16/1978 - 5/24/1988
Landis, David G.
  8/23/1988 - present
Leidy, Thomas K.
  10/22/1985 - present
Lindsay, Wanda
  1/1/2002 - present
Loux, Norman L.
  1/1/1955 - 11/13/1956;
  7/24/1984 - present

Meredith, Elizabeth B.
  10/22/1985 - 1/1/2004
Mininger, Harold M.
  1/1/1955 - 10/10/2003
Moyer, Curtis F.
  7/11/1968 - 12/31/1998
Moyer, J. Phillip
  6/28/1988 - present
Moyer, Merrill S.
  10/22/1985 - 12/31/2002
Moyer, Russell M.
  1/1/1955 - 1/1/1987
Pierce, John
  3/23/2004 - present
Rosenberger, Raymond H.
  1/1/1955 - 8/26/1980
Silverman, Ira
  10/22/1985 - 6/22/1993
Souder, Elvin R.
  1/1/1955 - 6/30/1996
Souder, Mahlon A.
  1/1/1955 - 8/26/1980
Souder, Paul F.
  1/1/1955 - 1/1/1990
Souder, Ronald
  1/1/1995 - present
Van Ommeren, Willard
  7/23/1988 - 1/1/1990
Washko, Carol D.
  1/1/1995 - 4/1/1998
Williams, Dorothy M.
  11/24/1981 - 3/1/2002
Yoder, Lloyd R.
  1/1/1955 - 11/1/1967
Zook, Margaret
  1/1/1997 - present

Appendix 3

PENN FOUNDATION EMPLOYEES

(through March 1, 2005; most recent position identified)

Abbas, Saleha *Psychiatrist* 9/20/1999 - 7/25/2000

Adamitis, Mark *Nurse* 7/1/1998 - 6/1/2004

Adams, Garry *Driver* 12/6/1997 - 1/5/1998

Adams, Helaine *Billing Clerk* 2/10/1994 - 5/22/1997

Adil, Thomas *Therapist* 7/6/2004 - present

Adkins, Susan *Account Clerk* 8/13/1999 - 8/1/2000

Afflerbach, Eric *Crisis Worker* 11/22/1999 - 5/23/2000

Aikey, Sandra *Secretary* 6/26/1990 - 12/1/1990

Aimaro, Marion *Patients Accounts Manager* 9/13/1982 - 1/14/1983

Akange, Margaret *Therapeutic Support Staff* 4/13/2004 - 6/7/2004

Albani, John *Therapeutic Staff Support* 3/7/2000 - 5/18/2000

Albert, Susan *Psychologist* 11/5/1996 - 4/16/1997

Albritton, Anne *Secretary/Receptionist* 7/28/2003 - 2/23/2005

Alcott, Kelly *Secretary* 4/17/2000 - 3/16/2001

Alderfer, Charis *Therapist, Partial Hospital* 2/28/2005 - present

Alderfer, Rachelle *Activity Leader* 4/17/1993 - 1/1/1996

Alderfer, Wesley *Maintenance Assistant* 4/27/1992 - 1/2/2002

Alexander, Debra *Fiscal Clerk/Secretary* 4/27/1992 - 6/29/1994

Alexander, Diane *EAP Evening Receptionist* 11/5/1990 - 9/21/1993

Alexander, Marjorie *Executive Secretary* 11/1/1957 - 6/6/1980

Alexander, Rosanne *Partial Hosp. Coordinator* 11/13/1989 - 6/4/1991

Allebach, Lynne *EAP Administrative Assistant* 1/9/1989 - 9/7/1990

Allebach, Rebecca *Residential Caseworker* 8/9/1983 - 11/17/1984

Allen, Harry *Mobile Therapist* 11/3/2004 - present

Alonge-Roe, Cynthia *MH Worker, Family Based Services* 2/28/2005 - present

Alpert, Linda *Social Worker* 12/6/1995 - 8/21/1996

Alston, Bobbie *Secretary/PRN* 1/9/1997 - 6/27/1997

Andreoni, Pamela *Nurse* 6/6/1988 - 1/2/1989

Angermann, Marcia *Social Worker* 11/8/1993 - 3/30/2005

Anthony, Nicole *Social Worker* 3/1/1997 - 7/24/2003

Anton, Jodi *Admissions Rep* 8/11/1997 - 12/30/1998

Appenzeller, James *Drive/PRN* 3/29/2000 - 11/1/2000

Appessos, Nicole *Residential Caseworker* 8/14/2000 - 6/18/2001

Applegate, Elizabeth *Psychiatric Patient Coordinator* 9/10/1982 - 6/22/1984

Appleman, William *Residential Advisor* 1/5/1998 - 2/23/1998

Aquilino, William *Residential Coordinator* 9/7/2004 - present

Ardecki, Linda *Managed Care/Medical Records Tech.* 5/4/1998 - 10/13/2000

Armstrong, Karen *Caseworker* 4/11/1994 - 11/1/1998

Armstrong, Theresa *Mobile Therapist* 9/14/2004 - present

Arnold, Anita *Mobile Therapist* 6/15/2004 - present

Arnwine, Eric *Therapeutic Staff Support* 3/3/2003 - present

Auckland, Mary *Medical Records Clerk (Temp.)* 6/24/1986 - 7/18/1986

Austin, Kelly *PRN Crisis Worker + On Call* 9/11/2000 - 7/30/2002

Baccari, Lois *Detox Coordinator* 8/22/1988 - 8/15/1989

Bachmeyer, Joan *Secretary* 5/17/1971 - 8/13/1971

Backer, Sharon *Intensive Community Counselor* 6/15/1998 - 9/4/1998

Baer, Richard *Driver* 6/4/2001 - 8/20/2002

Bahm, Christine *Intensive Community Counselor* 2/19/1997 - 6/19/1997

Bahner, Linda *Inpatient Counselor/Art Therapist* 1/2/2001 - 3/2/2001

Bailentine, Rebecca *Intensive Community Counselor* 7/31/1995 - 4/1/1996

Bailey, Beth *Outpatient Team Secretary* 2/23/1984 - 6/22/1984

Bailey, Ronald *Behavior Specialist* 5/20/1998 - 2/4/1999

Bailey, Sara *Supports Coordinator* 9/17/2001 - present

Bainhauer, Frederick III *Crisis Worker* 2/12/1997 - 2/28/1997

Bair, Robert *Social Worker* 12/6/1995 - 7/31/2001

Baird, Jade *Activity Therapist Asst.* 1/16/1988 - 4/24/1988

Baker, Emily *CRR/Drop-in Secretary* 10/6/1986 - 7/11/1990

Baker, Lynn *Med Review Nurse* 4/12/2000 - present

Baker, Nicole *Music Therapist* 3/22/1991 - 3/25/1992

Baker, Robbi *Medical Records Manager* 8/7/1995 - 3/6/1998

Baldwin, Zoe *Intensive Care Manager* 11/8/1999 - 1/28/2000

Bao, Lily *Intensive Community Counselor* 2/3/1999 - 5/31/1999

Barbadoro, Paul (Rob) *MR Case Manager* 9/2/1997 - 8/28/1998

Barbash, James *Psychologist* 7/1/1968 - 2/15/1980

Barlow, Debra *Medical Records* 6/6/1977 - 12/25/1981

Barlow, J. Todd *Director Drug and Alcohol Services* 4/1/1987 - present

Barndt, Kathleen *Psychiatric Patient Coord.* 3/4/1983 - 5/3/1985

Barndt, Rosemarie *Secretary/Receptionist* 5/23/1997 - 10/1/1998

Barnett, Stephanie *Dual Diagnosis Coordinator* 3/19/1999 - 2/19/2004

Barracano, Ralph *Psychologist* 3/26/1996 - 6/30/1997

Bartlett, RuthAnn *Stepping Stone Advisor* 4/7/1980 - 1/8/1991

Basmajian, Julie *Billing Clerk* 7/10/1995 - 7/18/1997

Batcha, Charlotte *Social Worker* 5/2/1995 - present

Batley, Jason *Addictions Technician* 6/7/1989 - 8/30/1993

Baurys, Dawn *Secretary* 3/9/1998 - 5/4/1998

Baxindine, Edna *SAP Coordinator* 3/17/1992 - 11/22/1994

Bayard, Aaron *House Case Mgr./Referral Coord.* 7/1/2002 - 10/28/2004

Baymor, Connie *Human Resource Assistant* 5/28/1996 - 7/6/1999

Bayon, Jose *Addictions Technician* 4/29/2003 - 4/4/2005

Bear, Michael *Business Manager* 7/20/1994 - 10/23/1996

Beattie, Kelly *Activities Worker* 12/19/2001 - 5/18/2004

Beaumont, Robin *Activities Worker* 12/12/2001 - 9/2/2002

Beauregard, Joanne *Intensive Comm. Counselor* 6/12/1996 - 10/24/1997

Beauvais, Danielle *EAP Counselor* 2/8/2005 - present

Bechtold, Lori *Wraparound Secretary* 5/24/1999 - 3/25/2000

Beck, Mary *Social Worker* 3/1/1997 - 6/1/1999

Bedford, Angela *Nurse* 9/8/1998 - present

Bedford, Robert *Addictions Technician II* 4/8/1998 - 1/14/2000

Beer, Angela *Therapeutic Staff Support* 12/21/2004 - present

Beese, Gary *Administrator* 7/19/1971 - 5/15/1978 - present

Beitz, Nancy *Outpatient Team Secretary* 3/28/1983 - 6/4/1984

Belke, Susan *Nurse Supervisor* 4/7/1994 - 8/17/2001

Bellucci, Carol *Art Therapist* 10/18/1993 - 9/19/2003

Bench, Ellen *Medical Records Manager/Quality Improvement Coord.* 12/15/1992 - 9/20/1996

Bender, Elizabeth *On Call Secretary* 3/8/1995 - 11/1/1995

Benjamin, Kathleen *Addictions Technician* 9/12/2000 - present

Benner, Julianna *Intensive Case Management* 4/22/2003 - 6/7/2004

Berardelli, Harry *MIS Coordinator* 3/23/2001 - present

Berg, Bernard *Psychiatric Patient Coordinator* 7/1/1980 - 3/31/1985

Berger, Cindy *Therapeutic Staff Support* 2/23/2000 - 3/24/2000

Bergey, Evon *Newtown Clinical Director* 6/24/1999 - 1/14/2000

Berke, Charlotte *Intake Representative* 11/23/1998 - 3/8/2000

Bernat, Virginia *Recovery Center Evening Secretary* 2/28/1991 - 3/15/1991

Bernd, Roger *Nurse* 3/1/1998 - present

Berner, Elaine *On-Call Secretary* 8/24/1993 - 9/1/1994

Bernstein, Mark *Assistant Medical Director; Psychiatrist* 5/28/1980 - 8/24/1989

Berrios, Barbara *Secretary* 10/6/1997 - 6/5/2003

Berry, Beverly *Activity Assistant* 10/28/1992 - 5/22/1993

Bhallo, Sajeda *Primary Inpatient Counselor* 10/2/2000 - 10/3/2003

Biehl, Rosanne *3A Inpatient Activities Assistant*
1/6/1990 - 7/1/1992
Biello, Carol *Nurse* 7/8/1998 - 10/28/1999
Bilofsky, Ira *Director/Langhorne* 3/1/1997 -
7/1/1998
Bincarovsky, Kristyna *Crisis Worker* 1/26/2000 -
1/11/2001
Bingaman, Brenda *Secretary/Receptionist*
10/26/1983 - 3/1/1985
Birky, David *Public Relations Director*
10/24/1983 - 7/6/1987
Bishop, Brandon *Therapeutic Staff Support*
4/26/1999 - 3/3/2000
Bishop, Terri *Fiscal & Statistical Asst.* 7/20/1981
- 12/23/1983
Bitner, Alan *Lead Addictions Technician II*
3/27/2002 - present
Black, Christine *Receptionist* 11/1/1999 -
6/29/2001
Blaxland, John *Crisis Worker* 5/17/1996 -
8/22/1997
Bleam, Joanne *File Clerk* 11/10/1998 -
3/23/1999
Bloom, Sandra *Psychiatrist* 12/26/1978 -
6/8/1979
Blumenthal, Cynthia *Outpatient Counselor*
8/1/2000 - present
Blumenthal, William *Associate Director, Recovery
Center* 11/4/1991 - present
Bochey, Mary Ann *Primary Therapist* 5/26/1993 -
12/9/1994
Boguslaw, Angela *Case Manager* 6/11/1984 -
11/15/1985
Bolish, Eileen *Inpatient Case Mgr.* 1/9/1988 -
11/8/2000
Booker-Carter, Cheryl *Psychiatrist* 9/22/1998 -
6/28/2001
Bordner, Linda *Secretary/Switchboard Operator*
4/12/1976 - 6/12/1978
Borowski, Barbara *Residential Assistant*
3/26/1990 - present
Boss, Michelle *Crisis Coord.* 6/9/1997 -
2/5/1999
Boswell, Lori *Wraparound Secretary* 6/16/2004 –
2/23/2005
Bower, Donald *TEP Residential Aide* 7/8/2004 -
10/2/2004
Bowman, Barry *Residential Instructor* 4/29/1989
- 9/26/1989
Boyer, Alyssa *Therapeutic Staff Support*
5/22/2003 - 8/31/2003
Bradford, Tedd *Therapist* 9/19/1996 - present
Bradley, James *Addictions Technician* 11/5/2001
- 1/30/2002
Bradley, Ursula *Nurse* 7/5/1988 - 7/31/1988
Brady, Nicole *Intensive Community Counselor*
8/20/1996 - 8/30/1996
Brady, Patricia *Cleaning Person (PT)* 6/11/1979 -
10/25/1979
Braken, Lawrence *Driver* 8/26/1991 - 6/1/1999

Brandt-Landy, Linda *D/A Therapist* 4/4/1988 -
10/26/1989
Brennan, Teres *Addictions Technician* 11/6/2001
- 9/13/2004
Brent, Jennifer *Managed Care Representative*
10/23/2000 - present
Breon, Robert *Residential Instructor* 7/29/1992 -
8/24/1993
Bresinger, Cynthia *Admissions Rep.* 1/27/1997 -
7/22/1999
Breslin, Maureen *Intensive Community Counselor*
4/8/1996 - 6/28/1996
Brewster, Justin *Crisis Worker* 8/14/2003 -
11/27/2003
Bright, Susan *Intensive Comm. Counselor*
6/9/1993 - 9/27/1996
Britt, Maria *Therapist* 3/26/1990 - 2/15/1991
Bromwell, Jennifer *PRN Crisis Worker* 1/3/2001 -
2/24/2002
Brong, Diane *Psychotherapist* 8/2/1988 -
5/27/1993
Brooks, Carol *Managed Care Representative*
11/27/2001 - 3/20/2003
Brower, Patricia *Intensive Case Manager*
10/12/1992 - 2/17/1995
Brown, Colleen *Medical Records Clerk*
12/4/2000 - 11/2/2001
Brown, Deidre *Intensive Community Counselor*
2/3/1999 - 8/13/1999
Brown, Janice *Case Manager* 8/7/1985 -
8/21/1986
Brown, Margaret *Admissions Representative*
9/20/1995 - 1/31/1997
Brown, Richard *Addictions Technician* 11/6/2000
- 8/31/2001
Brown, Timothy *Crisis Worker* 7/28/2003 -
3/15/2005
Browne, Joanne *Behavior Specialist* 9/18/1996 -
11/21/1996
Brunk, Elizabeth *EAP Director* 5/31/1989 -
7/21/1998
Brunk, Gayle *Residential Instructor/Intensive
Case Manager* 6/30/1992 - 3/3/1994
Bryans-Brennan, Barbara *Psychologist* 7/9/1996
- 9/15/1998
Buch, David *Psychiatrist* 10/1/1989 - 11/1/1993
Buchanan, Scott *EAP Counselor* 2/22/2000 -
5/25/2000
Bucher, Rachel *Therapeutic Staff Support*
12/17/2002 - 10/3/2003
Buckley, Renee *Fiscal Clerk* 3/1/1992 - 5/1/1992
Buehrle, Pamela *Stepping Stones Advisor*
2/1/1988 - 9/15/1988
Bukovec, Deborah *Psychotherapist* 11/12/1996 -
11/16/2000
Bullock, Peter *EAP Counselor* 1/4/1988 -
9/29/1989
Burak, Rhonda *Social Worker* 6/5/1995 - present
Burkholder, Jay *Psychotherapist* 1/27/1997 -
12/31/1997

Burns, Geraldine *Caseworker* 6/18/1979 - 3/7/1980

Burns, Raymond *Intensive Community Counselor* 4/8/1997 - 12/24/1997

Burwell, Barbara *Associate Administrator* 1/21/1985 - 4/30/1990

Butt-Polier, Melissa *Outpatient Counselor* 7/14/1997 - 6/17/2004

Byrd, Suzanne *Mobile Therapist* 10/9/1996 - 6/6/1997

Cahill, Cindy *Switchboard Receptionist* 2/11/1998 - 2/20/1998

Campbell, Catherine *Outpatient Team Secretary* 12/21/1981 - 8/20/1982

Campbell, Darene *Secretary/Receptionist* 10/12/1993 - 6/13/1996

Cannon, Kathleen *Addictions Technician* 9/21/1993 - 9/28/1993

Canouse, Janet 8/23/1971- 8/1/1972

Cappel, Cynthia *Female Residential Advisor* 7/2/2002 - 2/22/2004

Caputo, Yvonne *EAP Counselor* 9/18/1989 - 7/1/1998

Caraway, Vernon *Intensive Community Counselor* 1/7/1998 - 4/20/1998

Cardineau, Erika *Supports Coordinator* 6/23/2003 - present

Carlson, Cindy *Secretary* 9/5/2000 - 9/7/2000

Carlson, Louise *Residential Caseworker* 10/31/1990 - present

Caroff, Betty *Business Manager* 9/26/1978- 12/30/1988; *CFO* 5/3/1999 - 7/1/2004

Caroff, Bonnie *Computer Analyst II* 2/12/1981 - 9/25/1996

Caroff, Jessica *File Clerk* 6/12/2002 - present

Carraquillo, Karen *Intensive Community Counselor* 8/18/1997 - 9/11/1997

Carroll, Geri *Intake/Fiscal Caseworker* 8/31/1988 - 6/6/1990

Carver, Zoe *Mobile Therapist, Wraparound* 1/11/2005 - present

Cassel, Michele *EAP Counselor* 3/5/1986 - 10/29/1996

Castner, Kathleen *Intake Worker* 4/28/1986 - 2/10/1989

Castree, Laura *Behavioral Specialist/Mobile Therapist* 7/30/2003 - 12/23/2003

Catalanotti, Margaret *Admissions Worker* 7/15/1996 - 11/21/1996

Chadwick, Diana *Addictions Technician* 2/13/1995 - 6/19/1995

Chaikin, Ricki *Addictions Technician* 8/11/1998 - 6/30/1999

Chapman, Christine *Residential Caseworker* 4/1/2002 - present

Charles, Thomas *Residential Instructor* 2/19/1985 - 7/19/1985

Chasko, Joann *Mobile Therapist* 3/18/1996 - 5/10/1996

Chatzinoff, Kenneth *Psychologist* 4/11/2000 - 6/30/2000

Chau, Khuong *Therapeutic Staff Support* 12/28/1999 - 2/4/2000

Chernikovich, Kathy *Cleaning Person* 3/31/1980 - 6/3/1981

Chipley, Cathryn *Outpatient/Partial Hospital Prog. Coord.* 4/30/2001 - present

Chow, Traci *Scheduling Secretary* 7/7/2003 - present

Christian, Betty *EAP Counselor* 5/23/1991 - 7/1/1994

Cisick, Dennis *Addiction Technician* 6/4/1999 - 6/1/2000

Ciuitarese, Carolyn *Intensive Community Counselor* 1/5/1998 - 7/13/1998

Clark, Donna *Human Resources Assistant* 2/6/1995 - 4/12/1996

Clark, Ellen *Crisis Worker* 11/21/1990 - 6/20/1997

Clark, Juanita *Addictions Technician* 10/30/2003 - 12/21/2003

Clark, Lisa *Therapist* 1/28/2004 - present

Clayton, David *Psychologist* 2/5/1968 - 1/31/2005

Clayton, Nora *Registered Nurse* 10/25/1991 - 2/20/1995

Clemens, Rebekah *Therapeutic Staff Support* 9/14/1999 - 1/19/2001

Clemens, Terri *Medical Records Technician* 3/19/1998 - 6/14/2000

Clements, Richard *Mobile Therapist/Behavior Spec.* 4/29/1999 - 10/26/1999

Clifford, Peter *Occupational Therapist* 8/6/1986 - 7/31/1987

Clipp, Jay *Residential Aide* 12/4/1998 - 5/28/1999

Clymer, Gloria *Insurance Billing Clerk* 10/7/1996 - present

Cocron, Gloria *Resource Coordinator* 5/1/1978 - 9/4/1981

Colamarino, Gina *Intensive Community Counselor* 8/17/1998 - 2/4/2000

Cole, Ronald *PRN Driver* 3/22/2004 - present

Cole, Sally *Health Care Coordinator* 5/26/2004 - present

Coleman, Wanda *Clinical Assistant* 9/26/1994 - 12/30/1994

Colletti, Lynne *TEP Mail Clerk* 9/25/2001 - 2/1/2002

Collier, Charlotte *Behavioral Specialist* 9/11/1995 - present

Colonna, Suzanne *Administrative Assistant* 2/10/1997 - 12/8/2000

Comfort, Dorothy *Supports Coordinator* 5/22/1997 - present

Comparato, Cynthia *Social Worker* 9/30/1999 - 6/30/2000

Conboy, Michelle *Therapy Technician* 8/17/1989 - 2/4/1990

Connelly, Matthew *Intensive Community Counselor* 8/2/1993 - 8/25/1995

Coogan, Arthur *Residential Instructor* 9/23/1985 - 8/17/1986

Cope, Janine *PRN Crisis Worker* 6/13/2002 - present

Copel, Sidney *Psychologist* 6/11/1996 - 2/4/2000

Corcoran, Lisa *PRN TSS Trainer* 9/13/1999 - present

Cordisco, Linda *EI Service Coordinator* 5/27/1997 - 11/19/1999

Cormick, Karen *Accounts Payable/Payroll Clerk* 4/6/2000 - 10/30/2001

Corson, Pam *EAP Therapist* 5/15/1990 - 10/8/1993

Cotton, Amy *Receptionist/Secretary* 1/26/1998 - 8/30/1999

Coughlan, Jule *Switchboard Receptionist* 4/2/1998 - 3/4/1999

Coughlan,Timothy *Therapeutic Staff Support* 5/21/2001 - 11/15/2001

Cougle, Lynne *Receptionist/Intake Rep* 3/20/2000 - 4/18/2000

Covelens, Beverly *Data Entry* 6/9/1997 - 9/17/1998

Cramer, Lou Ann *Transcriptionist* 7/6/1992 - 4/28/1995

Crane, Carol *Crisis Worker* 11/23/1999 - 3/22/2000

Craven, Holly *Data Entry Clerk* 6/7/1999 - 6/15/2001

Crawford, Priscilla *Substance Abuse Counselor* 3/7/1977 - 7/5/1985

Creciun, Michael *Addictions Technician* 4/23/1996 - 5/19/1996

Crimbly, Dolly *Secretary/Receptionist* 7/17/1997 - 8/28/1998

Crites, Kathleen Hope *Psychotherapist* 2/13/1996 - 12/19/1996

Croll, Sandra *Intake Worker* 7/7/1986 - 5/24/1995

Crouthamel, Linda *Caseworker* 3/7/1980 - 7/29/1980

Crouthamel, Tracy *Lifeguard* 6/29/1993 - 9/2/1993

Crowthers, Melisssa *Receptionist* 8/25/1998 - 3/31/1999

Cruice, Esther *Secretary/Receptionist* 8/13/1984 - 12/1/1987

Cucchiaro, Nicholas *Intensive Community Counselor* 1/19/1999 - 3/23/1999

Cullen, Kathleen *Residential Advisor* 10/14/2004 - present

Cullen, Linda *Nurse* 7/22/1988 - 11/25/1988

Cundiff, Alice *Addictions Technician* 2/1/2000 - 3/1/2000

Cunningham, Gary *Assistant Counselor* 11/12/1990 - 9/16/1999

D'Agosta, Mehan *Case Manager* 5/9/1994 - 4/21/1995

D'Amico, Stephanie *Social Worker* 5/15/1995 - 8/31/1995

D'Ancona, Amy *Psychiatric Social Worker* 1/13/1990 - 6/20/1990

D'Antonio, Andrew *Addictions Technician* 2/8/2000 - 8/27/2001

D'Arcy, Kimberly *Intensive Community Counselor* 11/4/1997 - 9/4/1998

D'Zmura, Justine *Psychologist* 6/6/1994 - 2/29/1996

Dacey, Amisa *Mobile Therapist* 6/24/2003 - present

Dale, Sandra *Nurse* 6/26/1994 - present

Daly, Allan *Medical Records Clerk* 1/17/1998 - 2/1/1998

Daly, Terese *Mobile Therapist* 1/11/1999 - 2/4/2000

Damone, Andrea *Crisis Worker* 6/4/2003 - present

Dandurand, Kyle *Therapeutic Staff Support* 2/20/2004 - 7/1/2004

Daniels, Nancy *Stepping Stones Advisor* 12/7/1983 - 4/16/1984

Danner, Wafa *Accountant, BreakThrough* 11/14/1988 - 7/14/1989

Danzman, Robarn *Therapeutic Staff Support* 4/23/2003 - 4/1/2005

Darling, Jo-Ellen *Admissions Rep.* 7/9/1994 - 5/9/2000

Darrow, Laura *Crisis Worker* 8/5/2002 - 10/2/2002

Dattner, Laura *Intensive Community Counselor* 11/3/1997 - 11/6/1998

Daves, Anne *Case Manager* 3/9/1988 - 6/30/1988

Davidock, Jill *Residential Instructor* 4/14/1986 - 7/1/1988

Davidson, John *Clinical Supervisor* 3/27/1989 - 12/19/1995

Davis, Campbell *Psychiatrist* 7/19/1988 - 8/11/1995

Davis, Carol *Psychologist* 12/5/1995 - 1/25/1996

Davis, Molly *Executive Secretary* 5/13/1981 - 7/15/1982

Day, Jill *Admissions Representative* 2/23/2004 - 12/16/2004

Day, William *Social Worker* 11/4/1997 - 10/25/1999

Dayton, Lorita *Social Worker* 5/30/1999 - 8/15/1998

Deal, Julia *D&A Coordinator* 8/28/1989 - 12/15/1989

Degaitis, Stephanie *Case Management Supervisor II, Bucks* 5/10/1990 - present

Degezelle, Kendra *Clinical Assistant* 1/3/1995 - 1/24/2000

DeGroot, Heather *Mobile Therapist* 9/4/1996 - 3/31/1998

DeLuca, Linda *Office Coordinator* 3/1/1997 - 8/24/1999

Dembrosky, Lisa *Psychiatric Rehabilitation Specialist* 4/4/1994 - present

DeMott, Stacy *Secretary/Receptionist* 9/8/1998 - 9/25/1998

Denton, Joseph *Behavioral Specialist* 2/11/2003 - 2/23/2005

DeRivas, Carmela Psychiatrist 11/1970 - 7/1972

Derstine, Elaine *Psychiatric Patient Coord.* 12/9/1982 - 3/31/1985

Derstine, Janet *Admin. Secretary* 11/28/1988 - 11/3/1989

Derstine, Kenneth *Office Clerk, TEP* 3/6/2002 - 4/12/2002

Derstine, Lynette *Correspondence Secretary* 7/10/2000 - present

Derstine, Steven *File Clerk* 7/14/1998 - 1/15/1999

Derstine, Trina *Medical Records Clerk* 6/16/1998 - Unknown

Desai, Abhilash *Inpatient Medical Director* 11/3/2003 - 9/30/2004

Detweiler, Donald *Director* 3/14/1994 - present

Detweiler, Phyllis *Secretary* 3/22/1977 - 8/7/1978

Detweiler, Susan *Mail Clerk, TEP* 4/12/2000 - 9/1/2000

Detweiler, Tara *Administrative Case Manager, Montgomery* 6/9/2000 - present

Deuble, E'lise *Case Manager* 5/5/1982 - 6/28/1983

Deuchar, Rebecca *Crisis Worker* 6/8/2004 - present

Deutsch, Cheryl *BreakThrough Secretary* 4/3/1989 - 5/4/1989

Devlin, Diane *Director of Children's Community Based Services* 8/26/1996 - present

DeVoll, Donna *Secretary/Receptionist* 9/1/1993 - 9/16/1994

DeYoung, Annetta *Fiscal Assistant* 2/2/1981 - 2/20/1981

Diak, Kathleen *OP Therapist/Coordinator* 7/25/1988 - 6/30/1989

DiCiurcio, Gina *Social Worker* 5/2/1997 - 6/27/2001

Dickson, Dean *Clinical Supervisor* 3/1/1997 - 6/29/2001

DiDonato, Susan *Secretary* 2/24/2003 - 3/21/2003

Diehl, Joy *Admissions Representative* 1/11/1988 - present

Diehl, Peggy *Secretary* 6/12/1989 - 6/6/1990

Diehl, Susan *Admissions Representative* 2/9/1999 - 11/1/2000

Diener, Nancy *RN/Therapist* 11/7/1994 - 4/29/1998

Dietrich, Gretchen *Mobile Therapist* 8/7/2000 - 2/28/2001

Dillon, Janice *Switchboard Receptionist* 3/22/1999 - 7/9/1999

Diorio, Donna *Managed Care Rep.* 1/3/2000 - 8/3/2001

DiSciullo, Kim *Case Manager* 6/26/2000 - 12/29/2000

Distel, Janet *Social Worker* 5/20/1999 - 5/24/2000

DiTucci, Christine *Addictions Technician* 2/25/2004 - 2/26/2004

Dodson, Lois *School Services Coordinator* 9/22/1993 - present

Doheny, Barbara *Accounting Clerk* 2/26/1990 - 8/13/1993

Donahue, Stephen *Psychologist* 10/24/2003 - present

Donegan, Emily *Secretary* 5/26/1998 - 11/8/2000

Donnelly, Bernadette *Receptionist* 7/9/1984 - 1/25/1985

Dorsey, Dorthea *Residential Advisor* 12/6/1997 - 8/15/2004

Dougherty, Diane *Secretary- On Call* 4/21/1992 - 9/11/1993

Dougherty, Nancy *Crisis Worker* 5/10/2004 - 12/26/2004

Dougherty, Patricia *School Services Coordinator* 1/9/1995 - 11/1/2000

Douglas, Andrew *Intensive Community Counselor* 5/19/1994 - 6/1/1998

Doyle, Erma *Business Manager* 6/10/1996 - 6/13/1997

Doyle, Katherine *Case Manager/Therapeutic Staff Support* 7/6/2004 - 5/13/2005

Doyle, Sherry *Case Manager* 3/5/1990 - 4/19/1990

Draper, Carol *Activity Assistant* 2/17/1992 - 7/16/1994

Drennen, Timothy *Wraparound Counselor* 1/3/1994 - 7/12/1996

Dries, Theresa *Therapy Technician* 2/2/1990 - 2/17/1990

Driscoll, Kelly *Therapeutic Staff Support* 3/28/2001 - 4/10/2001

Droz, Luzma *Accounts Payable Clerk* 4/3/1995 - 3/7/1997

Drury, Cheryll *Secretary/Recovery Services* 12/29/1998 - 5/26/2000

Duffy-Bell, Donna *Director of Rehabilitation Services* 11/13/1984 - present

Dulin, Amy *Case Manager* 6/25/1996 - 6/30/2003

Dull, Barbara *Lifeguard* 6/28/1994 - 6/1/1997

Dunlap, Abby *Summer Camp Intern* 6/23/2004 - 7/23/2004

Dunlap, Kimberly *Mobile Therapist* 7/22/2003 - present

Dunn, John *Psychiatrist* 2/27/1960 - 6/5/1992

Dunning, Diane *Social/Recreational Aide* 7/3/1995 - present

Dunning, Robert *Inpatient Counselor* 1/31/1994 - present

Dupont, Pauline *RN, BreakThrough* 8/12/1988 - 2/13/1989

Dupper, Janice *Administrative Assistant II*
3/14/1988 - present

Eagan, Jennifer *Intensive Case Manager*
2/1/2001 - 11/10/2001

Earussi, Pamela *Activity Therapist* 12/3/1988 -
11/12/1992

Eastland, Patricia *Secretary* 7/17/1990 -
1/8/1993

Ebersole, Barbara *Admissions Coordinator*
5/26/1992 - 9/18/1992

Ebling, Deneen *Mobile Therapist* 4/19/1996 -
7/30/1997

Eckhart, Betty *Accountant* 8/12/1974 -
9/1/1978

Edelman, Terry *Insurance/Billing Clerk/Secretary*
2/20/1989 - 7/1/1993

Edmunds, Evelyn *Psychologist* 4/3/1984 -
7/17/1987

Edwards JR, Robert *Intensive Case Manager*
3/30/2001 - 8/3/2001

Efuwape, Joshua *Mobile Therapist* 9/28/2000 -
8/17/2004

Egan, Jeanette *EAP Counselor* 6/3/2003 -
10/17/2003

Egan, Wendy *Therapeutic Staff Support*
1/15/2001 - 8/28/2002

Ehrhorn, George *Nurse Practitioner* 9/2/2003 -
present

Ehst, Rhoda *Outpatient Therapist* 3/3/1986 -
4/4/1989

Elkins, Jennifer *Intensive Case Manager*
3/29/2004 - present

Elrod, Shirley *Crisis Worker* 9/15/1997 -
4/9/1998

Ely, Elaine *Residential Caseworker* 11/10/1986 -
12/17/1989

Emerick, Margaret *Executive Assistant* 3/8/1966
- present

Eng, Ruth *Outpatient Team Secretary* 8/17/1983
- 6/12/1987

Ennis, Donna *Addictions Technician* 10/22/1993
- 1/31/1999

Erb, Jeanne *Secretary* 6/12/1996 - 7/31/1996

Erhardt, Leslie *Managed Care Representative*
7/15/1998 - 8/5/1998

Erickson, Larry *Controller* 3/23/1998 - 9/30/1999

Ervin, Janet *Switchboard Operator* 12/1/1956 -
7/10/1979

Eschbach, Eugenie *Psychiatrist* 9/4/1990 -
7/17/1996

Etzrodt, Laurie *Clinical Director* 1/24/2000 -
12/29/2000

Eubanks, Kimberly *Secretary/Receptionist*
10/1/1994 - 6/15/2001

Evans, Holly *Therapeutic Staff Support*
7/23/2001 - 11/15/2001

Evans, Kimberly *Insurance Billing Clerk*
8/21/2000 - 6/11/2001

Evans, Marie *Psychiatric Rehab. Assistant*
10/20/1997 - present

Evans, William *Maintenance Coordinator*
4/9/1997 - 11/1/2000

Everitt, Sandra *Office Manager* 9/20/1982 -
12/1/1987

Ewing, Cindy *Therapeutic Staff Support*
5/1/2001 - 5/14/2001

Eyer, Gerry *Secretary/Receptionist* 3/5/1998 -
12/15/1998

Eyet, Christine *Aftercare Tech.* 11/17/1997 -
7/15/1998

Fadeley, Daniel *Addictions Technician* 6/26/1995
- 8/9/1995

Fake, Traci *Intensive Community Counselor*
7/7/1998 - 9/28/1998

Farber, Shirley *Psychiatric Nurse* 3/27/1984 -
3/31/1991

Farlow, Linda *Admissions/Triage Caseworker*
10/1/1992 - 12/29/1995

Fegely, Lois *Billing/Accounts Receivable*
9/15/1998 - 11/29/1999

Feliciano, Ronald *Addiction Technician*
2/18/1999 - 6/1/1999

Fell, Edward *EAP Counselor* 3/3/1988 -
9/29/1989

Fendler, Trudy *Nurse* 12/21/1988 - 4/23/1989

Fennell, Ronald *Social Worker* 3/9/1995 -
12/1/1994

Ferrell, Robert *Addictions Counselor* 1/3/1984 -
11/25/1988

Ferrence, Mark *EAP Counselor* 2/1/2002 -
2/20/2003

Ferrich, Cheryl *Medical Records Manager*
3/23/1998 - 5/22/1998

Ferrier, Frederick *Addictions Technician*
11/29/1996 - 2/15/1997

Ferrizzi, Jean *Nurse* 12/18/1997 -
10/16/1998

Fettig, Jamie *Outpatient Counselor* 10/1/2002 -
8/29/2003

Fingalsen, Randall *Addictions Technician*
8/24/1992 - 2/21/1993

Finnegan, Colleen *Addictions Technician*
1/3/2002 - 1/30/2002

Finnegan, Katherine *Case Manager/Therapeutic
Staff Support* 6/16/2003 - present

Finnegan, Melissa *Intensive Community
Counselor* 4/27/1998 - 5/26/1998

Firster, Gary *Program Coordinator* 7/10/1995 -
1/23/1998

Fischer, Ellen *Wraparound Coordinator*
6/10/2004 - present

Fischer, Michelle *Social Worker* 10/20/1998 -
11/17/1998

Fischer, Victoria *Psychotherapist* 2/6/1996 -
10/23/1996

Fisher, Andrea *Intensive Community Counselor*
5/20/1996 - 7/10/1996

Fisher, Tracy *Secretary/Receptionist* 11/4/1996 -
11/15/1996

Fithen, Edna *File Clerk* 7/6/1999 - 9/13/1999

Flango, Wendy *Executive Secretary* 6/16/1980 - 7/31/1980

Flederbach, Linda *EAP Counselor* 10/17/2003 - 12/29/2004

Fleischmann, Veronica *MR Case Manager* 6/22/1998 - 9/15/1999

Flore, Daniel *TEP Mail Clerk* 3/17/2003 - 10/7/2003

Fluck, Barbara *Medical Records Clerk* 11/25/1985 - 6/5/1986

Foderaro, Joseph *Social Worker* 12/26/1978 - 7/10/1979

Fong, Kai Heng (Elizabeth) *Social Worker* 3/20/1995 - 6/1/1999

Forsythe, Darryl *Mobile Therapist* 7/27/1999 - 2/4/2000

Foss, Wende *Addictions Technician II* 10/15/1997 - present

Fox, Brenda *Wraparound Case Manager* 4/4/1994 - 5/9/1996

Fox, Shannon *Intensive Case Manager* 3/22/2004 - 3/26/2004

Frank, Tracy *Transcriptionist/Secretary* 6/19/1996 - 4/3/1998

Frasco, Gina *Receptionist* 3/24/1997 - 5/27/1997

Fravel-Peck, Bonnie *File Clerk* 1/5/1998 - 2/15/1999

Fredrick, Nancy *Nurse/Rehab PRN* 8/20/1988 - 6/27/1989

Freeman, Tia *Receptionist/Secretary* 6/19/2001 - 4/14/2003

Friedman, Sondra *Social Worker* 11/29/1994 - 12/18/1996

Friesen, Victor *Psychologist* 3/1/1997 - 5/29/1997

Frisch, Paul *Mobile Therapist* 4/19/1996 - 2/4/2000

Frost, Paula *Social Worker* 4/9/1999 - 6/19/2000

Frye, Susan *Team Secretary Transitions* 9/8/1987 - 1/13/1989

Fulford, John *Crisis Worker* 1/24/2002 - 6/30/2002

Fulmer, Marjorie *Administrative Assistant* 9/8/1987 - 6/30/1989

Funchion, Dana *Addictions Counselor* 8/11/1994 - 11/19/1998

Gable, Jacob *Addictions Technician* 1/20/2000 - 9/29/2000

Gaenssle, Anne *Resource Coordinator* 5/17/1999 - 11/21/2000

Gallagher, Kathy *Therapy Tech.* 8/2/1989 - 9/30/1989

Gallagher, Margaret *Registered Nurse* 3/5/1990 - 6/23/1991

Gallo, Ralph *Pediatrician* 10/16/1975 - 5/31/1979

Galt, Catherine *Administrative Case Manager* 1/11/2001 - 4/12/2001

Gammon, Maureen *Intensive Community Counselor* 10/4/1993 - 7/1/1996

Garee, Joyce *Intensive Community Counselor* 3/1/1997 - 7/31/1997

Garges, Nicole *Intensive Case Manager* 9/18/2000 - 6/5/2002

Garges, Priscilla *Therapeutic Staff Support* 5/22/2003 - 6/4/2003

Garman, Stephanie *Addictions Technician* 2/23/1999 - 4/1/2000

Garner, Christine *Intensive Community Counselor* 11/21/1997 - 1/6/1999

Gartner, Jennifer *Data Entry Clerk* 3/16/1999 - 8/24/2000

Gatkar, Lois *Registered Nurse* 6/1/1993 - 2/15/1995

Gaumer, Eric *Maintenance Worker* 5/10/2000 - 4/12/2002

Gaumer, Jennifer *Wraparound Camp Counselor* 5/14/2001 - 5/1/2003

Gaumer, Kathy *Transcriptionist* 9/5/2000 - 11/15/2001

Gebhard, Margo *Addictions Counselor* 11/28/1994 - 9/20/2004

Gedrimas, Leslie *Crisis Worker PRN* 10/29/1998 - 11/9/1998

Gehman, Ann *Social Worker* 3/2/1998 - 6/25/2000

Gehman, Elaine *Administrative Assistant* 1/19/1981 - 10/14/1988

Gehman, Rebecca *Fiscal Case Manager* 12/21/1981 - 7/15/1991

Gehringer, Madeleine *Nurse Supervisor* 6/27/1995 - present

Geib, Dawn *Adult Intensive Case Manager* 10/16/1996 - 1/9/1998

Geiger, Valerie *Resource Coordinator/NSH Liaison* 5/8/1995 - 6/30/1997

Geiselman, Kimberly *Mobile Therapist* 8/30/2004 - present

Geissler, Emilie *Case Manager* 8/17/2004 - present

Gelsebach, Beth *Addictions Technician II* 10/5/1992 - present

Gensemer, Colleen *Intensive Community Counselor* 8/18/1997 - 7/16/1999

Gentry, John *Psychotherapist* 2/4/1997 - 6/1/1999

George, David *Residential Advisor* 6/24/2004 - present

Geraci, Linda *Case Manager* 5/16/1996 - 7/19/1996

Gerard, Adrianna *Intensive Case Manager, Bucks* 8/9/1999 - present

Gerena, Natanael *Wraparound Mobile Therapist* 4/26/1994 - 7/22/1997

Gerenser, Anne *Therapeutic Staff Support* 10/13/2003 - 4/30/2004

Gerhert, Kay *Psychiatric Patient Coord.* 8/31/1981 - 8/31/1982

Giamo, Patricia *Adolescent Partial Coord.* 8/16/1999 - 6/18/2004

Giddy, Jacqueline *Addictions Technician*
12/22/2004 - present
Gilles, Kimberly *Crisis Coordinator* 11/18/1999 -
6/15/2000
Gilliano, Lillian *PRN Nurse* 5/27/2003 - present
Gilson, Marianne *Director of Quality Improvement*
8/7/1989 - present
Glaskin, Carol *Psychiatrist* 8/9/1982 - 2/28/1983
Glass, Paul *Residential Aide* 1/24/2005 -
3/31/2005
Godshall, Carol *Residential Instructor* 9/27/1993
- 5/31/1995
Godshall, Norell *Residential Aide* 7/14/1998 -
6/24/2000
Gollon, John *PRN Mail Clerk* 12/1/2003 - present
Gonzalez, Wilson *Addictions Technician*
8/26/2003 - 10/1/2003
Good, Brian *Intensive Community Counselor*
11/13/1996 - 6/12/1998
Good, Deborah *Receptionist* 8/12/1981 -
12/5/1985
Good, Philip *Maintenance Coordinator*
10/9/2000 - present
Good, Philip Jordan *MIS Assistant* 5/12/2004 -
present
Gootman, Regina *Billing Clerk* 9/8/1999 -
6/8/2001
Gordon, Heidi *MES Level II Counselor/Outpatient*
Counselor 1/18/1999 - present
Gorski, Betsy *Social Worker* 5/30/1978 -
10/11/1979
Goshow, Janet *Secretary* 4/15/1980 - 12/1981
Goshow, Jennifer *On-Call Secretary* 5/24/1994 -
5/27/1997
Goshow, Jessica *Camp Counselor* 7/1/2002 -
present
Goshow, John *President* 10/10/1977 - present
Gould, Debra *Autism Resource Professional*
5/27/1997 - present
Gradel, Margaret *Mail Clerk* 1/5/2004 - present
Graham, Beverly *Addictions Technician*
7/11/2001 - present
Grajewski, Maureen *Managed Care*
Representative 6/7/1999 - present
Grant, Laura *Mobile Therapist* 10/18/1996 -
8/14/1998
Grasse, Lori *Back-Up, Secretary* 7/19/1996 -
12/22/1997
Gray, Kathleen *Residential Advisor* 5/14/2003 -
8/7/2003
Gray, Sarah *Residential Advisor* 3/20/2002 -
9/24/2002
Gray, Sharon *Residential Advisor* 5/14/2003 -
8/7/2003
Greaves, Linda *Intensive Community Counselor*
7/13/1998 - 9/14/1998
Green, Jack *Social Worker* 8/27/1990 -
10/24/1990
Greenberg, Sondra *Social Worker* 5/15/1995 -
7/28/2000

Greger, Michele *Medical Secretary* 3/3/1997 -
6/30/2000
Grida, Michele *Director of Client Registration*
8/17/1994 - present
Griffin, Elizabeth *Psychiatric Rehab.*
Specialist/MAP Unit Supervisor 11/9/2004 -
present
Grimes, Kelly *Crisis Worker* 1/26/1998 -
1/26/1998
Grimm, Vincent *Intensive Case Manager*
7/13/1990 - 12/9/1994
Groarke, Patrick *Residential Instructor* 6/19/1991
- 3/24/1992
Gross, Joellen *Therapy Technician* 8/10/1988 -
1/22/1991
Gross, Judy *Adjunctive Therapist* 8/10/1985 -
9/13/1986
Gross, Karl *File Clerk TEP* 3/13/2000 -
9/13/2000
Gross, Kenneth *Maintenance Assistant*
5/22/1989 - 12/26/1996
Grossman, Barry *Psychologist* 11/4/1998 -
10/6/2000
Grote, Gerard *Social Worker* 5/15/1995 -
11/16/1996
Grubb, Carol *Partial Hosp. Therapist* 8/25/1997 -
1/31/2005
Grubb, Sharon *Addictions Technician* 4/6/2000 -
10/21/2002
Gruss, Dawn *Administrative Manager, MH Case*
Management 2/17/1995 - 11/22/1995
Gruver, Julie *Admissions Rep.* 11/9/1998 -
1/5/1999
Guinther, Theodore *Therapy Technician* 4/4/1988
- 10/28/1988
Gulbis, Benita *Secretary* 4/4/1994 - 5/17/1996
Guntz, Patricia *Psychiatric Caseworker*
10/11/1982 - 11/17/1989
Guy, Cheryl *Family Based Mental Health*
Services Coordinator 7/19/2000 - present
Guy, Sharleen *Admissions Rep.* 2/11/1997 -
12/1/1997
Guy-Floyd, Dawn *Crisis Worker* 6/4/1998 -
5/30/2004
Gwozdz, Judith *Residential Instructor* 3/8/1986 -
9/1/1986
Gyenes, Margaret *Emergency Specialist*
9/10/1984 - 2/14/1986
Haas, Judith *Admissions/Fiscal Clerk* 3/2/1993 -
9/1/1994
Hafler, Jean *PRN Transcriptions* 7/15/1993 -
7/11/1996
Haggert, Kathleen *Secretary, Recovery Services*
11/24/1997 - 6/21/2000
Hahn, Laura *Therapeutic Staff Support* 2/3/2003
- 8/20/2004
Hain, Lisa *Intensive Community Counselor*
9/17/1997 - 10/20/1997
Haines, Sharon *Secretary/Receptionist* 1/6/2000
- 11/22/2000

Hakun, Karen *Mobile Therapist* 3/5/1996 - present

Halamar, Michael *Therapeutic Staff Support* 7/10/2000 - 8/29/2001

Haldeman, Joan *Transcriptionist* 9/16/1986 - 8/12/1988

Halewich, Stefania *Secretary Receptionist* 5/1/1995 - 6/15/2001

Hall, Alison *Program oordinator/Psychodramatist* 9/14/1992 - 10/27/2000

Halsel, Lois *Coordinator of Clinical Practices* 6/4/1986 - present

Halteman, Dea *Activity Leader* 12/6/1996 - 8/27/2000

Hambly, Bryan *Resource Coordinator, Bucks* 8/11/2003 - present

Hamburger, George *Maintenance Assistant* 7/9/1991 - 3/2/1992

Hamilton, Darren *Addictions Technician* 2/8/2005 - 2/23/2005

Hamilton, Erinn *Intensive Care Manager* 7/7/2003 - 2/23/2004

Hamm, Nancy *Fiscal Assistant* 3/2/1981 - 9/20/1982

Hamvas, Sandra *Early Intervention Service Coordinator* 6/7/2004 - present

Handzy, Alexandra *Psychotherapist* 1/3/1995 - 3/16/1999

Haney, Lorraine *Secretary* 11/29/2004 - present

Hansberry, Karen *Residential Advisor* 5/18/2004 - present

Hansen, Omar *TEP Office Clerk* 4/12/2002 - 2/20/2003

Hansen, Susan *Social Worker* 4/10/1995 - present

Hapeman, John *Mobile Therapist* 11/19/1996 - 2/4/2000

Hardcastle, James *TEP Residential Aide* 11/17/2003 - 3/15/2004

Hardstine, Kevin *Mail Clerk* 9/27/1999 - 4/14/2000

Harper, Nancy *Admissions Rep.* 10/20/1997 - 11/13/1998

Harrington, Linda *Administrative Assistant* 6/24/2004 - present

Harris, Christine *Oupatient Team Secretary* 12/28/1983 - 2/24/1984

Hartman, James *Detox Coordinator* 12/8/1986 - 5/29/1987

Hartman, Jeanette *Medical Records Clerk* 1/14/2002 - 2/27/2003

Hartwick, Kristen *Therapeutic Staff Support* 2/19/2002 - 2/22/2002

Hartzel, Robert *PRN Crisis Worker* 4/25/2001 - 6/26/2001

Hartzell, Leslie *Mobile Therapist* 11/23/2004 - 1/31/2005

Hartzell, Rebecca *Lifeguard* 6/17/1997 - 6/15/2000

Hauck, Karen *Berks Director* 5/20/1997 - 2/3/2000

Hawkes, Steven *Intensive Community Counselor* 4/11/1994 - 8/1/1999

Heckman, Harold *Psychiatrist* 2/12/1990 - 10/10/1991

Heebner, Cheri *Intensive Community Counselor* 9/18/1996 - 4/9/1997

Heller, Lois *Secretary/Receptionist* 12/4/2000 - 6/29/2001

Helsel, Beryl *Mental Health Technician* 7/26/1999 - 5/28/2002

Hendricks, Kimberly *Executive Secretary, PRN* 3/3/1997 - 11/1/2000

Hendrickson, Nancy *Counselor* 10/20/1995 - 10/10/1996

Hengey, Karen *Switchboard Receptionist* 7/18/2002 - present

Henkels, Brian *Addictions Technician* 1/17/2003 - 11/1/2003

Henry, Kelly *Residential Instructor* 2/9/1996 - 9/17/1997

Henry, Symantha *Case Manager* 5/6/1996 - 2/4/2000

Herman, Theodore *Addictions Technician II* 6/17/1998 - present

Hertzler, Laurel *Public Relations Asst.* 6/15/1982 - 12/3/1983

Hessinger, Betsy *Residential Instructor* 3/2/1986 - 6/28/1987

Heubach, Deborah *Addiction Technician* 3/13/2000 - 5/1/2000

Hild, Beverly *Psychologist* 5/2/1997 - 6/29/2001

Hill, Zoe *Social Worker* 6/1/1999 - 6/29/2001

Hilmer, Debra *Secretary* 10/7/1991 - 2/17/1992

Hines, Michelle *PRN Residential Instructor* 7/5/1995 - 5/14/2001

Hines, Pamela *Intensive Case Manager* 8/9/1993 - 3/21/1996

Hinkle, Krista *File Clerk* 1/5/1998 - 1/7/1998

Hinkle, Lorraine *Receptionist* 11/29/1976 - 8/12/1977

Hirsh, Gail *Residential Instructor* 9/23/1998 - 12/31/2000

Histand, June *Fiscal Assistant* 10/1/1975 - 1/23/1976

Histand, Linda *Caseworker* 10/25/1978 - 6/29/1979

Histand, Martene *Admin./Support Services Director* 9/2/1992 - 11/30/2000

Histand, Megan *Float Secretary, PRN* 6/8/1999 - 2/25/2000

Histand, Tonya *Secretary, PRN* 11/18/1998 - 2/23/2000

Hitchcock, Keith *Childrens Case Manager* 4/18/1994 - 3/19/1998

Hoffman, Dorothy *Medication Clinic Nurse* 7/30/1996 - 2/3/1999

Hoffman, Mark *Psychologist* 11/26/1996 - 3/28/1997

Hoffmayer, Trisha *Therapeutic Staff Support* 9/29/2004 - present

Hollenbach, Elizabeth *Administrative Case Manager, Bucks* 4/16/2001 - present

Holmes, Tommy *Maintenance Helper* 6/12/1989 - Unknown

Hooker, Jeanne *Case Manager* 5/3/1989 - 1/30/1990

Hoopes, Dawn *Recreation Therapist* 10/30/1995 - 11/21/1996

Hoover, Linda *Therapeutic Staff Support* 5/19/2003 - 11/30/2003

Hopkins, Cheryl *Intensive Community Counselor* 3/19/1996 - 3/28/1996

Hopkins, Kelley *TEP Mail Clerk* 11/4/2002 - 7/28/2003

Hopkins, Kelly *PRN Rec. Clerk* 11/4/2002 - 6/7/2004

Hoppe, William *MES Level I Worker* 11/16/1995 - 10/15/2002

Hornig, Germaine *Intensive Care Manager* 7/12/1985 - 8/25/1993; *Social Worker* 1/2/2001 - 5/1/2002

Hornig, Gordon *MES Coordinator* 11/9/1994 - present

Hornung, Ann *Social Worker* 6/29/1995 - 8/30/1999

Horowitz, Stuart *Residential Caseworker* 12/23/1985 - 11/25/1987

Hostetter, Joanne *Admin. Case Manager* 11/15/1995 - 1/19/2001

Houser, Kimberley *Lifeguard* 6/15/1995 - 9/1/1995

Houser, Mandi *Therapeutic Staff Support* 12/30/2002 - 6/6/2003

Howard, Nicole *Intensive Community Counselor* 2/3/1998 - 9/1/1998

Howes, Elizabeth *PRN Behavioral Specialist* 4/26/2004 - 5/15/2005

Hu, Sansan *Intensive Community Counselor* 9/9/1996 - 4/20/1998

Hu, Xin (Nancy) *Accountant* 7/8/1998 - 9/18/1998

Hubbard, Judith *Pre-School Teacher* 1/31/1972 - 6/26/1974

Hudson, Erin *Intensive Case Manager, Bucks* 6/12/2000 - 1/14/2005

Huff, Lucy *Therapist* 7/6/2004 - present

Huffman, Julie *Therapy Technician* 8/22/1989 - 10/28/1989

Hufnagle, Cheryl *Secretary* 6/10/1996 - 10/3/1997

Hufnagle, Henry *PRN Lifeguard* 6/22/2000 - 6/1/2002

Huggins, Brenda *Transcriptionist* 1/3/1989 - 1/13/1989

Hughes, Tara *Payroll Clerk* 8/3/1998 - 3/31/2000

Hummer, Irene *Crisis Worker* 2/2/1988 - 7/24/1988

Hunsberger, Christine *Fiscal Coordinator* 2/7/1998 - present

Hunsberger, Gladys *Secretary Substitute* 7/11/1983 - 6/30/1987

Hunsberger, Joanne *MR Case Manager* 4/22/1998 - 5/14/1998

Hunsberger, Patricia *TEP Office Clerk* 10/4/2004 - present

Hunsberger, Tracy *Residential Instructor* 6/2/1999 - 7/14/2000

Hunter, Danielle *Receptionist/Secretary* 11/1/1999 - 11/17/2000

Hunter, Natalie *Registered Nurse* 8/7/1989 - 9/28/1990

Hutchins, J. Ann *Therapy Technician* 4/4/1988 - 2/22/1990

Hutnick, David *Addictions Technician* 7/7/1994 - 4/4/1995

Iatarola, Rhonda *Medical Records Clerk* 11/5/2001 - 11/5/2001

Iezzi, Teresa *Crisis Worker* 9/9/2004 - present

Incollingo, Mary *Billing Clerk* 3/30/1998 - 1/14/2000

Irvin, Nicole *Mobile Therapist* 11/5/2001 - 4/26/2005

Isaak, Arthur *Recreational/Activity Therapist, Day Treatment* 5/29/1964 - 6/30/1992

Iskenderian, Kevork *Psychiatrist* 1/9/2000 - 12/3/2000

Iskra, Barbara *Secretary/Client Services Rep.* 11/11/1996 - 2/29/2000

Israel, Jessica *Intensive Case Manager/Female DD Advisor* 7/13/1998 - 5/31/2002

Jalil, Guillermo *Mobile Therapist* 7/25/1999 - 2/4/2000

James, Kathleen *Psych. Nurse/Social Worker* 8/26/1985 - 5/7/1986

Jankiewicz, Martha *Mobile Therapist* 2/17/2004 - 5/3/2004

Jantzi, Douglas *Primary Therapist* 9/10/1984 - 10/8/1988

Jantzi, Karen *Emergency Specialist* 5/12/1986 - 7/31/1988

Jaros, Justin *Residential Aide TEP* 6/8/1999 - 12/4/1999

Jefferson, Cynthia *Secretary/Receptionist* 2/1/1983 - 2/4/1983

Jellen, Diane *Addictions Technician* 5/13/1999 - 10/31/2000

Jenkins, Eric *Intensive Community Counselor* 7/7/1997 - 7/21/1997

Jenkins, Lesley *Admissions Rep.* 6/26/2000 - 6/11/2001

Jeruchim, Joan *Psychologist* 10/9/1998 - 3/26/2001

Johnson, George *Social Worker* 9/9/1999 - 8/18/2000

Johnson, Patrice *Psychiatrist* 3/17/1992 - 7/22/1992

Johnston, Christine *Intensive Community Counselor* 8/12/1997 - 3/31/1999

Jombe, Mary Anne *Mail Clerk, TEP* 2/26/2001 - 10/2/2002

Jones, Kathleen *Residential Advisor* 3/5/2002 - 2/13/2004

Jones, Kristine *Addictions Technician* 1/20/2000 - 3/1/2000

Jordan, Hanna *PRN Managed Care Specialist* 5/14/1997 - 8/1/1997

Juransinski-Urso, Colette *Intensive Community Counselor* 3/14/1997 - 4/20/1998

Jurciukonis, Elizabeth *Executive Secretary* 1/19/1981 - 4/24/1981

Jurin, Renee *Secretary* 4/21/2003 - 7/8/2003

Kachline, Evelyn *SAP Coordinator* 3/5/1990 - 9/30/1992

Kachmar, Kathleen *Data Entry Clerk* 10/1/1996 - 1/29/1997

Kadela, Kristine *Case Worker* 2/17/1975 - 10/17/1978

Kaercher, Jill *Secretary/Receptionist* 4/21/2003 - present

Kalb, Margaret *Social Worker* 4/7/1998 - present

Kalkstetin, David *Psychiatrist, Independent Contractor* 6/26/1997 - 4/6/2000

Kalstein, Deborah *Case Manager* 7/18/1988 - 11/29/1988

Karaisz, Juile *Intensive Community Counselor* 2/4/1999 - 11/11/1999

Karalis, John *Mail Clerk-TEP* 11/26/2001 - 12/7/2001

Kardon, Richard *D&A Specialist* 12/18/1973 - 1/12/1979

Karlovic, Dario *Weekend Supervisor* 12/6/1997 - 4/4/1999

Karver, Megan *Therapeutic Staff Support* 7/21/1999 - 9/10/1999

Kates, Joshua *Psychotherapist* 3/20/1997 - 3/26/1997

Kauffman, Lisa *Administrative Case Manager, Bucks* 12/5/1994 - present

Kaufman, Frances *PRN Activities Worker* 12/1/1992 - 6/30/2003

Keach, Debra *Residential Instructor* 9/26/2000 - 12/15/2002

Kearney, Carol *Registered Nurse* 10/30/1990 - 12/1/1994

Keefer, Jodi *Addictions Technician* 7/18/2002 - 12/11/2003

Keeley, Elaine *Transcriptionist* 2/22/1988 - 2/16/2004

Keemer, Gerald *Mobile Therapist* 3/15/1999 - 2/4/2000

Keener, Romayne *Nurse* 12/15/1988 - 4/29/1989

Keeney, Maureen *Stepping Stones Advisor (PT)* 2/26/1985 - 10/8/1986

Keim, Brian *Therapeutic Staff Support* 5/19/2003 - 6/3/2003

Keiper, Erin *Therapeutic Staff Support* 7/23/2001 - 8/25/2001

Keller, Debra *Receptionist* 10/8/1990 - 1/12/1993

Keller, Judith *EAP Counselor* 2/26/1988 - 5/31/1988

Keller, Lorie *Secretary* 8/8/1990 - 2/19/1994

Keller, Mary *Switchboard Receptionist* 3/24/1975 - present

Kellers-Kile, Laura *Accounting Clerk* 3/13/1989 - 11/17/1989

Kelly, Christi *PRN Crisis Worker + On-Call* 5/1/2001 - present

Kelly, Ellen Anne *Case Manager* 1/23/1978 - 11/3/1978

Kelly, Grace *Managed Care Representative* 8/9/1999 - 2/11/2000

Kenna, Melissa *Medical Records/Transcriptionist* 6/14/1989 - 8/23/1989

Kern, Ann *Creative Therapist* 10/6/1982 - 7/27/1989

Kern, Karen *Director of MH Clinical Services* 9/7/1971 - present

Kerner, Nancy *Addictions Counselor* 9/1/1998 - 4/20/2001

Kerns, Ernestine *Billing Clerk* 4/6/1998 - 9/15/1999

Kerr, Kimberly *Secretary/Receptionist/Transcriptionist PRN* 8/7/2000 - 6/21/2001

Kervick, Kevin *Director of Children and Adolescent Services* 1/1/1993 - 2/15/1996

Ketner, Robie *Wraparound Office Clerk* 7/7/1997 - 4/15/1999

Kichline, Ann *Residential Advisor* 2/4/1998 - 7/5/2002

Kidd, Beverly *Case Manager* 11/16/1988 - 12/1/1989

Kiefer, Shirley *Stepping Stones Advisor* 5/14/1981 - 2/7/1985

Kieffer, Rodney *Intensive Community Counselor* 6/17/1996 - 4/20/1998

Killgore, William *EAP Director* 1/9/1984 - present

Kimpton, Linda *Therapeutic Staff Support* 2/21/2000 - 2/9/2001

Kind-Rubin, Andrew *Psychologist-Unlicensed* 4/29/1988 - 1/6/1989

King, Brooke *PRN Medical Records Clerk* 12/10/2001 - 3/27/2003

King, Frank *BreakThrough D&A Director* 4/15/1987 - 6/17/1988

King, Joanne *Addictions Counselor* 7/10/1995 - 4/15/1999

King, John *Mobile Therapist* 5/23/1994 - 8/23/1995

Kingsbauer, LeeAnne *Secretary* 9/24/1975 - 3/30/1990

Kinsey, Jacqueline *Therapeutic Staff Support* 8/12/2004 - present

Kirby, Barbara *EI Service Cooridinator* 7/6/1995 - 5/30/1997

Kirkland, Martha *TEP Mail Clerk* 10/4/2004 - 4/8/2005
Kissinger, Ruth *Residential Instructor* 10/18/1982 - 7/31/1983
Klein, Jane *Registered Nurse* 7/18/1989 - 9/20/1990
Kline, Allison *Therapy Technician* 2/2/1990 - 4/23/1990
Kline, Amber *Therapeutic Staff Support* 9/27/2001 - 12/11/2003
Kling, Mark *Business Manager* 10/2/1996 - 6/25/1997
Klingman, Tracy *Administrative Assistant* 2/12/1990 - 10/26/1990
Klock, Sandra *Cash Poster* 2/17/1998 - 6/8/2001
Klose, Marilyn *Residential Advisor* 9/13/2002 - present
Klose, Stephanie *Residential Advisor, Wraparound* 1/14/2005 - present
Kluiter, Sara *Admissions Representative* 1/25/2005 - 2/10/2005
Knepp, Ryan *Resource Coordinator, Bucks* 6/20/2003 - present
Knieriem, Meg *Receptionist* 10/25/1988 - 6/13/1991
Knight, Joanna *Managed Care Rep.* 7/7/2000 - 6/11/2001
Knott, Patricia *Adjunctive Therapist* 1/1/1983 - 9/30/1986
Koch, Glenn *Addictions Technician* 7/31/2002 - 1/31/2005
Koch, Linda *Addiction Counselor* 12/5/1988 - 12/29/1989
Kochenderfer, Noreen *Managed Care Auth. Specialist* 11/18/1996 - 2/25/1997
Koehler, Gina *Penn School Counselor* 2/15/1993 - 5/22/1998
Koehler, Melanie *Secretary* 10/4/2004 - 11/5/2004
Koehler, Paul *Social Worker* 11/29/1994 - 9/30/1996
Kohl, Gail *Typist* 6/4/1984 - 6/22/1984
Kolb, Brenda *Administrative Assistant* 9/15/1986 - 9/28/1987
Kollet, Catherine *Admissions Representative* 7/10/1995 - 11/7/1996
Kopf, Deborah *Addictions Technician* 9/29/1993 - 4/24/1994
Kopystecki, Barbara *Mental Health Professional* 9/30/1996 - present
Kordelski, Edward *Driver* 4/5/2002 - present
Korr, Bethry *Psychiatric Patient Coordinator* 8/10/1982 - 6/22/1985
Kossman, Deborah *Behavior Specialist* 8/8/1994 - 12/29/1995
Kotwal, Neville *Psychiatrist Independent Contractor* 7/5/1995 - 9/24/1998
Koziupa, Diana *Psychiatrist* 3/5/1996 - present
Kramer, Stephanie *Case Manager* 7/11/1994 - 8/16/1996

Kratz, Charles *Maintenance Assistant* 5/28/1981 - 8/31/1984
Kratz, David *PRN Crisis Worker* 4/14/2004 - 10/11/2004
Kratz, Richard *Management Trainee* 8/17/1992 - 9/1/1994
Kratz, Vernon *Psychiatrist* 7/2/1973 - present
Kraybill, Donald *Psychologist* 7/1/1982 - 2/29/1988
Krell, Adele *Addiction Tech.* 2/17/1997 - 4/10/1997
Kriebel, Elizabeth *Mobile Therapist* 10/24/2000 - 10/31/2000
Krim, Michael *Therapy Tech.* 6/12/1989 - 6/13/1990
Kristel, Erin *Case Manager* 5/30/2000 - 6/8/2000
Krolikowski, Rhonda *PRN Social/Recreational Aide* 2/4/1991 - present
Kucas, Patrick *Case Management Supervisor I* 2/13/1995 - present
Kuhns, Cynthia *Executive Secretary* 9/15/1980 - 12/2/1980
Kuhns, Ryan *Intensive Case Manager* 5/23/2002 - 10/1/2004
Kulp, Elizabeth *Medical Records Clerk* 12/21/1981 - 2/26/1985
Kulp, Susan *Secretary/Receptionist* 8/7/2000 - 8/10/2000
Kulp, T. Joyce *Fiscal Assistant* 2/12/1979 - 1/23/1981
Kunkel, Jamie *Clinical Assistant* 7/24/1995 - 9/7/1995
Kupusnick, Tracy *Intensive Community Counselor* 7/30/1997 - 10/31/1998
Kuriger, Suzanne *MR Case Management* 9/8/1997 - 6/19/1998
Kurtz, Diana *Caseworker* 5/1/1976 - 3/30/1977
Kurtz, Richard *Maintenance Worker* 5/19/2003 - present
Kurz, Gina *PRN Nurse* 11/16/2004 - 1/31/2005
Kushner, Scott *Office Clerk* 3/29/1999 - 3/3/2001
Kuzmick, Robert *Intensive Community Counselor* 4/25/1994 - 5/18/1995
LaBadie, Brandon *Intensive Community Counselor* 7/2/1997 - 6/1/1999
Labs, Priscilla *Quakertown Secretary* 12/21/1981 - 9/3/1982
LaBuda, Melissa *Mobile Therapist* 10/1/1999 - 3/31/2000
Ladley, Curtiss *Psychologist, Medical Assistance Clients* 4/9/2001 - present
LaFerrara, Patricia *Secretary/Client Services* 5/12/1997 - 6/1/1999
Laincz, Betsy *Nurse* 7/7/2003 - present
Lally, Steve *Counselor Assistant* 9/5/1996 - 2/26/1999
Lamb, Janet *Intensive Community Counselor* 10/3/1997 - 7/13/1998
Lambert, Adina *Psychologist* 5/15/1995 - 6/29/2001

Landes, G. Lawrence *Social Worker* 5/1/1963 - 5/24/1985

Landes, Henry *Administrator* 7/24/1978 - 10/14/1988

Landes, Katrina *Therapeutic Staff Support* 1/15/1999 - 8/25/2000

Landis, Beryl *Mailings Coordinator* 10/18/1982 - 2/27/1987

Landis, Cynthia *Executive Secretary* 5/28/1980 - 2/24/1983

Landis, Dorothy *Sub. Team Secretary* 4/21/1988 - Unknown

Landis, Earl *Maintenance Supervisor* 8/28/1969 - 3/26/1999; *Maintenance Worker* 8/28/2000 – present

Landis, Jennifer *File Clerk, PRN* 5/26/1998 - 5/4/2001

Landis, Joyce *Receptionist* 12/4/1973 - 11/30/1976

Landis, Kathryn *Volunteer Coordinator* 4/6/1964 - 12/31/1976

Landis, Linda *Psychiatric Patient Coordinator* 8/16/1982 - 3/11/1983

Landis, Lois *Registered Nurse* 7/31/1989 - 1/21/1990

Landis, Michael *Maintenance Assistant* 5/19/1974 - 12/19/1986

Landis, Philip *Maintenance Worker* 5/15/1995 - 8/1/1997

Landis, Sandra *Director of Human Resources* 7/1/1969 - present

Landis, Wendy *Residential Instructor* 3/27/1987 - 8/6/1992

Langen, Gail *Asst. Business Manager* 7/14/1986 - 6/30/1994

Langsdorf, Connie *Secretary/Adult Services* 9/7/1999 - 9/7/1999

Lapp, Brian *Intensive Community Counselor* 5/9/1997 - 12/1/1997

Lapp, Nancy *Director Pastoral Services* 3/15/1996 - 11/30/1998

Lara, Nancie *Behavioral Specialist* 3/24/2004 - 4/13/2005

Larson, Sherry *Med. Review Nurse* 6/27/1995 - 6/19/1996

Laudenslager, Darlene *Therapy Technician* 5/18/1990 - 4/5/1992

Lavin, Lucia *Activities Worker* 9/17/2002 - present

Lavin, Virginia *Med. Review Nurse* 10/28/1997 - 5/1/2001

Lawler, Phyliis *Mobile Therapist* 10/22/1998 - 3/16/1999

Lawler, Virginia *Social Worker* 6/15/1995 - 11/16/1996

Lawrence, Robin *Residential Advisor* 6/24/2004 - present

Lawrence, Victor *Mobile Therapist* 8/9/1996 - 4/20/1998

Le, Y *TEP Mail Clerk* 4/12/2000 - 11/30/2001

Lechner, Jason *Therapeutic Staff Support* 10/28/1999 - 2/4/2000

Lederach, Brenda *Therapist* 7/19/1983 - 7/23/2004

Lederach, Vicki *Clerk Typist* 8/22/1977 - 12/25/1981

Leedom, Charlotte *Psychotherapist* 5/15/1995 - present

Leh, Lisa *Bucks County Resource Coord.* 7/10/2000 - 1/19/2001

Leister-Rice, Kelli *Admin. Asst.* 3/23/1989 - 12/28/1990

Lennon, Loretta *Managed Care Rep.* 4/28/1997 - 5/1/1997

Leonards, Jeffrey *Psychologist* 6/6/1984 - 5/29/1985

Lepley, Anne *Secretary/Receptionist* 3/12/2001 - present

Lerch, Michelle *Human Resources Assistant* 9/7/1999 - present

Lermitte, Peter *Therapist* 10/22/2003 - present

Lester, Richard *Therapy Technician* 10/25/1988 - 12/1/1989

Leutze, Pamela *Office Manager* 5/14/1997 - 10/12/2000

Lex, Eleanor *Social Worker* 8/4/2003 - 3/17/2005

Lindh, Deborah *Social Worker* 5/15/1995 - 11/16/1996

Lindsay, Wanda *TEP-Residential Aide* 7/24/2000 - 2/23/2001

Link, Abigail *Intensive Case Manager* 8/22/2001 - 6/27/2003

Linke, Brenda *Nurse* 6/7/2004 - 9/13/2004

Lipscomb, William *Addictions Technician* 4/14/1994 - 6/20/1994

Lister, Ryan *Addictions Technician* 9/13/2000 - present

Littleton, Christine *Receptionist* 10/24/1997 - 5/15/1998

Livezey, Christa *Therapeutic Staff Support* 6/24/2002 - 11/27/2002

Lizotte, George *Therapy Technician* 5/25/1988 - 7/18/1989

Lobron, Joanmary *TEP Mail Clerk* 6/26/2001 - 11/4/2002

London, Debra *Psychiatrist* 11/14/1988 - 4/28/1989

Long, Delores *Secretary* 9/1/1971 - 3/14/1975

Long, Patricia *Case Manager* 7/15/1999 - 7/14/2000

Loper, Amanda *Therapeutic Staff Support* 11/1/2004 - 4/22/2005

Loring, Gina *Secretary/Referral Coordinator* 9/3/2002 - 10/2/2002

Loris, Joanne *Secretary* 3/4/1968 - 5/1/1969

Lott, Drew *Administrative Case Manager* 1/2/1997 - 5/22/1998

Loughridge, Carol *EAP Secretary* 5/24/1999 - 6/12/2000

Loux, Norman *Psychiatrist* 9/1/1955 - 7/1/1984

Lowery, Susan *Receptionist* 7/17/1972 - 12/21/1973

Luna III, Israel *Intensive Community Counselor* 1/26/1998 - 9/7/1999

Lutchendof, Norma *Secretary* 7/14/1975 - 2/28/1977

Lyczkowski, Joseph *Addictions Technician* 3/19/1992 - 5/16/1992

Lynch, Jessica *Mail Clerk* 9/14/1998 - 3/19/1999

Lynn, Jennifer *Mobile Therapist, Wraparound* 2/21/2005 - present

Lynn, Kelly *Secretary/Receptionist* 8/28/1995 - 12/20/1996

Lyons, Wilbert *Psychiatrist* 7/1/1962 - 12/31/1978

Mack, Christa *Inpatient Social Worker* 4/7/1974 - 10/15/1999

Mack, Shannon *Mobile Therapist* 7/10/1996 - 8/28/1996

MacMullen, Jennifer *Intensive Community Counselor* 10/10/1994 - 10/10/1995

Maddux, Mary Jane *Admissions Rep.* 11/12/1998 - 2/4/1999

Madof, Frank *Psychologist* 5/15/1995 - 6/29/2001

Madtes, Dorothy *Crisis Worker* 11/17/2003 - 12/19/2004

Maitz-Parson, Ann *Social Worker* 12/8/1998 - 8/17/1999

Maldonado, Manuel *Addictions Technician* 9/14/1994 - 1/24/1995

Mallory, Phyllis *Switchboard Receptionist* 8/3/1999 - 1/31/2002

Maloney, Ann *Mobile Therapist* 10/18/2004 - 11/30/2004

Maloney, Lois *Pre-School Teacher* 9/10/1974 - 6/15/1978

Manahan, Hugh *Therapy Tech.* 11/16/1988 - 10/20/1990

Mancuso, Helene *Case Manager* 11/11/1999 - 2/4/2000

Manfredi, Alexandra (Sandy) *Intake Worker/Assessor* 1/6/1999 - present

Manning, Jennifer *Intensive Case Manager* 11/29/2004 - present

Mannino, Elizabeth *Summer Camp Intern* 6/23/2004 - 7/23/2004

Manns, Angela *Switchboard Receptionist* 5/12/1998 - 6/20/2002

March, Matthew *Intensive Community Counselor* 5/21/1996 - 6/20/1996

Marco, Melissa *Case Manager/Therapeutic Staff Support* 11/1/2000 - 8/20/2004

Margush, Elizabeth *Therapeutic Staff Support* 8/21/2000 - 6/15/2001

Mariner, Melissa *Resource Coordinator, Montgomery* 1/16/2002 - present

Markee, Robert *TEP Mail Clerk* 10/7/2003 - 4/18/2004

Marks, Christina *Accounts Payable Clerk* 9/18/1995 - 1/19/1998

Markus, Roslyn *Addictions Technician* 5/11/1992 - 9/6/1993

Marnell, Anthony *Mental Health Professional* 4/12/2004 - present

Marshall, Barbara *Patient Care Coordinator* 7/14/1997 - 12/5/1997

Marston, Brett *Social Worker* 2/2/2005 - present

Martin, Donna *Psychologist, MH Outpatient* 2/28/2005 - present

Martin, Joseph *Intensive Community Counselor* 4/23/1996 - 1/31/2000

Martin, Kathy *Medical Records Clerk* 7/5/1989 - 4/9/1999

Martin, Wilmer 3/1/1977 - Unknown

Marzano, Sharon *Secretary/Receptionist* 9/27/1999 - 9/7/2000

Masgai, Joseph *Therapeutic Staff Support* 6/11/1997 - 10/23/2000

Masin-Moyer, Melanie *Social Worker* 9/8/1997 - present

Massey Dietz, Donna *Administrative Assistant II* 7/14/2003 - present

Mastroni, Robin *Social Worker* 11/16/2000 - 7/31/2001

Matos, Elidad *Intensive Community Counselor* 5/1/1996 - 4/20/1998

Matthews, Kerri *Therapeutic Staff Support* 6/24/2004 - 8/23/2004

Matthews, Michael *Behavior Specialist* 3/28/1994 - 7/3/1996

Mattson, Lisa *Residential Advisor, Village of Hope* 1/14/2005 - present

Mauger, Laura *Wraparound Secretary* 8/13/1990 - 8/22/1997

Maurer, Robin *Clerk Typist* 3/20/1978 - 10/15/1979

Mauro, Lucille *Director of Clubhouse* 5/6/1993 - present

May, Corey *PRN On-Call Crisis Worker* 9/5/2001 - 2/1/2002

Mayberry, Sharon *Occupational Therapist* 9/8/1987 - present

McBride, Ginger *Clinical Supervisor* 4/1/1991 - 12/31/1992

McCafferty, Karen *Therapeutic Staff Support* 12/10/2001 - 8/14/2002

McCarthy, Tamara *Penn Gardens On-Site Staff* 3/1/1994 - present

McCauley, Diane *Secretary/Client Rep.* 8/19/1996 - 9/27/1996

McCauley, Floyce *Psychiatrist, Childrens Unit* 3/22/1995 - 7/12/1999

McCleery, Juliet *Addictions Technician* 9/14/1999 - 5/2/2000

McCloskey, Karen *Administrative Case Manager* 6/26/1995 - 6/30/1997

McConnell, Sharon *Assistant Teacher* 9/10/1974 - 6/15/1978

McCormack, Paul *Addictions Technician*
12/21/1990 - 7/24/1992

McCormick, Beverly *Nurse PRN* 8/4/1988 -
1/28/1990

McDermott, Patricia *TEP File Clerk* 9/18/2000 -
10/20/2000

McDonald, Carol *Administrative Assistant II*
10/10/1979 - present

McGahran, Matthew *Crisis Worker* 2/21/2000 -
9/5/2000

McGarvey, Leslie *Community Consultation
Director* 11/29/1982 - 6/16/1989

McGinn, Patricia *Mobile Therapist* 3/26/1996 -
present

McGlory, Katherine *Personal Coordinator*
6/28/1989 - 5/18/1990

McGowan, Heather *Wraparound Counselor*
5/10/1995 - 12/3/1998

McGrath, James *House Case Manager/Referral
Coordinator* 2/25/2004 - present

McGrath, Susan *Addictions Counselor*
10/6/1998 - 10/15/1998

McIlhenny, Paul *Child Psychiatrist* 8/3/1992 -
8/1/1997

McIntyre, Jacqueline *Mobile Therapist* 9/3/2003 -
present

McKendry, Brian *Crisis Worker* 11/23/1999 -
11/1/2000

McKeown, Lori *Addictions Technician* 8/1/2001 -
8/8/2001

McLain, Kelly *Intensive Community Counselor*
3/23/1998 - 4/15/1998

McLanahan, Holly *CRR/Drop-in-Secretary*
10/6/1986 - 1/4/1990

McLaughlin, Doris *Medical Secretary* 11/9/1981
- 12/11/1981

McLaughlin, Geri *Secretary* 9/12/2000 -
11/11/2002

McLaughlin, John *Driver II* 7/15/2000 -
present

McLaughlin, Meridith *Therapeutic Staff Support*
11/5/2002 - 4/11/2003

McLean, Nancy *Psychologist* 3/1/1997 -
6/1/1999

McLinden, Linda *Medical Records Manager*
7/10/1989 - 10/29/1992

McMasters, Jean *SAP Coordinator* 7/31/1987 -
1/26/1989

McMeekin, Kim *Sr. Managed Care Rep.*
2/3/1997 - 10/13/2000

McMullen, Jacqueline *Addictions Technician*
10/22/2002 - 9/1/2003

McMullen, Jacqueline *PRN Addictions Technician*
11/10/2004 - 2/1/2005

McNamara, Timothy *Addictions Technician*
6/14/2000 - 5/1/2001

McNicholas, Tara *Therapeutic Staff Support*
12/6/1999 - 12/13/1999

McQuarrie, Thomas *MES Worker* 12/3/2002 -
present

Medori, Janet *Psychiatric Social Worker*
7/1/1970 - 4/28/1972

Mellott, Francine *Chief Financial Officer* 8/1/2003
- present

Melo, Stefanie *MES/Outpatient Assessor*
10/4/2004 - present

Mendelman, Joanne *Psychologist* 4/29/1988 -
12/29/1989

Mervin, Craig *TEP Mail Clerk* 10/2/2002 -
3/16/2003

Messa, Michelle *Admissions Representative*
12/1/2003 - present

Messa, Patricia *Insurance Billing Clerk*
11/26/1990 - present

Metcalfe, Kristin *TEP Mail Clerk* 1/24/2002 -
10/24/2002

Methlie, Nancy *Residential Caseworker*
11/12/1985 - 7/14/2003

Michael, Deborah *Medical Recorder Secretary*
9/22/1997 - 11/30/2000

Michener, Jennifer *Nurse* 3/28/2000 - present

Michener, Martha *Nurse* 10/21/1997 - present

Miller, Amy *Resource Coordinator* 4/12/1999 -
4/19/1999

Miller, Colene *Crisis Worker* 8/19/2002 -
6/4/2003

Miller, Courtney *Mobile Therapist, Behavior
Specialist* 11/13/2000 - 11/7/2003

Miller, Gay *Outpatient Team Secretary* 4/16/1984
- 4/30/1988

Miller, Henry *Nurse* 7/18/2002 - 12/18/2002

Miller, Jean *Typist* 1/16/1984 - 1/3/1985

Miller, Jeffrey *Social Worker* 12/6/1995 -
7/31/1999

Miller, Megan *Intensive Community Counselor*
8/7/1996 - 8/14/1998

Miller, Megan *Therapeutic Staff Support*
9/11/1998 - 7/28/2000

Miller, Paul *Outpatient Therapist* 10/10/1983 -
7/2/1984

Miller, Paula *Admissions Rep.* 1/13/1997 -
8/22/1997

Miller, Richard *Activity Assistant* 9/27/1986 -
11/23/1987

Milnes, Megan *Psychiatric Rehab. Worker/Work
Unit Assistant* 10/25/2004 - present

Mininger, Phyllis *Stepping Stones Club Advisor*
6/19/1984 - 3/1/1988

Mitchell, Cindy *Intensive Community Counselor*
2/1/1999 - 9/1/1999

Mitchell, Russell *Residential Caseworker*
11/3/1994 - 5/5/2997

Mitchell-Lichtfus, Carolann *Switchboard
Receptionist* 4/7/1998 - 4/20/1998

Moehrle, Gretchen *Crisis Worker* 8/5/2002 -
11/18/2002

Monastero, Ann Marie *Secretary- On Call*
3/16/1992 - 1/12/1993

Monge, Susan *Addictions Technician* 4/28/2004 -
present

Monico, Joyce *Accountant* 11/2/1998 - present
Moog, Karen *Psychiatric Rehab. Worker/Clerical Unit Leader* 4/9/2001 - 9/15/2004
Moore, Amy *Float Secretary* 6/7/1999 - 6/15/2000
Moosbrugger, Joseph *Therapeutic Staff Support* 12/7/2001 - 4/16/2002
Mora, Pablo *IT Assistant* 2/9/2005 - present
Moran, Ann *Aftercare Coordinator* 7/8/1994 - 11/4/1994
Morgan, Doris *Social Worker* 2/13/1990 - 4/30/1998
Morgan, Jennifer *Insurance Clerk* 11/3/1997 - 6/9/1999
Morgan, Robin *Registered Nurse* 9/16/1969 - 9/13/1971
Morin, Sister Michelle *Chaplain* 2/13/2002 - present
Morris, Tara *Nurse* 3/29/2000 - 4/14/2000
Morrison, Evelyn *Intensive Community Counselor* 12/15/1997 - 5/27/1998
Morrow, Dorcas *Psychiatrist* 10/9/1989 - 2/7/1991
Moser, John *Intensive Community Counselor* 10/13/1997 - 8/27/1999
Mosher, Rose *Medical Secretary/Office Assistant* 8/2/1999 - 6/7/2000
Moyer, Andrea *Secretary/Asst.* 1/26/1998 - 9/15/1998
Moyer, Brenda *Secretary* 8/31/1994 - 4/19/1995
Moyer, Frank *Van Driver* 3/6/1989 - 9/1/1994
Moyer, Laurel *Secretary(PRN)* 8/20/1984 - 9/19/1985
Moyer, Leeanne *Accountant/Business Manager* 11/16/1987 - 11/2/1990
Moyer, Palma *Nurse, Rehab* 4/25/1989 - 6/10/1990
Moyer, W. Brooke *Public Relations Coordinator* 8/24/1992 - 4/23/1999
Mueller, Michelle *Medical Records Clerk II* 6/1/1998 - 8/4/1999
Mugrauer, Wayne *Deputy Administrator* 7/20/1981 - 5/23/1985
Mullin, John *Addictions Technician II* 11/8/1989 - Unknown
Mullin, Linda *Administrative Assistant* 12/18/2000 - 6/29/2001
Mumbauer, Heather *MR Case Management* 8/9/1993 - present
Muntzer, Eve *Intake Specialist* 5/18/1998 - 4/28/2000
Murphy, Cornelius *Addictions Technician* 2/21/2001 - 4/1/2001
Murphy, Stella *Receptionist/Switchboard* 5/22/1989 - 5/31/1990
Murphy, Teresa *Mobile Therapist* 6/2/2004 - present
Musselman, Danielle *PRN Secretary* 5/8/2000 - 3/10/2001

Musselman, Gerald *Psychologist* 7/7/1970 - 5/30/1979
Musselman, Jolene *Scheduling Secretary* 4/18/1994 - present
Muta, Cindy *Psychiatric Rehabilitation Specialist* 6/10/2002 - present
Myer, Rodney *Administrative Case Manager* 6/1/1998 - 6/1/1999
Myer, Sara *Managed Care Rep.* 5/26/1998 - 6/1/1999
Myers, Justine *Secretary* 2/6/1991 - 4/18/1996
Myers, Stephen *Driver* 10/4/2002 - 2/23/2005
Myrick, April *Resource Coordinator, Bucks* 7/27/2001 - 8/2/2001
Nagel, Deborah *Addictions Counselor* 1/24/2005 - present
Naimo, Nancy *Secretary/Receptionist* 5/1/1995 - 9/4/1997
Nang, Merrie *Managed Care/Intake Rep* 8/19/1999 - 8/20/1999
Nase, Bonnie *Supports Coordinator* 5/2/2000 - present
Nase, Holly *Therapeutic Staff Support/Case Manager* 9/1/1999 - 7/13/2001
Nathan, Joan *Triage Clinician* 1/25/1994 - present
Naylon, Anne *Nurse* 8/8/2000 - present
Nejako, David *Crisis Worker, PRN On-Call* 11/3/1999 - 2/13/2002
Nelson, Deborah *Behavior Specialist* 9/20/1994 - 1/21/2001
Nemeth, Andrew *Psychiatrist* 6/17/1997 - 6/29/2001
Ness, Carlton *Intensive Community Counselor* 3/7/1996 - 4/8/1996
Neville, Karen *Secretary* 3/22/2004 - present
Newton, Anne *Psychiatrist* 9/1/2001 - present
Ney, Aileen *Therapeutic Staff Support* 10/27/2004 - 2/23/2005
Nguyen, Elizabeth *Psychologist* 4/19/1999 - 5/18/1999
Nguyen, Thy *Mobile Therapist/Behavioral Specialist* 9/23/2004 – 11/15/2004
Nicholl, Patricia *Secretary/Receptionist* 11/2/1999 - 11/22/1999
Nicholson, Angelique *Acting Penn School Coordinator* 2/10/1997 - 1/14/2000
Nicholson, Jean *A/P Clerk* 1/22/1990 - 2/16/1990
Nogueira, Jose *Psychiatrist* 3/1/1997 - 6/29/2001
Nolan, Jocelyn *Social Worker* 5/1/1999 - 9/8/2000
Nulty, Catherine *RN* 2/28/1990 - 4/3/1990
Nusser, Margaret *Social Worker* 11/8/1999 - 1/30/2000
Nyce, Gwendolyn *Secretary* 10/11/1990 - 4/10/1991
Nyce, Phyllis *Clerk/Typist* 11/14/1973 - 6/30/1977

O'Brien, Barbara *Nurse-Psychiatric* 1/17/1979 - present

O'Brien, Elizabeth *Addictions Technician* 6/14/2000 - 4/1/2001

O'Brien, Gerald *Psychologist* 4/9/1986 - present

O'Hara, Sandra *Case Manager* 9/12/1990 - 5/7/1994

O'Neil, Mary Ann *Mobile Therapist* 10/16/1996 - 2/4/2000

Okun, Russell *Case Manager* 2/3/1997 - 5/12/1997

Oliveira, Kedma *MCC Exchange Worker* 8/12/1982 - 7/22/1983

Olkowski, Maryanne *Receptionist, EAP* 6/1/1993 - 2/7/1996

Olson, Emma *Administrative Assistant* 9/10/1979 - 5/25/1982

Ondra, Winona *Nursery School Assistant* 12/1/1970 - 7/1/1974

Oniskey, Trisha *Activities Worker* 3/7/2001 - 3/21/2001

Orth, Elizabeth *Outpatient Counselor/MES Level II Counselor* 5/3/2004 - 9/3/2004

Osmun, Wendy *Billing Clerk* 10/12/1999 - 6/20/2003

Oudinot, Vickie *Intensive Community Counselor* 12/17/1998 - 2/4/2000

Owens, Danielle *Secretary/Assistant* 1/23/1997 - 1/9/1998

Packard, Susan *Psychologist* 1/11/1996 - 2/5/2001

Paecht, Maureen *Collections Liaison* 12/13/2004 - 1/31/2005

Pagano, Anne Marie *Data Specialist* 8/31/1987 - 1/20/1989

Painter, Sharyn *Residential Advisor/Alumni Advisor* 9/3/1996 - present

Palcewski, John *Addictions Technician* 4/9/1992 - 6/21/1999

Palermo, Angela *Secretary* 4/24/2000 - 2/14/2003

Palmer, Jennifer *Public Relations Assistant* 5/19/2003 - present

Palumbo, Theresa *Secretary* 11/4/1996 - 11/22/1996

Papazian, Maura *Social Worker* 5/15/1995 - 6/29/2001

Papciak, Elaine *Team Secretary* 12/30/1992 - 8/12/1994

Parker, Lisa *Early Intervention Coordinator* 3/1/1992 - 3/24/1995

Patterson, Cathleen *Licensed Practical Nurse* 12/21/1992 - 1/19/1999

Patterson, Frances *EAP Therapist* 2/29/1988 - 2/16/1999

Patterson, Robert *Maintenance Assistant* 4/11/1988 - 4/28/1989

Paul, Cinthia *Intensive Case Manager* 7/6/1993 - 7/31/2001

Pavelcze, Louis *Van Driver* 2/20/1995 - 3/27/1995

Payton, Kirsten *Secretary/Receptionist* 11/27/2000 - 3/8/2001

Pearre, Theresa *Behavioral Specialist* 12/27/2004 - present

Pearson, Linda *Receptionist* 6/26/1990 - 7/1/1990

Peck, Anthony *TEP Residential Aide* 11/4/2002 - 11/15/2002

Peck, Nancy *Secretary/Receptionist* 2/17/1997 - 9/18/1997

Peck, Susan *Crisis Worker, Float* 10/9/1998 - 1/8/1999

Pendleton, Joanne *Clerical Unit Supervisor* 4/4/1994 - 1/31/1995

Penney, Paula *Social Worker* 7/19/2000 - 2/15/2001

Pennings, Kristen *Intensive Community Counselor* 9/29/1998 - 3/5/1999

Peperato, Cheryl *Transcriptionist* 8/17/1987 - 7/1/1988

Pepper, Cynthia *Secretary* 7/26/1999 - 7/28/1999

Pepper, Joyce *Outpatient Counselor* 10/4/2004 - present

Permar, Shaun *Therapeutic Staff Support* 5/28/2003 - present

Peterson, Elizabeth *Secretary* 4/16/1978 - 4/16/1979

Petrosini, Amy *Intensive Community Counselor* 10/29/1996 - 4/18/1997

Pfeiffer, Pamela *EAP Counselor* 2/27/2002 - 5/6/2003

Phillips, Anna *Psychologist* 9/24/2003 - 10/1/2003

Phillips, Debra *Transcriptionist* 11/1/1999 - 4/14/2000

Phillips, Heather *Partial Hospital Director* 11/17/2003 - present

Phillips, Lynn *Social Worker* 2/1/1994 - 4/11/1997

Pierce, Kelly *Addictions Technician* 8/11/1999 - present

Piffer, Nicole *Intensive Community Counselor* 8/5/1996 - 7/31/1997

Pillay, Sharlean *PRN Crisis Worker* 7/31/2001 - present

Pitkow, Avis *Outpatient Counselor* 2/2/2004 - present

Pizzollo, Tara *Patient Care Coordinator* 3/1/1997 - 8/13/1999

Plantholt, Michael *Therapeutic Staff Support* 2/18/2002 - 7/15/2002

Pliskin, Lisa *Receptionist, PRN* 5/15/1995 - 6/30/1997

Pobre-So, Josephine *Psychiatrist* 1/23/2002 - present

Podgornik, Sonia *Therapeutic Staff Support* 3/8/1999 - 8/13/1999

Polanczyk, Jill *Therapeutic Staff Support* 3/7/2000 - 8/4/2000

Polao, Rochelle *Newtown Licensed Social Worker* 12/4/1996 - 6/29/2001

Polier, John *Social Worker* 5/19/1997 - 7/21/2000

Pop, Janice *EAP Counselor* 3/26/1984 - 7/12/1985

Popal, Bashier *Intensive Community Counselor* 7/22/1997 - 5/31/1999

Pope, Ronald *Psychiatrist* 7/11/1994 - 7/4/1999

Poster Jr., Francis *Recreation Therapist* 6/4/1990 - 10/17/2003

Poster Sr., Francis *Support Technician* 5/7/2002 - present

Poster, Bryan *Intensive Community Counselor* 4/18/1996 - 1/4/1999

Poust, Barbara *Secretary/Case Management Services* 5/23/1988 - present

Powell, Allision *Therapeutic Staff Support* 9/3/2004 - 10/8/2004

Powell, John *Psychiatrist* 1/6/1992 - 1/6/1994

Powell, Kelly *Case Manager* 4/16/1991 - 2/17/1995

Pregler, Lawrence *Director Of BreakThrough* 2/9/1989 - 2/7/1990

Prehl, Kory *Driver* 5/22/1995 - 9/16/2000

Proctor, Robert *MES and Rehab at Home Counselor/Assessor* 5/21/1997 - present

Prusch, Nancy *Secretary* 6/16/1994 - 9/3/1991

Przyblowski, Mariln *Billing Consultant* 10/7/1998 - 6/30/1999

Przyuski, Donna *Outpatient Team Secretary* 5/9/1983 - 12/16/1983

Pummer, Anne *PRN Nurse* 8/9/2001 - 1/7/2004

Quay, Lisa *Managed Care Representative* 6/30/2003 - 1/2/2004

Querubin, Lynn *Primary Counselor* 7/31/2001 - 4/15/2004

Quier, Nelda *Registered Nurse* 6/26/2001 - 8/28/1991

Quinby, Trina *Secretary/Receptionist* 8/30/1993 - 12/30/1996

Raab, Andrea *Clerical Support* 1/27/1997 - 6/30/1997

Radice, Andrea *PRN Crisis Worker + On-Call* 3/7/2001 - present

Radzai, Sandra *Secretary* 1/21/1963 - 12/2/1964

Raichev, Iliana *Early Intervention* 3/13/1995 - 1/31/1996

Rajcan, Marie *Psychiatric Social Worker* 9/25/1991 - 6/12/1998

Ramirez, Cynthia *Psychotherapist* 5/18/1992 - 3/11/1993

Ramsden-Donahue, Karin *Behavioral Specialist* 9/15/1999 - present

Ramsey, Stephanie *Intensive Community Counselor* 7/10/1995 - 2/16/1996

Rankin, Melinda *Therapeutic Staff Support* 9/24/1999 - 1/3/2000

Rapkin, Bonnie *Psychotherapist* 5/14/1996 - 5/31/1998

Rapkin, Robert *Psychiatrist* 10/17/1994 - present

Rapp, Valerie *Addictions Technician* 9/13/1999 - 10/15/1999

Rappaport, Ellen *Counselor (Group Facilitator)* 11/2/1999 - 2/1/2000

Rawley, Dorothy *Psychologist* 3/1/1997 - 6/30/1998

Rawlins, Robert *L.P.N.* 10/6/1993 - 5/31/1996

Raynock, Lenore *Therapeutic Staff Support* 7/28/2003 - 12/22/2003

Reach, Elizabeth *Chemical Dependency Director* 8/5/1985 - 2/27/1987

Ream, Jamison *Mobile Therapist* 10/13/1997 - 7/8/1999

Reaser, Mary *Secretarial Staff Supervisor* 7/31/1990 - present

Recicar, Kristen *Addictions Technician* 12/13/2000 - 6/5/2001

Redko, Andrei *Intensive Case Manager* 5/3/2004 - 9/30/2004

Reed, Anna Mae *Quality Assurance Coord.* 5/5/1975 - 8/31/1988

Reeder, Linda *Secretary* 3/18/1991 - 12/31/2000

Reese, Cindy *Music Therapist* 3/16/1992 - 9/30/1993

Reeves, Charlotte *Administrative Case Manager* 8/11/2004 - present

Reith, Loretta *Behavioral Specialist* 11/9/2000 - present

Rembolt, Penny *Mobile Therapist* 6/9/1999 - 8/13/1999

Renner, Kim *Receptionist* 7/5/1978 - 8/14/1981

Renner, Lynn *Residential Assistant* 3/20/2000 - present

Repa, Beverly *Data Entry* 9/1/1993 - 1/30/1998

Resh, Daniel *Clinical Supervisor* 6/19/1995 - 6/14/1996

Respes, Maurice *Addiction Technician* 1/25/2002 - 4/25/2003

Rest, Anna Marie *Supports Coordinator* 6/5/2000 - 2/19/2003

Rest, Shyrl *Accounts Payable/Paryoll Clerk* 9/30/2002 - present

Rezeli, Ryan *TEP Mail Clerk* 10/27/2003 - 4/6/2004

Riccitelli, Jeanne *Billing Supervisor* 2/7/2000 - 5/11/2000

Rice, Kelly *Inpatient Counselor* 6/14/1999 - 8/25/2000

Richard, Emma *Therapy Technician* 10/25/1988 - 8/30/1989

Richards, John *Psychiatrist* 7/1/1964 - 2/28/1977; 8/12/1992 - 6/30/1993

Richman, Carol *Psychologist* 1/23/1996 - 12/22/2000

Richwine, Liesl *Administrative Assistant, EAP* 9/5/1990 - 11/1/1995

Rickert, Shannon *Mobile Therapist* 10/23/2003 - 12/26/2003

Ricketts, Mary Joyce *Employment Education Specialist* 9/14/1998 - 4/26/2002

Ridgway, Marjorie *Therapy Technician* 7/12/1989 - 4/3/1992

Ridgway, Stephen *Primary Therapist* 2/25/1991 - 2/18/1993

Riedel, Faye *Secretary* 9/16/1975 - 9/11/1986

Riegel, Barbara *Residential Caseworker* 1/3/1986 - 6/27/1995

Rigel, Christine *Activity Leader* 9/27/1986 - 10/1/1989

Riley, Rita *Advancement Assistant* 10/17/1988 - present

Riman, Jill *Temporary Help, Business Office* 4/1/1987 - 4/22/1987

Riniker, Andrew *Maintenance Worker* 6/8/1998 - 2/25/2000

Riordan, Theresa *Detoxification Coordinator* 6/8/1984 - 6/20/1986

Rittenhouse, Stephanie *Addictions Technician* 2/26/2001 - 10/18/2002

Ritter, Elaine *PRN Nurse* 7/23/1990 - 5/31/1996

Ritter, Samantha *Case Manager* 7/6/1998 - 2/11/2000

Ritter, Thomas *Addictions Technician* 1/20/2000 - present

Rivard, Michele *Social Worker* 3/28/2000 - 12/7/2001

Roberts, Pamela *Client Registration Coordinator* 10/2/1995 - 11/30/1998

Rochlin, Barbara *Addictions Counselor* 10/23/1989 - 4/22/1999

Rodriquez, Jorge *Addictions Technician* 8/18/1998 - 10/15/1998

Rohl, Marguerite *Van Driver* 1/5/2000 - present

Rohl, Pamela *File Clerk* 1/5/1998 - 7/1/1998

Rohrbach, Kimberly *Marketing Assistant* 11/6/1989 - 2/3/1995

Rohrman, Clarice *EI Service Coordinator* 3/20/1995 - 6/20/1995

Rolston, David *Residential Instructor* 3/10/1997 - 3/21/1998

Romm, Kyle *Addictions Technician* 5/23/2000 - 9/6/2000

Rook, Michelle *Social Worker* 7/13/1999 - 5/4/2000

Rooney, James *TEP Residential Aide* 8/18/2003 - 10/27/2003

Roper, Allison *Therapeutic Staff Support* 8/30/1999 - 2/4/2000

Rosefeldt, Paul *Mobile Therapist* 4/26/1996 - 3/13/1998

Rosenberg, Matthew *Mobile Therapist* 1/29/1998 - 8/29/1999

Rosenberger, Karen *Psychologist* 4/1/2002 - present

Rosenberger, Nancy *Crisis Worker* 4/17/2000 - 3/22/2001

Rosenberger, Suzi *File Clerk* 6/28/1999 - 6/28/2000

Roskow, Alan *Therapy Technician* 5/10/1990 - 8/13/1990

Roskow, Nan *Therapy Technician* 2/6/1990 - 1/1/1991

Ross, Emil *Admissions Rep.* 7/10/1995 - 8/25/1995

Rossman, Christine *Intensive Case Manager* 2/16/1998 - 8/17/2001

Roth, Bonnie *File Clerk, TEP* 8/25/1998 - 3/10/2000

Roth, Brenda *Intensive Community Counselor* 9/15/1997 - 6/1/1998

Roth, George *Addictions Technician* 11/18/1994 - 11/21/1994

Roth, Kelly *Secretary/Receptionist* 3/30/1999 - 6/14/1999

Roth, Vale *Intensive Community Counselor* 12/1/1994 - 2/1/1996

Rothenberger, Melissa *Supports Coordinator* 10/14/2002 - present

Roush, Ella *Public Relations/Communications Director* 11/1/2004 - present

Rudolph, Dorothy *Art Therapist/Child Therapist* 7/17/1989 - 11/25/1991

Rueffer, Robert *Addictions Technician* 4/10/1991 - 11/1/1991

Ruggiero, Frances *Secretary/Receptionist* 10/18/1999 - present

Ruggiero, Linda *Therapy Technician* 11/7/1988 - 2/28/1989

Ruppert, John *Residential Advisor* 5/19/1997 - present

Rush, Barak *Primary Counselor* 12/18/2002 - 4/17/2003

Rush, Karen *ON-Call Transcriptionist* 5/21/1991 - 9/15/1995

Rushannon, Kathleen *Intensive Community Counselor* 8/21/1997 - 4/15/1998

Rusiewicz, Barbara *Social Worker/ Mobile Therapist* 8/15/1995 - 6/6/2002

Ruth, Beth *Communications Specialist* 6/8/1987 - 7/29/1988

Rutherford, Lisa *Social Worker* 11/28/2000 - present

Ryan, Debra *Crisis Coordinator* 3/16/1987 - present

Ryan, Stephen *PRN Addictions Technician* 8/22/2002 - 12/18/2002

Sadler, Rebecca *Business Office* 8/22/1969 - 4/16/1979

Salazar, Salvador *Program Resource Representative* 7/1/1992 - 2/15/1993

Salguero, Anne *Admissions Representative* 12/7/1998 - 12/9/1998

Samony, Geraldine *Secretary* 3/22/1999 - 9/9/1999

Sanchez, Raphael *Intensive Community Counselor* 1/13/1998 - 5/12/1998

Sandow, Robert *Therapy Technician* 1/31/1990 - 2/18/1991

Sandy, Loretta *Acting Director Breakthrough* 6/8/1987 - 6/20/1989

Santaniello, Shirley *Addictions Technician* 5/25/1994 - 1/1/1995

Santiago-Collazo, Daisy *Mobile Therapist* 1/16/1997 - 7/22/1997

Sarangoulis, Linda *Intensive Community Counselor* 8/5/1996 - 7/30/1997

Satek, Jane *Residential Instructor* 4/19/1998 - 2/16/2000

Savage, Nicole *Administrative Case Manager* 6/1/1998 - 6/1/1999

Savanick, Martha *Crisis Intervention Team* 8/6/1975 - 4/30/1976

Scally, Karen *Therapy Technician* 5/18/1988 - 9/28/1990

Schaff, Joseph *Addictions Technician* 3/19/1990 - 9/26/1993

Schaible, Troy *Case Management Support Technician* 9/19/2000 - 10/28/2002

Schairer, James *Social Worker/Behavioral Specialist* 5/5/1997 - 4/19/2001

Schantzenbach, Wayne *Social Worker* 8/1/1979 - 7/5/1988

Schaper, Heather *Intensive Community Counselor* 4/7/1998 - 6/12/1998

Schauer, Jennifer *PRN Student, Summer Camp* 6/25/2001 - 5/1/2002

Scheetz, Cheryl *Activity Assistant* 3/16/1991 - Unknown

Scheetz, Kathleen *Intensive Community Counselor* 11/11/1996 - 7/13/1998

Scheffler, Robert *Social Worker* 6/2/1999 - 6/15/2000

Schell, Harold *Chief Financial Officer* 3/30/1990 - 5/1/1998

Schell, Joy *Secretary/Client Services Rep* 3/3/1997 - 7/8/1999

Schell, Rebecca *Wraparound Records Auditor* 5/16/1994 - 1/1/1996

Schellenberger, Jeffrey *Intensive Community Counselor* 11/21/1997 - 9/14/1998

Schelling, Karen *Addictions Counselor* 9/14/1999 - 3/1/2000

Schenk, Deborah *Residential Coordinator* 4/18/1994 - 11/19/1997

Scherr, Andrew *Addictions Technician I* 4/13/1993 - 9/6/1994

Schiavone, Vanessa *Residential Caseworker* 10/23/2000 - present

Schlegel, Jacqueline *R.C.O.P./Partial Hosp. Coordinator* 10/28/1989 - 7/31/2001

Schleicher, Katherine *Mobile Therapist* 8/31/2004 - present

Schlosser, Dawn *Activity Leader* 5/19/1992 - 5/19/1992

Schmalbruch, Erika *Intake Rep.* 5/15/1995 - 10/31/2000

Schmell, Norma *Clerk Typist* 1/11/1988 - 12/27/1988

Schmitt, Kelly 12/7/2004 - 3/15/2005

Schmitz, Janet *EAP Counselor* 9/28/1993 - present

Schneider, Chester *Psychiatrist* 7/9/1973 - 4/1/1974

Schneider, Laurie *Intensive Community Counselor* 9/20/1997 - 8/14/1998

Schneider, Meryl *Addictions Technician* 5/15/1999 - 9/25/2000

Scholl, Nadine *Receptionist* 6/15/1970 - 11/23/1970

Scholl-Moore, Marnie *Mobile Therapist* 2/17/2004 - 4/19/2005

Schoneker-Shaw, Lori *EAP Counselor* 5/17/1989 - 3/5/1991

Schrag, Meghan *Mental Health Professional* 8/20/2002 - present

Schram, Cheryl *Social Worker* 11/18/1999 - 12/1/1999

Schreck, Mary Ann *Caseworker* 1/29/1976 - 2/20/1979

Schreiber, William *TEP Mail Clerk* 4/19/2004 - 9/27/2004

Schuck, Jeanne *Admin. Secretary/Transcriptionist* 9/12/1988 - 9/14/1989

Schultz, Ericka *Medical Records* 4/28/1997 - 4/30/1997

Schultz, Gary *Residential Aide-TEP* 10/2/2001 - 4/23/2002

Schulze, Christopher *Admissions Worker* 5/15/1995 - 6/3/1996

Schuman, Nancy *Intensive Community Counselor* 1/16/1998 - 3/12/1998

Schunke, Kimberly *Intensive Case Manager* 1/19/1998 - 3/27/1998

Schurr, Kirsten *Inpatient Case Manager/Crisis Worker* 7/27/1998 - 11/9/1998

Schutt, Margaret *Administrative Case Manager* 7/28/1997 - 5/22/1998

Schwartz, James *Van Driver* 4/10/1995 - 11/30/1997

Schwartz, Janice *Mobile Therapist/Creative Arts Therapy/Wraparound* 8/13/1999 - 12/17/1999

Schwenk, Donna *Addictions Technician* 10/27/1998 - 2/28/1999

Scott, Sherry *Transcriptionist* 3/4/1985 - 7/3/1986

Scully, Susan *Mobile Therapist* 11/24/1999 - 10/3/2000

Seamans, Lyn *Social Worker* 1/2/2002 - present

See, James *Driver* 5/9/1998 - present

Sefing, Kristie *EAP Counselor* 9/13/2001 - 12/22/2003

Segletes, Jennifer *Activity Assistant* 7/11/1992 - 10/1/1993

Seifert, Paul *EAP Director* 10/12/1992 - 6/4/1999

Selkow, Murray *Behavioral Specialist* 10/17/2003 - present

Sell, Patti *Penn Assoc., Secretary* 2/27/1989 - 2/2/1990

Sellers, Tarah *Crisis Worker* 10/30/2001 - 5/7/2002

Seneko, Constance *PRN Nurse* 9/12/2000 - 8/31/2001

Sergent, Debra *Residential Caseworker* 10/16/1995 - 4/18/1996

Serianni, Marilynn *Nurse* 12/8/1988 - 12/18/1989

Serino, Donna *Secretary* 7/6/2004 - 10/12/2004

Session, Betty *Admissions Representative* 12/1/2004 - present

Sessions, Timothy *EAP Counselor* 6/7/2001 - present

Shaffer, Marc *Chief Financial Officer* 7/31/2000 - 4/30/2001

Shank, Rowland *Psychologist* 10/15/1984 - 11/14/1985

Shannon, Christine *Director of Residential Services* 9/10/1981 - present

Sheeran, Beth *EAP Counselor* 9/1/1994 - 7/22/2003

Shelly, Renee *Medical Records Clerk* 11/22/1982 - 9/13/1985

Shelly, Samantha *Medical Records Clerk* 4/26/1985 - 7/4/1985

Shenk, Christine *Mobile Therapist/Beh. Specialist* 12/8/1999 - 11/1/2000

Sheridan-McANdrew, Ann *Case Manager* 10/5/1998 - 3/17/2000

Shield, David *Intensive Community Counselor* 6/29/1998 - 8/14/1998

Shipman, Mark *Addictions Technician* 8/1/1988 - present

Shisler, Lisa *Fiscal Assistant* 6/27/1977 - 6/29/1979

Shockley, Silvana *Intensive Community Counselor* 4/19/1996 - 2/4/2000

Shortridge, Bret *Addictions Technician* 9/14/1999 - 2/27/2002

Shosh, Eva *Nurse* 6/20/1988 - 4/21/1989

Showalter, James *Medical Director* 1/20/2000 - present

Showers, Lisa *Secretary/Receptionist* 12/9/1996 - 1/31/1997

Shreiner, Mary Ann *Nurse* 7/3/1989 - 2/26/1990

Shubert, Shirley *Addictions Technician* 5/7/2002 - 5/16/2002

Side, Lorraine *Psychiatric Nurse Coordinator* 6/24/1981 - 10/6/1982

Sidorov, Esther *Caseworker* 6/1/1972 - 1/23/1985

Silva-Burke, Gustine *Administrative Assistant* 10/20/1999 - 4/23/2004

Siman, Dawn *Therapeutic Staff Support* 5/12/2003 - 11/1/2004

Simmons, Wendy *Director of Dual Diagnosis and Housing Development* 3/1/1992 - 1/11/2002

Simonds, Barbara *Switchboard Receptionist* 7/12/2001 - 10/4/2001

Simonetti-Cowgill, Mary *Psychotherapist* 12/3/1996 - 6/1/1999

Simononis, Joyce *Clinical Coordinator* 5/15/1995 - 6/27/1996

Simpson, A. Ruth *Day Care Coordinator* 7/1/1962 - 5/29/1973

Sine, Melissa *Therapeutic Staff Support* 2/12/1999 - 3/2/2004

Siracusa, Janice *Residential Instructor* 1/6/1992 - 6/25/1992

Sitko, Mandy *Therapeutic Staff Support* 4/26/1999 - 6/27/2002

Slater, Amy *Inpatient Billing Clerk* 6/19/1989 - 7/24/1998

Slater, Elaine *Medical Records Clerk* 10/5/1992 - 11/2/2000

Slot, Rebecca *Intensive Community Counselor* 1/25/1999 - 9/1/1999

Slotter, Lisa *Secretary* 2/13/1989 - 8/3/1990

Smith, Albert *TEP Residential Aide* 2/12/2003 - 8/15/2003

Smith, Alicia *Activity Therapist* 10/4/1986 - 6/22/1987

Smith, Carrie *Therapeutic Staff Support* 9/11/1998 - 3/12/2003

Smith, Connie *Office Coordinator* 3/1/1997 - 9/23/1997

Smith, Gary *Mobile Therapist* 4/19/1996 - 10/3/1997

Smith, Heather *Mobile Therapist* 8/29/1994 - 2/7/1996

Smith, Joan *Caseworker* 7/28/1975 - 9/1/1978

Smith, Karen *Office Clerk, TEP* 3/13/2001 - 5/25/2001

Smith, Karoyle *Residential Advisor* 5/19/2003 - 8/7/2003

Smith, Kathleen *Recept./Sec* 10/14/1997 - 1/13/1998

Smith, Lamar Gregory *Inpatient Counselor* 10/19/1990 - present

Smith, Lauren *Administrative Case Manager* 6/28/2004 - 7/13/2004

Smith, Lesley *Mental Health Professional* 4/5/1999 - present

Smith, Lorraine *Medical Records Clerk* 9/9/1985 - 11/5/1990

Smith, Margaret *Medical Records Clerk* 10/1/2003 - 10/20/2003

Smith, Tina *Medical Records Clerk* 12/27/1988 - 7/19/1995

Smith, Whitney *MR Case Manager* 9/12/1995 - 8/22/1997

Smoot, C. Thomas *Psychologist* 7/21/1999 - 2/4/2000

Smoyer, Karen *Case Management Coordinator* 8/23/1982 - 7/1/1988

Snisky, Lisa *Crisis Coordinator* 6/5/2000 - 6/30/2000

Snow, Barbara *Data Entry Clerk* 10/7/2003 - present

Snyder, John *EAP Counselor* 7/31/1972 - present

Snyder, Kathy *Secretary/Client Services Rep.*
9/2/1997 - 11/26/1997

Snyder, Lisa *Managed Care Representative*
4/13/1998 - 4/21/1998

Soffin, Jean *Outpatient Therapist* 5/13/1991 -
12/16/1992

Sokoloff, Teri *Residential Advisor* 10/15/2003 -
1/24/2004

Solomon, Shirley *Secretary* 2/21/2003 -
2/13/2004

Somers, Donna *Partial Hospital Coordinator*
6/5/1989 - 6/21/1996

Sousa, Mildred *Administrative Secretary*
12/15/1986 - 8/28/1987

Spade, Timothy *Addictions Technician* 3/8/2004 -
present

Spencer, Cynthia *Teachers Aide* 8/20/1976 -
6/13/1977

Spengler, Lois *Secretary/Receptionist* 5/15/2000
- 11/22/2000

Spenthal, Linda *PRN Crisis Worker* 2/27/1996 -
6/15/2000

Spinato, Margaret *Advisor of Stepping Stones
Clubs* 2/26/1985 - 1/31/1988

Stancick, Randall *MR Case Manager* 3/31/1992
- 11/1/1999

Standish, Angela *Receptionist/Secretary*
6/29/1998 - 3/3/1999

Stanger-Copeland, Holly *Psychotherapist*
4/27/1992 - 8/3/1994

Stantee, Jessica *Addictions Technician*
7/19/1999 - 12/20/1999

Stanton, Molly *Outpatient Counselor w/Adm.
Duties* 7/16/2002 - present

Starnes, Valerie *Residential Advisor* 8/5/2002 -
11/11/2004

Stasiw, Gail *EI Service Coordinator* 3/18/1996 -
present

Stauffer-Moyer, Lori *PRN Psychologist/Behavioral
Specialist* 5/19/1997 - 4/16/2004

Stehel, Mary *Receptionist* 4/6/1999 - 4/14/1999

Stein, Jennifer *Dual Diagnosis* 12/8/1997 -
5/14/1999

Stein, Margie *Psychotherapist* 2/5/1996 -
4/18/1996

Steklenski, William *Driver* 1/22/2004 - 11/24/2004

Stelts, Sharon *Psychiatric Patient Coordinator*
10/17/1983 - 3/31/1985

Stevenson, Dana *Receptionist/Secretary*
3/23/2000 - 8/29/2000

Stevenson, Deborah *Director* 3/1/1992 - present

Stewart, Megan *Supports Coordinator* 6/7/2004 -
present

Stewarts, Christine *Admissions Rep.* 11/17/1997
- 1/12/1998

Stingle, Kathleen *Secretary* 12/7/1989 - 9/1/1994

Stone, Erica *Addictions Technician* 7/31/2000 -
8/10/2000

Stonebraker, Gail *Accts. Payable Clerk* 7/1/1997
- 11/30/1999

Stork, Ronald *Intensive Community Counselor*
5/20/1998 - 1/6/1999

Stout, Marilyn *File/Ins. Clerk* 3/24/1997 -
12/19/1997

Stover, Tania *Correspondence Secretary*
10/6/1998 - 6/23/2000

Straw, Janet *Intensive Case Manager* 12/6/2004
- present

Streapy, Julie *Activities Worker* 10/2/2001 -
11/12/2001

Strehle, Julianne *Supports Coordinator*
3/21/2000 - present

Streib, Stefanie *Intensive Case Manager, Adult*
10/29/2001 - present

Striba, Eric *Intensive Community Counselor*
9/24/1993 - 9/1/1994

Strouse, Deborah *Inpatient Counselor* 10/1/2003
- present

Sturtevant, Robert *Behavioral Specialist*
4/11/1996 - present

Suarez, Rosemary *On-Call Support* 6/21/1989 -
2/26/1991

Suloff, Julie *Nurse* 11/13/2001 - 6/27/2003

Swartley, Elizabeth *Clerk* 4/23/1974 -
9/25/1975

Swartley, Kris *Therapeutic Staff Support*
10/10/2002 - 9/12/2003

Swartley, Nancy *Pre-School Teacher* 6/13/1971 -
5/5/1972

Swartzendruber, Patricia *Psychiatric Patient
Coordinator* 5/26/1982 - 8/11/1982

Swartzendruber, William *Social Worker* 8/1/1967
- 6/30/1978

Swayne, Ann *Nursery School Teacher* 12/1/1970
- 6/9/1971

Swider, John *Therapeutic Staff Support* 5/7/2002
- 6/16/2003

Swome, Kimberly *Receptionist/Secretary*
1/27/1992 - 9/1/1994

Swope, William *MIS Director* 3/20/1995 -
10/2/1998

Symons, Diane *Scheduling
Secretary/Receptionist* 3/16/1998 -
3/18/1998

Synder, Lisa *Clerical Work Unit Supervisor*
3/20/1995 - 11/30/1995

Szasz-Boyce, Monika *PRN Crisis Worker*
10/9/2002 - 6/1/2003

Taccalozzi, Tara *Therapeutic Staff Support*
4/25/2001 - 5/10/2001

Talarico, Gina *Crisis Worker* 8/2/2000 -
6/30/2003

Talone, Janice *Clerk Stenographer* 10/25/1978 -
6/29/1979

Taylor, Barbara *Mobile therapist/Behavioral
Specialist* 6/7/1994 - 8/1/2001

Taylor, Denise *Case Manager* 6/17/1996 -
7/1/1997

Taylor, Dennis *Custodial/Maintenance* 8/20/1984
- 12/18/1987

Taylor, Lori *Supports Coordinator* 10/11/1999 - 5/4/2005

Tench III, John *Addictions Technician* 11/13/2001 - 1/9/2002

TenEyck, Sheila *Family Therapist* 7/17/1989 - 6/21/1990

Terpening, Sally *Addictions Technician* 12/28/2000 - 2/20/2004

Terrell, Cory *Intensive Community Counselor* 5/16/1996 - 6/25/1998

Theesfeld, Chad *MIS Coordinator* 4/14/1998 - 2/23/2001

Thelwell, Kezzy *PRN Crisis Worker* 6/12/2002 - 11/3/2004

Thinnes, Kathleen *Registered Nurse* 7/5/1989 - 6/10/1990

Thomas, Holly *EAP Counselor* 6/5/2000 - 2/7/2002

Thomas, John *Psychiatrist* 3/9/1997 - 6/30/1999

Thomas, Michele *Intensive Case Manager* 7/27/1999 - 8/30/2000

Thomas, Natilee *Mobile Therapist, Wraparound* 1/13/2005 - 5/15/2005

Thomas, Terri *EI Service Coordinator* 11/1/1999 - present

Thompson, Amy *QI/UR Specialist* 4/8/1996 - present

Thompson, Debra *EAP Counselor* 1/19/2004 - present

Timins, Grace *Addictions Counselor* 1/14/1986 - 10/14/1988

Tirjan, Nancy *Intensive Community Counselor* 9/20/1994 - 10/25/1996

Tobash, Michelle *Intensive Community Counselor* 7/30/1997 - 10/31/1998

Tobey, John *Mobile Therapist/Behavior Therapist, Wraparound* 8/10/1999 - 8/30/1999

Tobias, Stephen *Psychodramatist* 12/1/2000 - present

Toia, Amanda *Social Worker* 1/5/2981 - 2/10/1984

Toland, Cheryl *Admin. Case Manager, Bucks* 3/5/2001 - 1/31/2002

Tomlin, Angela *Inpatient Counselor w/Admin. Duties* 1/28/2002 - present

Tongue, Sharee *PRN Secretary* 11/15/1999 - 6/15/2000

Tonrey, Donna *Behavior Specialist* 5/2/1994 - 11/30/1995

Torres, Laurie *Secretary* 5/17/1999 - 9/17/2004

Trakat, Sandra *Geriatric Coordinator* 5/29/1973 - 3/10/2003

Transue, Denise *Adolescent Activity Therapist* 6/12/1995 - 10/20/1995

Trauger, Cindy *Medical Records* 6/16/1997 - 5/26/1999

Trauger, Patricia *Medical Review Secretary* 9/1/1959 - present

Trauger, Paul *Intake Manager/Assistant Counselor* 10/27/1997 - present

Treffinger, Lewis *Addictions Technician* 4/9/1996 - 4/10/1998

Trenholm, Patricia *Social Worker* 10/25/1994 - present

Trinkle, Ian *Addictions Technician* 2/4/2002 - 8/27/2002

Trinkle, Stephen *Inpatient Counselor* 8/27/1992 - present

Trout, Laurie *Marketing Rep* 6/19/1989-7/10/1992

Trumbauer, Beverly *Business Office* 6/16/1975 - 5/6/1981

Truver, Keith *Addictions Therapist* 9/27/1988 - 4/19/1989

Tucker, Karen *Managed Care Rep.* 1/18/1999 - 6/25/1999

Tumolo, Gerald *Therapeutic Staff Support* 5/31/2001 - 2/1/2002

Turner, Diane *Residential Caseworker* 10/8/1987 - present

Tust, Roseann *Addictions Technician* 5/8/1995 - 6/16/1995

Tweed, Christina *Intensive Case Manager, Childrens* 8/13/2001 - present

U'Selis, Gertrude *Receptionist* 6/18/1992 - 6/26/1992

Uhrich, Jennifer *PRN Secretary/Receptionist* 5/10/1999 - 3/10/2001

Ulmer, Maria *Alumni Case Manager/ Admin. Coordinator* 12/17/2001 - present

Undercuffler, Christine *Supports Coordinator* 7/6/2004 - present

Unger, Barry *Intensive Community Counselor* 9/16/1996 - 10/31/1996

Van Buren, Agnes *Psychologist* 9/27/1996 - 12/21/2000

Vandegrift, Patricia *Inpatient Program Director* 8/4/1980 - 7/7/1989

VanderVeur, Barbara *Med. Rec. Clerk II* 9/17/1985 - 6/7/2001

VanHoove, Rebecca *Intensive Community Counselor* 6/8/1998 - 6/1/1999

Vasconez, Lois *Partial Hospital Team Secretary* 7/18/1983 - 5/18/1984

Vasey, Lisa *Mental Health Worker* 9/7/1999 - present

Vella, Diane *Mobile Therapist/Behavioral Specialist* 11/10/1998 - 5/31/1999

Vereneck, Sandra *Medical Records Coordinator* 9/3/1996 - present

Verrilli, Michael *Addictions Technician* 2/6/2002 - 8/16/2002

Victor, Constance *Speech Therapist* 10/15/1973 - 6/15/1978

Vinson, Megan *Data Entry Clerk* 8/13/1996 - 9/12/1996

Vitelli, Philip *Psychiatrist* 1/1/2005 - present

Vivian, Rebecca *Therapeutic Staff Support* 8/7/2003 - present

Vocaturo, Christina *Adolescent Partial Coordinator* 8/16/2004 - present

Vogel, April *Crisis Worker* 10/20/2003 - present

Vogel, April *PRN Crisis Worker* 1/19/2000 - 2/24/2003

VonSchondorf, Susan *Nurse* 11/2/2004 - present

Voth, Barbara *Partial Hospital Director* 1/30/1995 - 1/15/2004

Voth, James *Maintenance Worker* 8/31/1998 - present

Voth, Scott *Maintenance Assistant* 7/5/1979 - 8/30/1979

Walbert, Jennifer *Therapeutic Staff Support* 12/2/1999 - 2/4/2000

Walgrove, Norma *Psych. Patient Coordinator* 2/2/1981 - 9/2/1981

Walker, Janet *Social Worker* 12/8/1995 - 6/21/1996

Walker, Kathleen *Residential Advisor* 1/7/2002 - 3/31/2003

Walker, Shannon *Intensive Community Counselor* 5/14/1996 - 1/12/1998

Wallace, Heather *Business Office* 8/6/1996 - 8/13/1996

Walsh, Muriel *Managed Care Auth. Specialist* 4/21/1997 - 4/17/1998

Walter, Charles *Addictions Technician* 3/12/1991 - 8/14/1992

Walters, Carol *Accountant* 11/3/1997 - 10/1/1999

Walthofer, Mark *Psychotherapist* 3/21/1997 - 5/12/1998

Wampole, Cindy *Secretary/Receptionist* 9/23/1999 - 4/12/2000

Ward, Cindy *Insurance Billing Clerk* 9/26/1996 - 3/17/1997

Ward, Lynn *Billing Clerk* 7/17/2000 - present

Ware, Richard *Psychotherapist* 6/1/1993 - 6/2/2000

Warinner, Deborah *Therapeutic Staff Support* 8/21/2000 - 10/13/2000

Washko, Carol *Director of Advancement* 11/28/1988 - 6/30/1992; 10/1/2001 - present

Wassmer, Seema *Mobile Therapist* 4/19/2004 - present

Watanabe, Gail *D/A Therapist* 3/14/1988 - 5/16/1988

Watchous, Andrew *Addictions Technician* 2/9/2004 - present

Watson, Elizabeth *Secretary* 11/13/1980 - 4/23/1984

Watson, Kenneth *Driver* 2/6/2002 - 3/8/2002

Weaver, Jennifer *Clinical Assistant* 9/14/1995 - 7/2/1998

Weaver, Marie *Billing/Insurance Clerk* 2/14/1983 - 7/30/1999

Weaver, Pamella *Referral Coordinator/RC, Bucks & Montg.* 5/25/1999 - 4/29/2005

Weaver, Shari *Secretary (Administration)* 7/7/1986 - 11/3/1986

Webb, Cristyn *Intensive Community Counselor* 6/17/1996 - 7/9/1997

Webb, Viola *Case Manager* 5/31/2001 - 4/17/2003

Weidemann, Janet *EAP Counselor* 10/7/1985 - 1/31/1988

Weinberg, Michelle *Social Worker* 7/1/2003 - present

Weiss, John *Aftercare Coordinator* 1/20/1989 - present

Weiss, Keith *Therapy Technician* 2/27/1990 - 7/3/1990

Weitzel, Rachel *Wraparound Billing Clerk* 7/7/1997 - 3/9/1999

Weller, Mary *Van Driver* 1/10/1974 - 9/28/1979

Welliver, Nicole *PRN Residential Instructor* 7/29/1998 - 5/10/2002

Welsh, Margaret *Relief Secretary, Floater* 5/5/1983 - 7/1/1987

Wenger, Warren *Adjuctive Therapist, Woodshop Activities Aide PT* 6/6/1983 - 7/1/1985

Wenig, Jennifer *Medical Records/Receptionist* 12/17/2000 - 6/29/2001

Wenrich, Kacey *Case Manager* 7/28/1997 - 2/4/2000

Wentz, Doris *Medical Records Clerk* 8/20/1990 - 7/31/2003

Werbeck, Timothy *Case Management Support Technician, Bucks* 11/11/1999 - present

Werner, Jessica *Intensive Case Manager, Adult/Children* 5/21/2002 - present

Wetzel, Kathleen *Residential Instructor* 3/7/1989 - 8/31/1990

Whaley, Christopher *TEP Mail Clerk* 4/19/2004 - 12/3/2004

Wheat, Claire *Medical Records Technician* 9/7/1999 - 7/28/2000

White, Jean *Nurse, Recovery Center Inpatient* 5/24/1999 - 12/1/1999

White, Suzanne *Intensive Community Counselor* 11/23/1998 - 11/18/1999

Whitechair, Judith *D/A Therapist, BreakThrough Rehab.* 4/6/1987 - 2/18/1991

Whitfield, Robin *Secretary/Receptionist* 9/24/1996 - 10/11/1996

Whitmire, Catherine *Data Entry Clerk* 8/11/1997 - 11/25/1998

Whittington, Gary *Intensive Community Counselor* 12/11/1996 - 2/4/2000

Wicen, Susan *Intake Worker* 2/26/1990 - 1/8/1993

Wiediger, Deborah *Secretary, PRN* 12/3/1998 - 6/15/2000

Wietecha, Judy *BreakThrough Secretary* 5/18/1987 - 5/29/1987

Wilhelm, Christy *Secretary/Receptionist* 11/10/1998 - 7/28/2000

Williams, Erin *Data Entry Clerk* 6/30/1997 - 6/15/2000

Williams, Inga *Therapeutic Staff Support* 4/12/2004 - present

Williams, John *Personal Choice Billing Specialist* 5/15/1995 - 10/31/1995

Williams, Lu Ann *Wraparound Coordinator* 12/12/1994 - 11/1/2000

Williams, Shirl *Mail Clerk* 9/14/1998 - 3/19/1999

Williamson, Karen *EAP Counselor* 11/5/1990 - present

Williamson, Nicholas *PRN Targeted Case Manager* 6/10/2004 - present

Williamson, Nicholas *Resource Coordinator* 6/5/2001 - 8/8/2003

Wills, Steven *SEP File Clerk* 5/22/2001 - present

Willson, Kathleen *Mobile Therapist* 4/25/2001 - 6/6/2001

Wilson, Bryan *Detox Coordinator* 11/23/1994 - 1/2/1998

Wilson, Sherry *Secretary* 12/3/1975 - 3/21/1978

Wilson, Susan *Behavioral Specialist* 7/30/2003 - present

Winfree, John *Addictions Technician* 1/4/1999 - 8/27/1999

Winters, Verdie *Data Entry Coordinator* 11/8/1999 - present

Wischusen, Nancy *Mobile Therapist/Behavioral Specialist* 6/10/1999 - 2/2/2001

Wise, Susan *Secretary/Referral Coordinator* 12/2/2002 - present

Wisser, Kathy *Recovery Center Director/Quality Improvement Coord.* 6/7/1988 - 12/20/2000

Witmer, Jean *MR Caseworker* 9/3/1974 - 10/27/1978

Woelk, Lamont *Pastoral Services* 10/5/1981 - 7/28/1993

Wolff, Wallace *Therapist* 4/23/2003 - present

Wolfgang, Stacy *Intensive Community Counselor* 8/28/1996 - 6/12/1997

Wood, Wendy *Activity Therapist, Day Treatment* 8/26/1953 - 9/4/1979

Woodhouse, Sharon *Secretary/Receptionist* 3/16/1998 - 5/5/1998

Woodman, Cary *Intensive Community Counselor* 7/1/1996 - 7/22/1997

Woodrow, Joan *Crisis Worker* 9/29/2000 - 1/31/2001

Woodside, Heather *Therapeutic Staff Support* 9/28/2003 - 3/14/2001

Woody, Leah *Therapeutic Staff Support* 9/10/2003 - present

Woolsey, Ann *Addictions Technician* 9/23/1991 - present

Worley, Annette *PRN Medical Review Nurse* 8/16/1995 - 2/8/2005

Worman, Linda *Patient Accounts Manager* 2/1/1982 - 8/20/1982

Worman-Stengel, Michelle *Special Projects Coordinator* 4/1/1998 - present

Worthington, Carrie *Addictions Technician* 10/15/1999 - 11/30/1999

Wright, Vincent *Addiction Technician* 12/2/1994 - Unknown

Wrobel, Richard *Assoc. Director MR Case Management* 11/7/1996 - 7/11/1997

Wurtz, Kelly *Crisis Worker* 4/2/2003 - present

Wyatt, Thomas *Van Driver* 4/7/1997 - 10/10/1997

Wykoff, Aimee *Resource Coord./State Hosp. Liaison* 1/13/1997 - 8/27/1999

Yakovich, Donna *Billing/Insurance Clerk* 5/2/1988 - 1/27/1989

Yeasted, Judith *Intensive Community Counselor* 3/1/1999 - 12/22/1999

Yerk, Nancy *MR Caseworker* 3/7/1977 - 6/11/1979

Yerkes, Margaret *Nurse* 6/8/1988 - 6/30/1988

Yoder, Christine *Registered Nurse* 3/28/1990 - 11/30/1990

Yoder, Dixie *Therapeutic Staff Support* 11/10/2003 - 12/31/2003

Yoder, Doris *Computer Consultant* 12/2/1994 - 4/3/1995

Yoder, Sheldon *Computer Consultant* 12/2/1994 - 4/3/1995

Yoder, Valerie *County Billing Clerk/Fiscal Technician* 3/17/1997 - present

Youells, Warren *Mental Health Assistant* 10/28/1985 - 6/12/1986

Young, Barbara *Medical Records Manager* 8/3/1998 - 3/29/1999

Young, Dalton *Inpatient Counselor* 4/1/1999 - present

Young, Heather *Residential Advisor* 1/7/2002 - 3/5/2002

Young, Nathan *Addictions Technician* 9/10/1999 - 1/16/2002

Youtz, Jerome *Addictions Counselor* 2/5/2002 - 10/3/2002

Yusavitz, Carl *Director of Pastoral Services* 10/2/2000 - present

Zancolli, Frances *PRN Nurse* 8/9/2001 - 11/1/2001

Zanger, Judith *Social Worker* 4/30/1997 - 6/15/2000

Zazow, Betsy *Social Worker* 12/28/1999 - 11/16/2000

Zazow, Paul *Psychiatrist* 5/22/1985 - 4/28/2005

Zehr, Krista *Childrens ICM* 6/1/1994 - 10/4/1996

Zemlan, Natalie *Psychologist* 11/10/2003 - 2/2/2004

Zeppenfelt, Kelly *Managed Care Rep.* 3/27/2000 - 6/16/2000

Zick, Margaret *Acting Co-Director Client Registration* 2/12/1996 - 5/10/1999

Ziegler, Karen *Secretary/Receptionist* 9/7/2000 - 12/5/2000

Zola, Gloria *Psychiatric Social Worker GVH3A* 11/26/1990 - 6/15/1992

Zwart, Nancy *Quakertown Office Secretary* 7/11/1984 - 6/3/1985

Zweizig, Jennifer *Mobile Therapist* 6/17/1996 - 4/1/1998

Index
